sixth edition

Medical Dosage Calculations

June Looby Olsen, R.N., B.S., M.S.
Professor of Nursing
The College of Staten Island
Staten Island, New York

Leon J. Ablon, B.A., M.S., M.A.
Associate Professor of Mathematics, Emeritus
The College of Staten Island
Staten Island, New York

Anthony Patrick Giangrasso, B.S., M.S., Ph.D.
Professor of Mathematics
LaGuardia Community College
Long Island City, New York

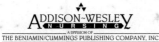

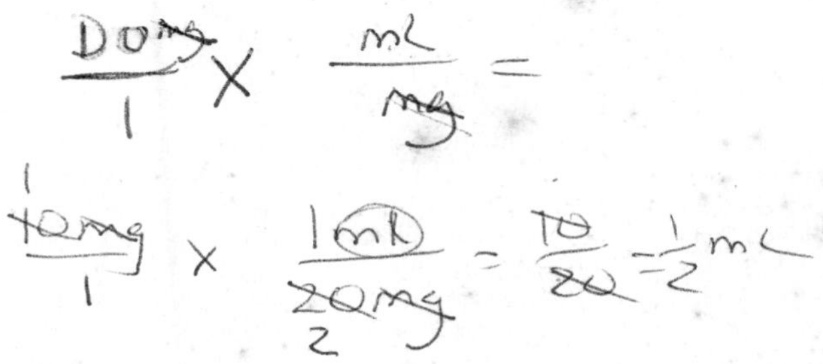

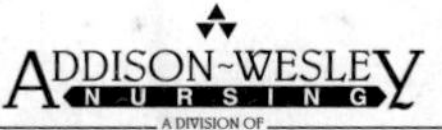

A DIVISION OF
THE BENJAMIN/CUMMINGS PUBLISHING COMPANY, INC.

Redwood City, California ¶ Menlo Park, California ¶ Reading, Massachusetts
New York ¶ Don Mills, Ontario ¶ Wokingham, U.K. ¶ Amsterdam
Bonn ¶ Paris ¶ Milan ¶ Madrid ¶ Sydney ¶ Singapore ¶ Tokyo ¶ Seoul
Taipei ¶ Mexico City ¶ San Juan

Executive Editor: *Patricia L. Cleary*
Developmental Editor: *Mark F. Wales*
Editorial Assistant: *Kendra Hurley*
Outside Services Supervisor: *Rani Cochran*
Project Manager: *Joan Keyes, Jonathan Peck Typographers*
Text Designer: *Patrick Devine, Jonathan Peck Typographers*
Cover Art Director: *Yvo Riezebos*
Cover Designer and Illustrator: *Terry Hight/Terry Hight Design*
Text Illustrators: *Valerie Taylor, Jonathan Peck Typographers; Kathy Lloyd, Lynx Graphics*
Copy Editor: *Luana Richards*
Senior Manufacturing Coordinator: *Merry Free Osborn*
Composition and Film Coordinator: *Vivian McDougal*
Compositor: *Jonathan Peck Typographers*
Printer: *Banta Company*

Library of Congress Cataloging-in-Publication Data
Olsen, June Looby.
Medical dosage calculations / June Looby Olsen, Leon J. Ablon, Anthony Patrick Giangrasso.—6th ed.
p. cm.
Rev. ed. of: Medical dosage calculation / June Looby Olsen . . . [et al.]. 5th ed. c1991.
ISBN 0-8053-5605-3
1. Pharmaceutical arithmetic. 2. Pharmaceutical arithmetic—Problems, exercises, etc. I. Ablon, Leon J. II. Giangrasso, Anthony Patrick. III. Title
[DNLM: 1. Drugs—administration & dosage. QV 748 052m 1995]
RS57.M425 1995
815′.14—dc20
DNLM/DLC 94-33488
for Library of Congress CIP

Care has been taken to confirm the accuracy of information presented in this book. The authors, editors, and publisher, however, cannot accept any responsibility for errors or omissions or for consequences from application of the information in this book and make no warranty, express or implied, with respect to its contents.

The authors and publisher have exerted every effort to ensure that drug selections and dosages set forth in this text are in accord with current recommendations and practice at the time of publication. However, in view of ongoing research, changes in government regulations, and the constant flow of information relating to drug therapy and drug reactions, the reader is urged to check the package inserts of all drugs for any change in indications of dosage and for added warnings and precautions. This is particularly important when the recommended agent is a new and/or infrequently employed drug. Mention of a particular generic or brand name drug is not an endorsement nor an implication that it is preferable to other named or unnamed agents.

The names of clients appearing in this book are fictitious, and the resemblance of these names to any person living or deceased is purely coincidental.

Nomogram from Behman, RE and Vaughn, VC. *Nelson Textbook of Pediatrics*, 13th ed., Philadelphia, WB Saunders Co. 1987. Reprinted by permission.

ISBN 0-8053-5605-3
1 2 3 4 5 6 7 8 9 10—BAH 98 97 96 95 94

Addison-Wesley Nursing
A division of The Benjamin/Cummings Publishing Company, Inc.
390 Bridge Parkway
Redwood City, California 94065

d e d i c a t i o n

June Looby Olsen
To my wonderful husband, Bill;
my children, Michelle and Keith; and my son-in-law, Ralph Keefe

Leon J. Ablon
To Dixie Piver Ablon, my wife

Anthony Patrick Giangrasso
To my beautiful wife, Susan,
and my children, Anthony, Michael, and Jennifer

preface

In a growing range of health-care settings, nursing and allied health professionals are assuming increasing responsibilities in every aspect of drug administration. The first step in assuming this responsibility is learning to calculate drug dosages accurately. Dosage calculation is not just about math skills, it is an introduction into the **professional context** of drug administration. Calculation skills and the reason for their application—this is what *Medical Dosage Calculations* has taught thousands of students with admirable success through five editions.

Medical Dosage Calculations is a combined text and workbook designed for the student of dosage calculations. Its consistent focus on safety, accuracy, and professionalism make it a valuable part of a dosage calculation course for nursing or allied health-care programs. It is also highly effective for independent study and may be used as a refresher to dosage calculation skills or as a professional reference.

Topics introduced and developed in *Medical Dosage Calculations* include:

- basic arithmetic skills
- systems of measurement
- dosage calculations for all common forms of drug preparations
- IV and specialized calculations

In addition to these topics, this edition includes substantially more information about basic drug administration. Readers will learn how to interpret actual drug labels, package inserts, and various forms of medication orders, as well as how to recognize a wide variety of syringes.

Key Features of *Medical Dosage Calculations*

We have built on the strengths of the previous editions by continuing to provide the thoroughness of a textbook with the practicality and convenience of a workbook. Here are the important features that have made *Medical Dosage Calculations* an effective and popular book through five editions.

- *Dimensional Analysis Calculation Method.* Dimensional analysis is a technique in which the units on the drug package are systematically converted to the units on the drug order. Rapidly becoming the primary dosage calculation technique among nursing and allied health educators, this method helps assure safety while eliminating the need to memorize formulas.
- *Learn by Example.* Each chapter unfolds basic concepts and skills through a series of examples:

Example 7.3

How many tablets should you give a patient if the order is for grain $\frac{1}{2}$ of codeine sulfate and each tablet contains grain $\frac{1}{4}$?

In this problem you want to convert the order grain $\frac{1}{2}$ to tablets.

$$\text{gr}\ \frac{1}{2} = ?\ \text{tab}$$

You want to cancel the grain and determine the equivalent amount in tablets.

$$\text{gr}\ \frac{1}{2} \times \frac{?\ \text{tab}}{?\ \text{gr}} = ?\ \text{tab}$$

Since 1 tab = gr $\frac{1}{4}$, the fraction is $\dfrac{1\ \text{tab}}{\text{gr}\ \frac{1}{4}}$.

$$\cancel{\text{gr}}\ \frac{1}{2} \times \frac{1\ \text{tab}}{\cancel{\text{gr}}\ \frac{1}{4}} = \frac{1\ \text{tab}}{\frac{2}{4}} = 1\ \text{tab} \div \frac{2}{4} = 1\ \text{tab} \times \frac{4}{2} = 2\ \text{tab}$$

So grain $\frac{1}{2}$ is equivalent to 2 tablets, and you should give the patient 2 tablets of codeine sulfate.

⊕ ⊕ ⊕

This method teaches concepts by *showing* the application.

- *Problem Sets.* This text/workbook offers learners over 1000 practice opportunities. Each chapter's practice opportunities are grouped into four problem sets:
  - Try These for Practice
  - Exercises
  - Additional Exercises
  - Cumulative Review Exercises

When applicable, each problem set reinforces skills in interpreting drug labels and medication orders and in recognizing syringes.

- *Case Studies and Comprehensive Self-Tests.* Realistic case scenarios that are part of each comprehensive self-test allow the student to apply concepts and techniques presented in the text to a clinical setting. Answers to three case studies and three comprehensive self-tests are in the text.

Organization. The skills mastered in *Medical Dosage Calculations* are arranged into four basic learning units:

- Unit 1: Basic Calculation and Administration Skills
  After a review of basic number skills, this section introduces the essentials of drug administration. A separate chapter introduces dimensional analysis using a friendly, commonsense approach.
- Unit 2: Systems of Measurement for Dosage Calculations
  This section covers the three systems of measurement that nurses and other allied health professionals must understand to interpret medication orders and calculate dosages. Readers learn to convert measurements between and within measurement systems.
- Unit 3: Common Medication Preparations
  The heart of the book, the chapters in this unit prepare readers to calculate oral and parenteral medication dosages and introduce the preparation of solutions. A new chapter has been included to familiarize students with syringes and their measurements.
- Unit 4: Specialized Medication Preparations
  This important final section provides a solid base for calculating IV and enteral flow rates as well as pediatric dosages.

Benefits of using *Medical Dosage Calculations*

- Constant skill reinforcement through frequent practice opportunities.
- Over 1000 problems for students to solve.
- Commonly used medications featured.
- Syringe illustrations and actual drug labels, drug package inserts, and medication orders in every applicable problem set and therefore more realistic, relevant dosage problems.
- Ample work space on every page for note-taking and problem-solving.
- Answers to Try These For Practice, Exercises, and Cumulative Review Exercises at the end of the text.
- Detachable Pocketminder to be carried on the job as a quick reference for essential dosage calculation information.

Instructor's Guide Available

This combined Instructor's Guide/Testbank (0-8053-5606) provides extra test questions, answers to test questions, answers to Additional Exercises, answers to Case Studies and Comprehensive Self-Tests 4–6, a list of Key Terms, possible teaching approaches relevant to each chapter, an overview of chapter missions, and a 50-question comprehensive examination with answers. This guide helps instructors prepare lectures and examinations quickly.

Summary of Reviewers

Deborah Dalrymple
Montgomery Community College
Warrington, Pennsylvania

Barbara Goodkin, MSN
Washtenaw Community College
Ann Arbor, Michigan

Maxine Goos, RN, MSN
Cumberland County College
Vineland, New Jersey

Anna Miller, MSN
Ball State University
Indianapolis, Indiana

Claire Mortensen, MSN
Skagit Valley College
Mount Vernon, Washington

Acknowledgments

Our special thanks to the faculty and students at the College of Staten Island, who have participated with support and suggestions for the past 22 years, especially Eugenia Borgia Murray. Special thanks also to our editor, Mark Wales, and his assistant, Kendra Hurley, at Benjamin/Cummings; our project manager, Joan Keyes, at Jonathan Peck Typographers; our copy editor, Luana Richards; and finally to Jessica Peralta, who, with her dedication and professionalism, assisted us in the preparation of this text.

My loving thanks and warmest regards to my daughter, Michelle Olsen Keefe. With her assistance and research, this text developed into its sixth edition.

To our friend and former co-author, the late Helen Siner Weisman, we thank you. You honored our writing group by your professional attitude and knowledge. We miss you.

We are pleased to acknowledge the following pharmaceutical companies that granted us permission to reproduce their labels:

Abbott Laboratories
Astra Pharmaceutical Products Inc.
Barr Laboratories, Inc.
Baxter Incorporated
Beecham Laboratories
Bolar Pharmaceutical Company, Inc.
Bristol-Myers Squibb Company
Burroughs Wellcome Co.
DuPont Pharmaceuticals
Geneva Pharmaceuticals, Inc.
Hercon Laboratories Corporation
Eli Lilly and Company
Knoll Pharmaceuticals
Lederle Laboratories
Marion Merrell Dow Inc.
Pfizer Incorporated
Roerig Division,
Pfizer Incorporated
Schein Pharmaceutical, Inc.
Smith Kline Beecham
The Upjohn Company

June Olsen
Leon Ablon
Anthony Giangrasso

table of contents

unit One Basic Calculation and Administration Skills

unit Two Systems of Measurement for Dosage Calculations

chapter 4 The Metric System 62

chapter 5 The Apothecary and Household Systems 73

chapter 6 Converting from One System of Measurement to Another 89

unit Three Common Medication Preparations

chapter 7 Calculating Oral Medication Doses 110

chapter 8 Preparation of Solutions 141

chapter 9 Syringes 159

chapter 10 Parenteral Medications 179

unit Four Specialized Medication Preparations

chapter 11 Calculating Flow Rates for Intravenous Infusions and Enteral Solutions 202

chapter 12 Calculating Pediatric Dosages 230

Case Studies/Self-Tests 253

Appendices A-1

Name: ______________________ **Date:** ______________

Class: ______________________ **Instructor:** ______________

Diagnostic Test of Arithmetic

Answers to the Diagnostic Test of Arithmetic can be found on page A-21 in Appendix A.

1. Write 0.625 as a fraction. ________

2. Write $\frac{2750}{1000}$ as a decimal number. ________

3. Round 4.781 to the nearest tenth. ________

4. Write $\frac{2}{3}$ as a decimal number rounded to the nearest hundredth. ________

5. $\frac{8.4}{0.21} =$ ________

6. $3.267 \times 100 =$ ________

7. $42.51 \div 10 =$ ________

8. $65 \div 0.05 =$ ________

9. $\frac{10}{21} \times 7 \times \frac{3}{5} =$ ________

10. $4\frac{2}{3} \div 21 =$ ________

11. $\frac{3}{4} \div \frac{9}{16} =$ ________

12. $\frac{\frac{3}{4}}{12} =$ ________

13. Write 35% as a fraction. ________

14. Write 2.5% as a decimal number without using the % symbol. ________

15. Write $4\frac{3}{5}$ as an improper fraction. ________

Unit One

Basic Calculation and Administration Skills

chapter 1

Review of Arithmetic for Medical Dosage Calculations

Objectives

After completing this chapter, you will be able to

- *convert decimal numbers to fractions.*
- *convert fractions to decimal numbers.*
- *round decimal numbers to a desired number of places.*
- *multiply and divide decimal numbers.*
- *multiply and divide fractions.*
- *simplify complex fractions.*
- *write percentages as decimal numbers.*
- *write percentages as fractions.*

Medical dosage calculations can involve whole numbers, fractions, decimal numbers, and percentages. Your results on the Diagnostic Test of Arithmetic, page A-21, will have identified your areas of strength and weakness. You can use Chapter 1 to improve your math skills or simply to review the kinds of calculations you will encounter in this text.

Changing Decimal Numbers and Whole Numbers to Fractions

A decimal number represents a fraction with a denominator of 10, 100, 1000, etc. Each decimal number has three parts: the whole-number part, the decimal point, and the fraction part. Table 1.1 shows the names of the decimal positions.

Reading a decimal number will help you to write it as a fraction.

Decimal Number		Read		Fraction
4.1	⟶	four and one tenth	⟶	$4\frac{1}{10}$
0.3	⟶	three tenths	⟶	$\frac{3}{10}$
0.07	⟶	seven hundredths	⟶	$\frac{7}{100}$
0.231	⟶	two hundred thirty-one thousandths	⟶	$\frac{231}{1000}$
0.0025	⟶	twenty-five ten thousandths	⟶	$\frac{25}{10,000}$

A number can be written in many different forms. For example, the decimal number 3.5 is read as *three and five tenths.* In fraction form it is $3\frac{5}{10}$ or $3\frac{1}{2}$. You can also write $3\frac{1}{2}$ as an *improper fraction,* as follows:

$$3\frac{1}{2} = \frac{3 \times 2 + 1}{1} = \frac{7}{2}$$

Table 1.1 *Names of Decimal Positions*

Whole-Number Part **Fraction Part**

0 0 0 0 . 0 0 0 0

thousands
hundreds
tens
ones
decimal point
tenths
hundredths
thousandths
ten thousandths

Notes/Workspace

precede decimals with a 0. so that it's visible ex — .125 0.125

Notes/Workspace

Example 1.1
Write 2.25 as an improper fraction.

The number 2.25 is read *two and twenty-five hundredths* and written $2\frac{25}{100}$. You can simplify:

$$2\frac{25}{100} = 2\frac{\overset{1}{\cancel{25}}}{\underset{4}{\cancel{100}}} = 2\frac{1}{4} = \frac{2 \times 4 + 1}{3} = \frac{9}{4}$$

> **Note**
>
> Simplify $\frac{25}{100}$ to $\frac{1}{4}$ by dividing both numerator and denominator by the same number, 25. This is called *canceling*.

Changing Fractions to Decimal Numbers

To change a fraction to a decimal, think of the fraction as a division problem. For example:

$$\frac{2}{5} \quad \text{means} \quad 2 \div 5 \quad \text{or} \quad 5\overline{)2}$$

Here are the steps for this division.

Step 1 Replace 2 with 2.0 and then place a decimal point directly above the decimal point in 2.0.

$$\begin{array}{r} . \\ 5\overline{)2.0} \end{array}$$

Step 2 Perform the division.

$$\begin{array}{r} 0.4 \\ 5\overline{)2.0} \\ \underline{2\ 0} \\ 0 \end{array}$$

So $\frac{2}{5} = 0.4$.

Example 1.2

Write $\frac{5}{2}$ as a decimal number.

$$\frac{5}{2} \quad \text{means} \quad 2\overline{)5}$$

Step 1 $\quad 2\overline{)5.0}$ (decimal point placed above)

Step 2

$$\begin{array}{r} 2.5 \\ 2\overline{)5.0} \\ \underline{4} \\ 1\,0 \\ \underline{1\,0} \\ 0 \end{array}$$

So $\frac{5}{2} = 2.5$.

Example 1.3

Write $\frac{193}{10}$ as a decimal number.

$$\frac{193}{10} \quad \text{means} \quad 10\overline{)193}$$

Step 1 $\quad 10\overline{)193.0}$ (decimal point placed above)

Step 2

$$\begin{array}{r} 19.3 \\ 10\overline{)193.0} \\ \underline{10} \\ 93 \\ \underline{90} \\ 30 \\ \underline{30} \\ 0 \end{array}$$

So $\frac{193}{10} = 19.3$.

There is a quicker way to do this problem. To divide any decimal number by 10, you move the decimal point in the number one place to the left. Notice that there is one zero in 10.

$$\frac{193}{10} = \frac{193.}{10} = 19.3. = 19.3$$

Notes/Workspace

Pg A22 - will be tested 2nd quiz

Notes/Workspace

To divide a number by 100, move the decimal point in the number two places to the left, since there are two zeros in 100. So, the quick way to divide by 10, 100, 1000, etc., is to count the zeros and then move the decimal point to the left the same number of places. The answer should always be a smaller number than the original. Check your answer to be sure.

Example 1.4

Write $\frac{9.25}{100}$ as a decimal number.

There are two zeros in 100, so move the decimal point in 9.25 two places to the left and fill the empty position with a zero.

$$\frac{9.25}{100} = 9.25 = 0.0925$$

Rounding Decimal Numbers

Sometimes it's convenient to round answers—that is, to find an approximate answer rather than an exact one. To round 0.257 to the nearest tenth—that is, to round the answer to one decimal place—you do the following:

> Look at the hundredths (second) decimal place digit. Since this digit is *5 or more*, round 0.257 by adding 1 to the tenths (first) decimal place digit. Finally, drop all the digits after the tenths place. So 0.257 becomes 0.3 when rounded to the nearest tenth.

To round 6.4345 to the nearest hundredth—that is, to round the answer to two decimal places—you do the following:

> Look at the thousandths (third) place digit. Since this digit is *less than 5*, round 6.4345 by leaving the hundredths digit alone. Finally, drop all the digits after the hundredths place. So 6.4345 becomes 6.43 when rounded to the nearest hundredth.

Example 1.5

Round 4.8075 to the nearest hundredth, tenth, and whole number.

4.8075 rounded to the nearest: hundredth = 4.81
tenth = 4.8
whole number = 5

Multiplying and Dividing Decimal Numbers

Notes/Workspace

To multiply two decimal numbers, first multiply, ignoring the decimal points. Then count the total number of decimal places in the original two numbers. That sum equals the number of decimal places in the answer.

Example 1.6

$304.2 \times 0.16 = ?$

```
 304.2    ←—  1 decimal place  }  Total of 3
×0.16     ←—  2 decimal places }  decimal places
 18252
 3042
48.672
  ↑
  |______  There are 3 decimal places in the answer.
           Place the decimal point here.
```

So $304.2 \times 0.16 = 48.672$.

Example 1.7

$304.25 \times 10 = ?$

```
 304.25   ←—  2 decimal places }  Total of 2
   ×10    ←—  0 decimal places }  decimal places
3042.50
    ↑
    |____  There are 2 decimal places in the answer.
           Place the decimal point here.
```

So $304.25 \times 10 = 3042.50$ or 3042.5.

There is a quicker way to do this problem. To multiply any decimal number by 10, move the decimal point in the number being multipled one place to the right. Notice that there is one zero in 10.

$$304.25 \times 10 = 304.\underset{\smile}{2},5 \quad \text{or} \quad 3042.5$$

To multiply a number by 100, move the decimal point in the number two places to the right, since there are two zeros in 100. So, the quick way to multiply by 10, 100, 1000, etc., is to count the zeros and then move the decimal point to the right the same number of places. The answer should always be a larger number than the original. Check your answer to be sure.

Notes/Workspace

Example 1.8

$23.597 \times 1000 = ?$

There are three zeros in 1000, so move the decimal point in 23.597 three places to the right.

$$23.597 \times 1000 = 23.5\,9\,7. \quad \text{or} \quad 23{,}597$$

So $23.597 \times 1000 = 23{,}597$.

Example 1.9

Write $\frac{106.8}{15}$ as a decimal number to the nearest tenth; that is, round the answer to one decimal place.

$$\frac{106.8}{15} \quad \text{means} \quad 15\overline{)106.8}$$

Step 1 $15\overline{)106.8}$ (with the decimal point placed above, in the quotient)

Step 2 Since you want the answer to the nearest tenth (one decimal place), do the division to two decimal places and then round the answer. Since the second place digit in the answer is *less than 5*, leave the first decimal place digit alone. Finally, drop the digit in the second (hundredths) decimal place.

```
     7.12
15)106.80
   105
    18
    15
     30
     30
      0
```

So $\frac{106.8}{15}$ is 7.1 to the nearest tenth.

Notes/Workspace

Example 1.10
$\frac{48}{0.002} = ?$

Note that there are three decimal places in 0.002, so move the decimal points in both numbers three places to the right.

$$\frac{48}{0.002} \text{ means } 0.002\overline{)48.} \text{ or } 0.0.0.2.\overline{)48.0.0.0.}$$

$$\begin{array}{r} 24000. \\ 2\overline{)48000.} \\ \underline{4} \\ 8 \\ \underline{8} \\ 0 \end{array}$$

So $\frac{48}{0.002} = 24{,}000.$

Multiplying and Dividing Fractions

To *multiply* fractions, multiply the numerators to get the new numerator and multiply the denominators to get the new denominator.

Example 1.11
$\frac{3}{5} \times 6 \times \frac{1}{5} = ?$

A whole number can be written as a fraction with 1 in the denominator. In this example, write 6 as $\frac{6}{1}$.

$$\frac{3}{5} \times \frac{6}{1} \times \frac{1}{5} = \frac{3 \times 6 \times 1}{5 \times 1 \times 5} = \frac{18}{25}$$

Example 1.12
$\frac{4}{5} \times \frac{3}{10} \times \frac{20}{7} = ?$

It is often convenient to cancel before you multiply.

$$\frac{4}{5} \times \frac{3}{\cancel{10}_{1}} \times \frac{\cancel{20}^{2}}{7} = \frac{24}{35}$$

To *divide* fractions, change the division problem to an equivalent multiplication problem by inverting the second fraction.

Notes/Workspace

Example 1.13

$1\frac{2}{5} \div \frac{7}{9} = ?$

Write $1\frac{2}{5}$ as the fraction $\frac{7}{5}$. Division $\left(\frac{7}{5} \div \frac{7}{9}\right)$ becomes the multiplication $\left(\frac{7}{5} \times \frac{9}{7}\right)$.

$$\frac{\overset{1}{\cancel{7}}}{5} \times \frac{9}{\underset{1}{\cancel{7}}} = \frac{9}{5} = 1\frac{4}{5}$$

Sometimes you must deal with whole numbers, fractions, and decimal numbers in the same multiplication and division problems.

Example 1.14

$\frac{1}{300} \times 60 \times \frac{1}{0.4} = ?$

$$\frac{1}{\underset{5}{\cancel{300}}} \times \frac{\overset{1}{\cancel{60}}}{1} \times \frac{1}{0.4} = \frac{1}{5 \times 0.4} = \frac{1}{2}$$

Note

Avoid canceling decimal numbers. It is a possible source of error.

Sometimes you will need to calculate an answer in a fractional form that contains no decimal numbers.

Example 1.15

$0.35 \times \frac{1}{60} = ?$

$$\frac{0.35}{1} \times \frac{1}{60} = \frac{0.35}{60}$$

The numerator of this fraction is 0.35, a decimal number. You can write an equivalent form of the fraction by multiplying the numerator and denominator by 100.

$$\frac{0.35}{60} \times \frac{100}{100} = \frac{0.35}{60.00} = \frac{35}{6000} = \frac{7}{1200}$$

Example 1.16

Give the answer to the following problem in a fractional form containing no decimal numbers.

$$0.88 \times \frac{1}{2.2} = ?$$

$$\frac{0.88}{1} \times \frac{1}{2.2} = \frac{0.88}{2.2}$$

Multiply the numerator and the denominator of this fraction by 100 to eliminate both decimal numbers.

$$\frac{0.88}{2.2} \times \frac{100}{100} = \frac{0.88}{2.2} = \frac{88}{220} = \frac{2}{5}$$

You can do this problem a different way by dividing 0.88 by 2.2.

$$2.2\overline{)0.88}\ \text{gives}\ 0.4 \quad \text{and} \quad 0.4 = \frac{2}{5}$$

Complex Fractions

Fractions that have numerators or denominators that are fractions are called *complex fractions.* The longer fraction line separates the numerator from the denominator and indicates division.

$$\frac{1}{\frac{2}{5}} \text{ means } 1 \div \frac{2}{5} \text{ or } 1 \times \frac{5}{2} \text{ which is } \frac{5}{2}$$

$$\frac{\frac{1}{2}}{5} \text{ means } \frac{1}{2} \div 5 \text{ or } \frac{1}{2} \times \frac{1}{5} \text{ which is } \frac{1}{10}$$

$$\frac{\frac{3}{5}}{\frac{2}{5}} \text{ means } \frac{3}{5} \div \frac{2}{5} \text{ or } \frac{3}{\cancel{5}_1} \times \frac{\cancel{5}^1}{2} \text{ which is } \frac{3}{2}$$

Notes/Workspace

Notes/Workspace

Example 1.17

$$\frac{\frac{1}{25} \times 500}{\frac{1}{4}} = ?$$

Convert to a simpler form.

$$\left(\frac{1}{25} \times \frac{500}{1}\right) \div \frac{1}{4} = ?$$

$$\left(\frac{1}{\overset{}{\underset{1}{\cancel{25}}}} \times \frac{\overset{20}{\cancel{500}}}{1}\right) \div \frac{1}{4} =$$

$$\frac{20}{1} \div \frac{1}{4} =$$

$$\frac{20}{1} \times \frac{4}{1} = 80$$

Example 1.18

$$\frac{2}{3} \times \frac{1}{\frac{3}{4}} = ?$$

Convert to a simpler form.

$$\frac{2 \times 1}{\frac{3}{1} \times \frac{3}{4}} = ?$$

$$\frac{2}{\frac{9}{4}} =$$

$$\frac{2}{1} \div \frac{9}{4} = \frac{2}{1} \times \frac{4}{9} = \frac{8}{9}$$

This problem could be done another way:

$$\frac{2}{3} \times \frac{1}{\frac{3}{4}} = ?$$

$$\frac{2}{3} \times \left(1 \div \frac{3}{4}\right) =$$

$$\frac{2}{3} \times \left(\frac{1}{1} \times \frac{4}{3}\right) =$$

$$\frac{2}{3} \times \frac{4}{3} = \frac{8}{9}$$

Percentages

Percent (%) means parts per 100 or *divided by 100.* In calculations dealing with a percentage, you drop the % symbol, divide the number by 100, and write it as a fraction or a decimal number.

$$13\% \quad \text{means} \quad \frac{13}{100} \quad \text{or} \quad 0.13$$

$$100\% \quad \text{means} \quad \frac{100}{100} \quad \text{or} \quad 1$$

$$12.3\% \quad \text{means} \quad \frac{12.3}{100} \quad \text{or} \quad 0.123$$

$$6\frac{1}{2}\% \quad \text{means} \quad 6.5\% \quad \text{or} \quad \frac{6.5}{100} \quad \text{or} \quad 0.065$$

Example 1.19

Write 0.5% as a fraction.

$$0.5\% = \frac{0.5}{100} = \frac{5}{1000} = \frac{1}{200}$$

There is another way to get the answer. You know that $0.5 = \frac{1}{2}$. So

$$0.5\% = \frac{1}{2}\% = \frac{1}{2} \div 100 = \frac{1}{2} \times \frac{1}{100} = \frac{1}{200}$$

Notes/Workspace

Notes/Workspace

Homework
14-15-16-17-18

xiii - check
that you know
problems - that
you can do every
problem in
under 20 minutes

memorize
lists on A:22

Practice Sets

You will find the answers to Try These for Practice and Exercises Practice Sets in Appendix A at the back of the book. Your instructor has the answers to the Additional Exercises.

Try These for Practice

Test your comprehension after reading the chapter.

1. Write $\frac{7}{8}$ as a decimal number. ________

2. $\left(\frac{5}{12} \times \frac{8}{25}\right) \times \frac{2}{5} =$ ________

3. $\frac{3.46 \times 4.5}{0.3} =$ ________

4. $\frac{\frac{2}{5}}{\frac{6}{15}} =$ ________

5. Write 7.5% as a decimal number. ________

Exercises

Reinforce your understanding in class or at home.

Convert the decimals to fractions.

1. 0.24 = ________

2. 3.24 = ________

Convert the fractions to decimals.

3. $\frac{5}{8} =$ ________

4. $\frac{4}{25} =$ ________

5. $\frac{1}{10} =$ ________

6. $\frac{1}{200} =$ ________

Notes/Workspace

7. $\frac{1}{300} =$ ________
(nearest thousandth)

8. $\frac{4500}{100} =$ ________

9. $\frac{6.25}{1000} =$ ________

10. $\frac{142.6}{7} =$ ________
(nearest tenth)

Convert to decimals.

11. $\frac{7.2}{0.06} =$ ________

12. $\frac{72}{0.006} =$ ________

Multiply the decimals.

13. $123.4 \times 100 =$ ________

14. $5.125 \times 1.3 =$ ________

15. $36.42 \times 1000 =$ ________

Divide the decimals.

16. $85 \div 0.05 =$ ________

17. $8.5 \div 0.5 =$ ________

Write the answers to Problems 18–22 in fractional form.

18. $\frac{4}{15} \times 30 \times \frac{1}{2} =$ ________

19. $6\frac{1}{2} \div 3 =$ ________

20. $26 \div 3\frac{1}{4} =$ ________

21. $4.25 \times \frac{1}{5} =$ ________

22. $\frac{1}{250} \times 125 \times \frac{1}{0.5} =$ ________

Write the answers to Problems 23–26 in fractional form and in decimal form to the nearest tenth.

23. $4.75 \times \frac{1}{1.5} =$ ________

24. $\frac{3}{\frac{5}{10}} =$ ________

Notes/Workspace

25. $\dfrac{\frac{1}{4}}{6} \times 8 =$ ________

26. $\dfrac{\frac{1}{4} \times 160}{\frac{5}{8}} =$ ________

Write the percentages as decimals.

27. $38\frac{2}{5}\% =$ ________

28. $35\% =$ ________

Write the percentages as fractions.

29. $6.75\% =$ ________

30. $1.5\% =$ ________

Additional Exercises

Now, on your own, test yourself! Ask your instructor to check your answers.

Write the decimals as fractions.

1. $0.015 =$ ________

2. $1.06 =$ ________

Write the fractions as decimals.

3. $\dfrac{6}{15} =$ ________

4. $\dfrac{9}{50} =$ ________

5. $\dfrac{3}{200} =$ ________

6. $\dfrac{1}{150} =$ ________ (nearest thousandth)

7. $\dfrac{1}{240} =$ ________ (nearest thousandth)

8. $\dfrac{264}{1000} =$ ________

Convert the following to decimals.

9. $\dfrac{43.5}{100} =$ ________

10. $\dfrac{503.8}{15} =$ ________
(nearest tenth)

11. $\dfrac{6.3}{0.07} =$ ________

Multiply the decimals.

12. $630 \times 0.007 =$ ________

13. $56.18 \times 7.2 =$ ________

14. $8.277 \times 100 =$ ________

15. $63.2 \times 10 =$ ________

Divide the decimals.

16. $2.61 \div 0.3 =$ ________

17. $261 \div 0.003 =$ ________

Write the answers to Problems 18–23 in fractional form.

18. $\dfrac{5}{12} \times 10 \times \dfrac{1}{15} =$ ________

19. $8\dfrac{1}{2} \div 6 =$ ________

20. $39 \div 3\dfrac{1}{4} =$ ________

21. $9.45 \times \dfrac{1}{15} =$ ________

22. $\dfrac{4}{200} \times 50 \times \dfrac{1}{0.2} =$ ________

23. $8.35 \times \dfrac{0.25}{0.5} =$ ________

Write the answers to Problems 24–26 in fractional form and in decimal form to the nearest tenth.

24. $\dfrac{\frac{1}{3}}{2} =$ ________

25. $\dfrac{4}{\frac{5}{3}} \times \dfrac{2}{9} =$ ________

26. $\dfrac{\frac{7}{10} \times 150}{2} =$ ________

Notes/Workspace

Notes/Workspace

Write the percentages as decimals.

27. 20.5% = ________ **28.** 42% = ________

Write the percentages as fractions.

29. 20.5% = ________ **30.** 24% = ________

chapter 2

Drug Administration

Objectives

After completing this chapter, you will be able to

- *identify the parts of a medication order.*
- *describe the information listed on a physician's order sheet and a medication administration record.*
- *identify the routes of drug administration.*
- *describe the forms in which medication is supplied.*
- *interpret information found on medication labels and package inserts.*
- *understand the "five rights" concerning medication administration.*
- *identify the trade name and the generic name of a drug.*
- *understand the legal implications involved in the administration of drugs.*

This chapter presents the components of the drug order, drug label, physician's order sheet, and the medication administration record. Each will be discussed in the context of their use in an institutional health-care setting such as a hospital or extended-care facility.

Notes/Workspace

Who Administers Drugs?

To a patient, drugs can be life-saving, therapeutic, or life-threatening. Physicians and dentists can legally prescribe medications. In many states, physician's assistants and nurse practitioners can also prescribe a range of medications related to their areas of practice.

The registered professional nurse (RN), licensed practical nurse (LPN), and the vocational nurse (VN) are responsible for administering drugs ordered by the prescriber. Of course, physicians can also administer drugs to patients.

In most cases, however, drug administration is a process involving a chain of health-care professionals. The prescriber *writes* the drug order, the pharmacist *fills* the order, and the nurse *administers* the drug to the patient. Everyone involved is equally responsible for the accuracy of the order and the safety of the patient.

In order to ensure patients' safety, health-care professionals who administer medications must understand how drugs act. This knowledge helps them determine when a drug should not be administered or when it should be used cautiously. Understanding drug actions is also important in determining whether a prescribed drug will interact with another drug that the patient is receiving. Drug actions are discussed in pharmacology textbooks and drug handbooks.

The Drug Administration Process

As someone who will be responsible for administering drugs to clients, you must know how to administer them safely. In particular, you must know the classic *Five "Rights" of Medication Administration.* These are the

- right drug
- right dose
- right route
- right time
- right patient

The Right Drug A drug is a substance that acts therapeutically on the physiologic processes of the human body. For example, the drug insulin is given to patients whose bodies do not manufacture insulin for the metabolism of food. Some drugs have more than one therapeutic property. Aspirin, for example, is an antipyretic (fever reducing), analgesic (pain relieving), and anti-inflammatory drug and has anticoagulant properties (decreases the viscosity of blood). It may be taken for any one, or all, of its therapeutic properties.

A drug can be prescribed using either its *generic* name or its *trade* name. For example, many companies manufacture the anticancer drug, cyclophosphamide (Figure 2.1). Cyclophosphamide is the drug's generic name. As the drug label in the figure shows, the manufacturer calls this drug Cytoxan. So, in this case, Cytoxan is the drug's trade name. A drug has only one generic name but can have many trade names. Each trade name is patented by the particular manufacturer of the drug.

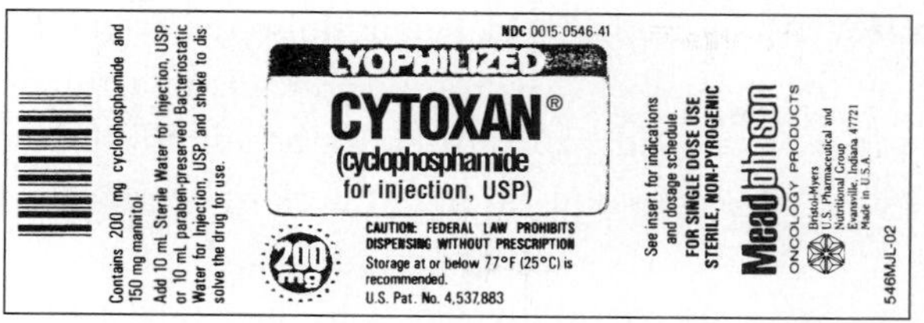

Figure 2.1 *A drug's trade name and generic name. The trade name (Cytoxan) appears in capital letters and can be identified by the raised ® to the right of the name. The drug's generic name (cyclophosphamide) usually appears in lowercase letters. The manufacturer (Mead-Johnson) chose the name Cytoxan for its version of this anticancer drug.*

Notes/Workspace

The drug's trade name usually has the symbol ™ or ® printed to the right of the name (for example, Cytoxan®). This is the drug's trademark or registration symbol. In addition, the trade name is usually printed in uppercase letters, while the generic name is printed in lowercase letters (see Figure 2.1). If the prescriber writes an order for Cytoxan, then the brand Cytoxan **must** be used, and no substitutions are allowed. But if the order uses the drug's generic name (for example, cyclophosphamide) or if the order indicates a trade name but states "substitution permitted," then cyclophosphamide made by any manufacturer can be administered.

Warning

Read drug names carefully! Many drugs have similar looking names. For example, digoxin is *not* digitoxin, and cefotetan is *not* cefoxitin.

The Right Dose There are many drug references available. They indicate the correct dose for a specific patient. These resources include pharmacology texts and drug handbooks, *The United States Pharmacopeia*, the *Physicians' Desk Reference*, and manufacturers' package inserts. Those prescribing and administering medications must learn the correct dose. It is their **legal responsibility** to know this information.

The right dose can be affected by the patient's weight or body surface area (BSA). Many drug doses administered to children or for cancer therapy are calculated based on BSA.

Body surface area is determined by formulas or by the use of a BSA nomogram. Body surface area is the actual measurement of the total skin area of a person measured in meters squared (m^2). The average adult is considered to have a BSA of 1.7 square meters. We can measure the BSA of a child or an adult if we know their height and weight. See the pediatric nomogram in Appendix F.

Notes/Workspace

The Right Route Medications must be administered in the form and via the route specified by the prescriber. Medications are manufactured in a variety of forms: liquids, vapors, and solids. Each drug can be administered by one or more routes: by injections, by absorption through the skin, or mucous membranes, or orally.

Parenteral medications are administered by inserting a hypodermic needle attached to a syringe into a body part. The syringe contains the drug that is to be administered. The most common parenteral drug administration sites are listed in Table 2.1. Learn these abbreviations for the major routes of drug administration.

Table 2.1 ***Major Parenteral Drug Administration Routes***

Route	Abbreviation	Meaning
Intramuscular	IM	into the muscle
Subcutaneous	sc	into the subcutaneous tissue
Intravenous	IV	into the vein
Intracardiac	IC	into the cardiac muscle
Intradermal	ID	beneath the skin

Medications can also be administered *cutaneously*—that is, through the skin or mucous membrane. This route includes topical administration on the skin surface; inhalation through the nose or mouth; and solutions and ointments applied to the mucosa of the eyes, nose, ears, and mouth. A nitroglycerin patch and the now-familiar nicotine patch, which are applied to the skin, are examples of cutaneously administered drugs. Suppositories containing medications are inserted into the appropriate orifice (vagina, rectum, or urethra).

Oral drugs are administered *by mouth* (po). These drugs are manufactured in many forms: tablets, capsules, and caplets (Figure 2.2); oral suspensions; elixirs; tablets for buccal administration (absorbed by the mucosa of the oral cavity);

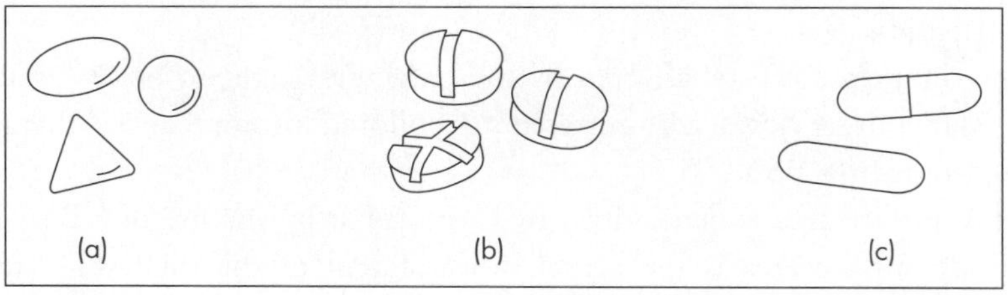

(a) (b) (c)

Figure 2.2 *Tablets, capsules, and caplets are manufactured in various shapes and forms: (a) unscored and enteric-coated tablets (should not be broken); (b) scored tablets, usually in halves (may be broken); (c) capsules and caplets (should not be broken).*

tablets for sublingual administration (absorbed under the tongue); and sustained-release (SR) capsules. SR capsules slowly release a controlled amount of medication over a period of hours (usually 24 hours).

Notes/Workspace

Note

The prescriber specifies the drug's route of administration. You cannot substitute one route of administration for another.

The Right Time The prescriber will indicate when and how often a medication should be administered: po (by mouth) medications, for example, can be given either before or after meals, depending on how the drug acts. A drug's frequency of administration may be stated specifically; for example, once a day (qd), twice a day (bid), three times a day (tid), and four times a day (qid). Also, medications can be ordered at varying times in a 24-hour day; for example, q4h (every four hours), q6h, q8h, q12h.

The Right Patient In a hospital setting, the identification bracelet identifies the patient. The name on the drug order form and the name on the patient's identification bracelet **must** match. Some patients are allergic to certain drugs or have an idiosyncratic (unusual) reaction to a drug. Therefore, patients must always be questioned concerning allergies, and this information must be recorded.

Warning

Anticipate side effects! A side effect is an undesired physiological response to a drug. For example, codeine relieves pain. But its side effects include constipation, nausea, drowsiness, and itching. Record any side effects noted and discuss them with the prescriber.

Drug Orders

A drug order (prescription) includes the patient's name, name of the drug, the dose, route of administration, and frequency of administration. This order must be written by a health professional licensed by the state to practice as a physician, dentist, advanced nurse practitioner, or a physician's assistant. This book uses the title "prescriber" to designate anyone with the authority to write a prescription. The pharmacist who fills the order by providing the medication ordered by the prescriber is also licensed by the state. A pharmacist cannot write an order or administer medications to patients.

Notes/Workspace

A drug order can take various forms. Figure 2.3 is an example of a physician's order sheet. Note the following information:

Date order written:	1/12/94
Time order written:	9:30 A.M.
Name of drug:	digoxin
Dose:	0.125 mg (milligram)
Route of administration:	po (by mouth)
Frequency of administration:	qd (once a day)
Name of prescriber:	J. Olsen M.D.

In addition, the physician's order sheet provides basic patient information:

Name of patient:	John Camden
Patient's registration number:	602412
Address:	23 Jones Ave., New York, NY 10024
Physician:	J. Olsen
Birth date:	2/11/55
Date of admission:	1/11/94

ordered by amt. of ingredients

GENERAL HOSPITAL

PRESS HARD WITH BALLPOINT PEN. WRITE DATE & TIME AND SIGN EACH ORDER

DATE	TIME	A.M. (circled) / P.M.
1/12/94	9:30	
digoxin 0.125 mg po qd		

SIGNATURE J. Olsen M.D.

IMPRINT
602412 1/11/94
John Camden 2/11/55
23 Jones Ave. RC
New York, NY 10024 BCBS
J. Olsen, M.D.

ORDERS NOTED
DATE 1/12/94 TIME 10 A.M. (circled) P.M.
❑ MEDEX ❑ KARDEX
NURSE'S SIG. A. Giangrasso

FILLED BY DATE

PHYSICIAN'S ORDERS

Figure 2.3 *Physician's order sheet*

Religion: Roman Catholic

Insurance: Blue Cross, Blue Shield

You will find a list of the most common abbreviations that might appear on a drug order in Appendix B. Now, try interpreting the physician's order sheet in Figure 2.4. Record the following information:

Date order written: 1-13-94

Time order written: 10:00 pm.

Name of drug: Xanax

Dose: 0.5 mg.

Route of administration: po by mouth

Frequency of administration: twice a day

Name of prescriber: A Giangrasso, MD

Name of patient: Catherine York

Patient's registration number: 422934

Address: 40 Addison Ave Rutland, Vt 05701

Physician: A, Giangrasso

Birth date: 12/1/62

Notes/Workspace

GENERAL HOSPITAL

PRESS HARD WITH BALLPOINT PEN. WRITE DATE & TIME AND SIGN EACH ORDER

DATE	TIME	A.M. / P.M.
1/13/94	10	(P.M.)
Xanax 0.5 mg po bid		

SIGNATURE A. Giangrasso M.D.

IMPRINT
422934 1/13/94
Catherine York
12/1/62
40 Addison Ave. Prot
Rutland, VT 05701 GHI-CBP

ORDERS NOTED

DATE 1/13/94 TIME 10:05 A.M. (P.M.)

❑ MEDEX ❑ KARDEX

NURSE'S SIG. J. Olsen

FILLED BY DATE

PHYSICIAN'S ORDERS

Figure 2.4 *Physician's order sheet*

Notes/Workspace

Date of admission: 1/13/94

Religion: protestant

Insurance: GHI – CBP

Here is what you should have found:

Date order written: 1/13/94

Time order written: 10 P.M.

Name of drug: Xanax

Dose: 0.5 mg

Route of administration: po (by mouth)

Frequency of administration: bid (twice a day)

Name of prescriber: A. Giangrasso M.D.

Name of patient: Catherine York

Patient's registration number: 422934

Address: 40 Addison Ave, Rutland, VT 05701

Physician: A. Giangrasso

Birth date: 12/1/62

Date of Admission: 1/13/94

Religion: Protestant

Insurance: GHI-CBP

Note that just under the patient "imprint" there is a small section entitled "Orders Noted." This section indicates the date and time that the order was transcribed to the medication administration record (discussed later in this chapter). The signature belongs to the nurse who transcribed this order from the physician's order sheet to the medication administration record.

Drug Labels

You will need to understand the information found on drug labels in order to calculate drug dosages and to ensure that a drug is prepared and administered safely. Every drug label provides the same kinds of information. Study the parts of the label in Figure 2.5 for chlorpropamide, a drug that lowers blood glucose. Follow the numbers on the label.

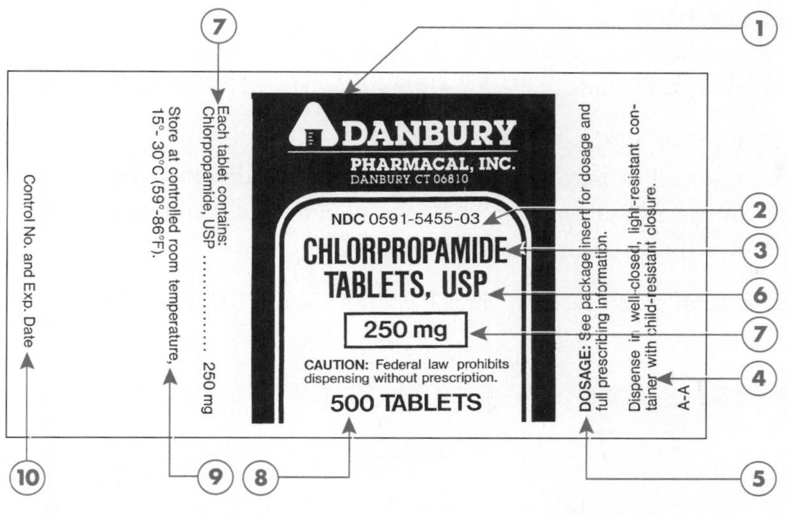

DANBURY
PHARMACAL, INC.
DANBURY, CT 06810
NDC 0591-5455-03
CHLORPROPAMIDE
TABLETS, USP
250 mg
CAUTION: Federal law prohibits dispensing without prescription.
500 TABLETS
Each tablet contains:
Chlorpropamide, USP .... 250 mg
Store at controlled room temperature,
15°- 30°C (59°-86°F).
Control No. and Exp. Date
DOSAGE: See package insert for dosage and full prescribing information.
Dispense in well-closed, light-resistant container with child-resistant closure.
A-A
1
2
3
4
5
6
7
8
9
10

Figure 2.5 *Drug label for chlorpropamide; see text for explanation.*

1. The manufacturer:
   Danbury Pharmacal, Inc.

2. National drug code (NDC) number:
   An identifying number assigned to this drug by the Drug Enforcement Agency (DEA).

3. Name and form of drug:
   The container holds tablets of chlorpropamide. Chlorpropamide is the drug's generic name, indicated by the fact that there is no ® or ™ following the drug's name.

4. Dispensing instructions:
   This tells the pharmacists to provide a light-resistant, child-proof container when filling this prescription.

5. Dosage recommendations:
   Instead of printing dosage information directly on the label, this manufacturer has printed them on an insert packed with the drug container. You will learn more about drug package inserts shortly.

6. USP:
   This means that the drug is prepared according to the standards set by the *United States Pharmacopeia,* which specifies the accepted formulations of drugs available in the U.S.

7. Amount of drug per dose (shown in two places):
   Each tablet contains 250 milligrans of chlorpropamide.

8. Number of tablets per container:
   The container holds 500 tablets.

Notes/Workspace

Notes/Workspace

9. Storage directions:
   Some drugs have to be stored under controlled conditions if they are to retain their effectiveness. This drug should be stored at room temperature.

10. Control number and expiration date:
    Drugs are mixed in batches—the control number identifies the batch. If a quality-control problem is detected, the manufacturer will recall defective batches of drugs by their control numbers.

    The expiration date specifies when the drug should be discarded.

Warning

Always read the expiration date! After the expiration date, the drug may lose its potency or act differently in the patient's body. Discard expired drugs. **Never** give them to patients!

Study the major kinds of information provided in Figure 2.6 for sucralfate (Carafate).

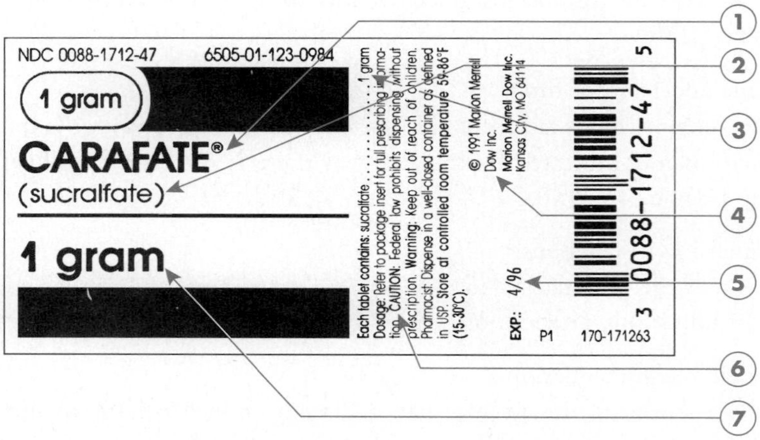

Figure 2.6 *Drug label for Carafate:*

1. *Trade name: Carafate*
2. *Generic name: sucralfate*
3. *Drug form: 1 gram tablets*
4. *Manufacturer: Marion Merrell Dow Inc.*
5. *Expiration date: April 1996*
6. *Caution: Federal law prohibits dispensing without prescription. Warning: Keep out of reach of children.*
7. *Dose: 1 gram*

Many drug labels contain detailed dosage information and important directions for mixing, administering, and storing a drug. These categories of information

Notes/Workspace

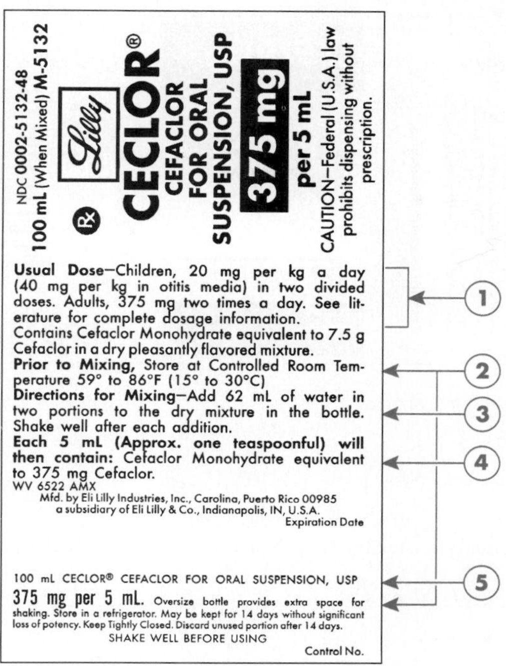

Figure 2.7 *Drug label for Ceclor; see text for explanation.*

are shown on the side of the drug label in Figure 2.7 for cefaclor (Ceclor), an anti-infective drug:

1. Usual dose:
   Separate doses for adults and children are specified. Children with otitis media (an ear infection) need twice the normal children's dose.

2. Storage (two places on label):
   Prior to mixing, the drug should be stored at room temperature. After mixing, it should be stored in a refrigerator and may be kept 14 days.

3. Directions for mixing:
   Ceclor is packaged as a powder within the bottle. Before administering this medication, you need to add 62 milliliters of water and shake the mixture.

4. Amount of drug per dose after mixing:
   Five milliliters of the prepared solution will contain 375 milligrams of Ceclor.

5. Volume of drug after mixing:
   When mixed as directed, the bottle will contain 100 milliliters of Ceclor solution.

You will learn more about preparing drug solutions in Chapter 8.

Notes/Workspace

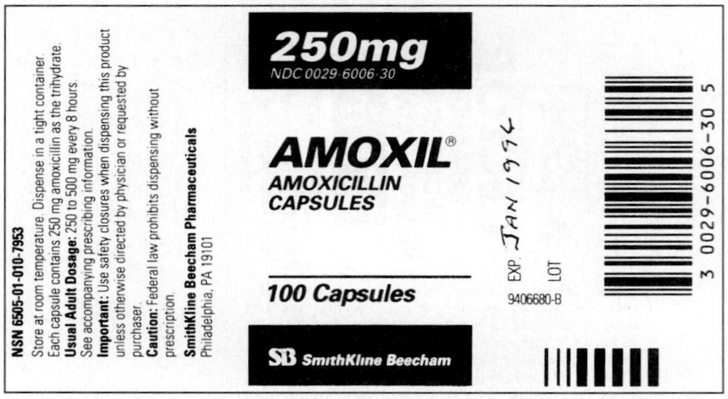

Figure 2.8 *Drug label for Amoxil*

Example 2.1

Examine the label shown in Figure 2.8 and record the following information:

Trade name: amoxil

Generic name: amoxicillin

Form: Capsules)

Dosage or strength: 250 mg.

Amount of drug in container: 100

Usual dosage: 250 mg. per capsule

Expiration date: Jan 1994

Storage temperature: room temperature

Here is what you should have found:

Trade name: Amoxil

Generic name: amoxicillin

Form: capsules

Dosage or strength: 250 mg per capsule

Amount of drug in container: 100 capsules

Usual dosage: 250–500 mg every 8 hours

Expiration date: January 1996

Storage temperature: at room temperature

Note the label for Amoxil does not have a control number. This number would be on the box that holds the bottle of capsules.

NDC 0002-5057-68
150 mL (When Mixed) M-5057

Rx

Lilly

CECLOR®

CEFACLOR FOR ORAL SUSPENSION, USP

125 mg per 5 mL

CAUTION—Federal (U.S.A.) law prohibits dispensing without prescription.

Usual Dose—Children, 20 mg per kg a day (40 mg per kg in otitis media) in three divided doses. Adults, 250 mg three times a day. See literature for complete dosage information.
Contains Cefaclor Monohydrate equivalent to 3.75 g Cefaclor in a dry pleasantly flavored mixture.
Prior to Mixing. Store at Controlled Room Temperature 59° to 86°F (15° to 30°C)
Directions for Mixing—Add 90 mL of water in two portions to the dry mixture in the bottle. Shake well after each addition.
Each 5 mL (Approx. one teaspoonful) will then contain: Cefaclor Monohydrate equivalent to 125 mg Cefaclor.
WV 6461 AMX

Mfd. by Eli Lilly Industries, Inc., Carolina Puerto Rico 00985
a subsidiary of Eli Lilly & Co., Indianapolis, IN, U.S.A.

Expiration Date

150 mL CECLOR® CEFACLOR FOR ORAL SUSPENSION, USP
125 mg per 5 mL. Oversize bottle provides extra space for shaking. Store in a refrigerator. May be kept for 14 days without significant loss of potency. Keep Tightly Closed. Discard unused portion after 14 days.
SHAKE WELL BEFORE USING

Control No.

Figure 2.9 *Drug label for Ceclor*

Notes/Workspace

Example 2.2

Examine the label shown in Figure 2.9 and record the information below:

Trade name: ______

Generic name: ______

Form: ______

Dosage or strength: ______

Amount after mixing: ______

Usual dosage: ______

Directions for mixing: ______

Here is what you should have found:

Trade name: Ceclor

Generic name: cefaclor

Form: oral suspension

Dosage or strength: 125 mg per 5 mL

Amount after mixing: 150 mL when mixed

Usual dosage: adults—250 mg three times a day
children—20 mg/kg a day in three divided doses

Directions for mixing: add 90 mL of water in two portions;
shake well after each addition

Drug Package Inserts

Sometimes the information you need to safely prepare, administer, and store medications is not located on the drug label. In such cases, you may need to read the *package insert.* The package insert is included with each container of a prescription drug and is prepared by the pharmaceutical manufacturer.

The information on a drug package insert is intended for the physician, pharmacist, or drug administrator. It contains complex descriptions of a drug's chemistry and how it acts in the body. Figure 2.10 shows an example of two pages from a drug package insert for nitroglycerin transdermal system. Despite the complexity of the description, always consult the package insert when you need detailed information about

- mixing and storing a drug
- preparing a drug dose
- when the drug should **not** be used
- side effects and adverse reactions

NITROGLYCERIN TRANSDERMAL SYSTEM

Prescribing Information

DESCRIPTION

Nitroglycerin is 1,2,3-propanetriol trinitrate, an organic nitrate whose structural formula is:

$$H_2CONO_2 \; | \; HCONO_2 \; | \; H_2CONO_2$$

and whose molecular weight is 227.09. The organic nitrates are vasodilators, active on both arteries and veins.

The Nitroglycerin Transdermal System is a flat unit designed to provide continuous controlled release of nitroglycerin through intact skin. The rate of release of nitroglycerin is linearly dependent upon the area of the applied system; each cm^2 of applied system delivers approximately 0.02 mg of nitroglycerin per hour. Thus, the 10-, 20-, and 30-cm^2 systems deliver approximately 0.2, 0.4 and 0.6 mg of nitroglycerin per hour, respectively.

The remainder of the nitroglycerin in each system serves as a reservoir and is not delivered in normal use. After 12 hours, for example, each system has delivered 4% of its original content of nitroglycerin.

The Nitroglycerin Transdermal System contains nitroglycerin in a laminated matrix composed of polyvinyl chloride/polyvinyl acetate copolymer, di-(2-ethylhexyl) phthalate, isopropyl palmitate, colloidal silicon dioxide, aluminum foil laminate, polyethylene foam and acrylic adhesive. The 10-, 20- and 30-cm^2 systems contain 62.5 mg, 125.0 mg and 187.5 mg of nitroglycerin, respectively.

Cross section of the system:

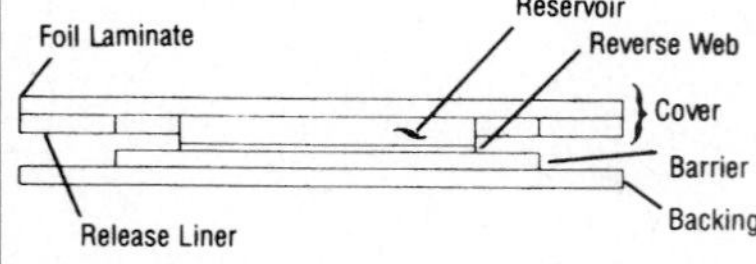

CLINICAL PHARMACOLOGY

The principal pharmacological action of nitroglycerin is relaxation of vascular smooth muscle and consequent dilatation of peripheral arteries and veins, especially the latter. Dilatation of the veins promotes peripheral pooling of blood and decreases venous return to the heart, thereby reducing left ventricular end-diastolic pressure and pulmonary capillary wedge pressure (preload). Arteriolar relaxation reduces systemic vascular resistance, systolic arterial pressure, and mean arterial pressure (afterload). Dilatation of the coronary arteries also occurs. The relative importance of preload reduction, afterload reduction, and coronary dilatation remains undefined.

Dosing regimens for most chronically used drugs are designed to provide plasma concentrations that are continuously greater than a minimally effective concentration. This strategy is inappropriate for organic nitrates. Several well-controlled clinical trials have used exercise testing to assess the anti-anginal efficacy of continuously-delivered nitrates. In the large majority of these trials, active agents were indistinguishable from placebo after 24 hours (or less) of continuous therapy. Attempts to overcome nitrate tolerance by dose escalation, even to doses far in excess of those used acutely, have consistently failed. Only after nitrates have been absent from the body for several hours has their antianginal efficacy been restored.

Pharmacokinetics: The volume of distribution of nitroglycerin is about 3 L/kg, and nitroglycerin is cleared from this volume at extremely rapid rates, with a resulting serum half-life of about 3 minutes. The observed clearance rates (close to 1 L/kg/min) greatly exceed hepatic blood flow; known sites of extrahepatic metabolism include red blood cells and vascular walls.

The first products in the metabolism of nitroglycerin are inorganic nitrate and the 1,2- and 1,3-dinitroglycerols. The dinitrates are less effective vasodilators than nitroglycerin, but they are longer-lived in the serum, and their net contribution to the overall effect of chronic nitroglycerin regimens is not known. The dinitrates are further metabolized to (non-vasoactive) mononitrates and, ultimately, to glycerol and carbon dioxide.

To avoid development of tolerance to nitroglycerin, drug-free intervals of 10-12 hours are known to be sufficient; shorter intervals have not been well studied. In one well-controlled clinical trial, subjects receiving nitroglycerin appeared to exhibit a rebound or withdrawal effect, so that their exercise tolerance at the end of the daily drug-free interval was *less* than that exhibited by the parallel group receiving placebo.

In healthy volunteers, steady-state plasma concentrations of nitroglycerin are reached by about two hours after application of a patch and are maintained for the duration of wearing the system (observations have been limited to 24 hours). Upon removal of the patch, the plasma concentration declines with a half-life of about an hour.

Clinical trials: Regimens in which nitroglycerin patches were worn for 12 hours daily have been studied in well-controlled trials up to 4 weeks in duration. Starting about 2 hours after application and continuing until 10-12 hours after application, patches that deliver at least 0.4 mg of nitroglycerin per hour have consistently demonstrated greater anti-anginal activity than placebo. Lower-dose patches have not been as well studied, but in one large, well-controlled trial in which higher-dose patches were also studied, patches delivering 0.2 mg/hr had significantly *less* anti-anginal activity than placebo.

It is reasonable to believe that the rate of nitroglycerin absorption from patches may vary with the site of application, but this relationship has not been adequately studied.

The onset of action of transdermal nitroglycerin is not sufficiently rapid for this product to be useful in aborting an acute anginal episode.

INDICATIONS AND USAGE

Transdermal nitroglycerin is indicated for the prevention of angina pectoris due to coronary artery disease. The onset of action of transdermal nitroglycerin is not sufficiently rapid for this product to be useful in aborting an acute attack.

CONTRAINDICATIONS

Allergic reactions to organic nitrates are extremely rare, but they do occur. Nitroglycerin is contraindicated in patients who are allergic to it. Allergy to the adhesives used in nitroglycerin patches has also been reported, and it similarly constitutes a contraindication to the use of this product.

WARNINGS

The benefits of transdermal nitroglycerin in patients with acute myocardial infarction or congestive heart failure have not been established. If one elects to use nitroglycerin in these conditions, careful clinical or hemodynamic monitoring must be used to avoid the hazards of hypotension and tachycardia.

A cardioverter/defibrillator should not be discharged through a paddle electrode that overlies a nitroglycerin transdermal patch. The arcing that may be seen in this situation is harmless itself, but it may be associated with local current concentration that can cause damage to the paddles and burns to the patient.

PRECAUTIONS

General: Severe hypotension, particularly with upright posture, may occur with even small doses of nitroglycerin. This drug should therefore be used with caution in patients who may be volume depleted or who, for whatever reason, are already hypotensive. Hypotension induced by nitroglycerin may be accompanied by paradoxical bradycardia and increased angina pectoris.

Nitrate therapy may aggravate the angina caused by hypertrophic cardiomyopathy.

Figure 2.10 *A typical drug package insert*

As tolerance to other forms of nitroglycerin develops, the effect of sublingual nitroglycerin on exercise tolerance, although still observable, is somewhat blunted.

In industrial workers who have had long-term exposure to unknown (presumably high) doses of organic nitrates, tolerance clearly occurs. Chest pain, acute myocardial infarction, and even sudden death have occurred during temporary withdrawal of nitrates from these workers, demonstrating the existence of true physical dependence.

Several clinical trials in patients with angina pectoris have evaluated nitroglycerin regimens which incorporated a 10-12 hour nitrate-free interval. In some of these trials, an increase in the frequency of anginal attacks during the nitrate-free interval was observed in a small number of patients. In one trial, patients demonstrated decreased exercise tolerance at the end of the nitrate-free interval. Hemodynamic rebound has been observed only rarely; on the other hand, few studies were so designed that rebound, if it had occurred, would have been detected. The importance of these observations to the routine, clinical use of transdermal nitroglycerin is unknown.

Information for Patients: Daily headaches sometimes accompany treatment with nitroglycerin. In patients who get these headaches, the headaches may be a marker of the activity of the drug. Patients should resist the temptation to avoid headaches by altering the schedule of their treatment with nitroglycerin, since loss of headache may be associated with simultaneous loss of antianginal efficacy.

Treatment with nitroglycerin may be associated with lightheadedness on standing, especially just after rising from a recumbent or seated position. This effect may be more frequent in patients who have also consumed alcohol.

After normal use, there is enough residual nitroglycerin in discarded patches that they are a potential hazard to children and pets.

A patient leaflet is supplied with the systems.

Drug Interactions: The vasodilating effects of nitroglycerin may be additive with those of other vasodilators. Alcohol, in particular, has been found to exhibit additive effects of this variety.

Carcinogenesis, Mutagenesis, and Impairment of Fertility: Studies to evaluate the carcinogenic or mutagenic potential of nitroglycerin have not been performed. Nitroglycerin's effect upon reproductive capacity is similarly unknown.

Pregnancy category C: Animal reproduction studies have not been conducted with nitroglycerin. It is also not known whether nitroglycerin can cause fetal harm when administered to a pregnant woman or whether it can affect reproductive capacity. Nitroglycerin should be given to a pregnant woman only if clearly needed.

Nursing Mothers: It is not known whether nitroglycerin is excreted in human milk. Because many drugs are excreted in human milk, caution should be exercised when nitroglycerin is administered to a nursing woman.

Pediatric Use: Safety and effectiveness in children have not been established.

ADVERSE REACTIONS

Adverse reactions to nitroglycerin are generally dose-related, and almost all of these reactions are the result of nitroglycerin's activity as a vasodilator. Headache, which may be severe, is the most commonly reported side effect. Headache may be recurrent with each daily dose, especially at higher doses. Transient episodes of lightheadedness, occasionally related to blood pressure changes, may also occur. Hypotension occurs infrequently, but in some patients it may be severe enough to warrant discontinuation of therapy. Syncope, crescendo angina, and rebound hypertension have been reported but are uncommon.

Extremely rarely, ordinary doses of organic nitrates have caused methemoglobinemia in normal-seeming patients; for further discussion of its diagnosis and treatment see **Overdosage**.

Allergic reactions to nitroglycerin are also uncommon, and the great majority of those reported have been cases of contact dermatitis or fixed drug eruptions in patients receiving nitroglycerin in ointments or patches. There have been a few reports of genuine anaphylactoid reactions, and these reactions can probably occur in patients receiving nitroglycerin by any route.

In two placebo-controlled trials of intermittent therapy with nitroglycerin patches at 0.2 to 0.8 mg/hr, the most frequent adverse reactions among 307 subjects were as follows:

	placebo	patch
headache	18%	63%
lightheadedness	4%	6%
hypotension and/or syncope	0%	4%
increased angina	2%	2%

OVERDOSAGE

Hemodynamic Effects: The ill effects of nitroglycerin overdose are generally the results of nitroglycerin's capacity to induce vasodilatation, venous pooling, reduced cardiac output, and hypotension. These hemodynamic changes may have protean manifestations, including increased intracranial pressure, with any or all of persistent throbbing headache, confusion, and moderate fever, vertigo; palpitations; visual disturbances; nausea and vomiting (possibly with colic and even bloody diarrhea); syncope (especially in the upright posture); air hunger and dyspnea, later followed by reduced ventilatory effort; diaphoresis, with the skin either flushed or cold and clammy; heart block and bradycardia; paralysis; coma; seizures; and death.

Laboratory determinations of serum levels of nitroglycerin and its metabolites are not widely available, and such determinations have, in any event, no established role in the management of nitroglycerin overdose.

No data are available to suggest physiological maneuvers (e.g., maneuvers to change the pH of the urine) that might accelerate elimination of nitroglycerin and its active metabolites. Similarly, it is not known which — if any — of these substances can usefully be removed from the body by hemodialysis.

No specific antagonist to the vasodilator effects of nitroglycerin is known, and no intervention has been subject to controlled study as a therapy of nitroglycerin overdose. Because the hypotension associated with nitroglycerin overdose is the result of venodilatation and arterial hypovolemia, prudent therapy in this situation should be directed toward increase in central fluid volume. Passive elevation of the patient's legs may be sufficient, but intravenous infusion of normal saline or similar fluid may also be necessary.

The use of epinephrine or other arterial vasoconstrictors in this setting is likely to do more harm than good.

In patients with renal disease or congestive heart failure, therapy resulting in central volume expansion is not without hazard. Treatment of nitroglycerin overdose in these patients may be subtle and difficult, and invasive monitoring may be required.

Methemoglobinemia: Nitrate ions liberated during metabolism of nitroglycerin can oxidize hemoglobin into methemoglobin. Even in patients totally without cytochrome b_5 reductase activity, however, and even assuming that the nitrate moieties of nitroglycerin are quantitatively applied to oxidation of hemoglobin, about 1mg/kg of nitroglycerin should be required before any of these patients manifests clinically significant ($\geq$10%) methemoglobinemia. In patients with normal reductase function, significant production of methemoglobin should require even larger doses of nitroglycerin. In one study in which 36 patients received 2-4 weeks of continuous nitroglycerin therapy at 3.1 to 4.4 mg/hr, the average methemoglobin level measured was 0.2%; this was comparable to that observed in parallel patients who received placebo.

Notwithstanding these observations, there are case reports of significant methemoglobinemia in association with moderate overdoses of organic nitrates. None of the affected patients had been thought to be unusually susceptible.

Methemoglobin levels are available from most clinical laboratories. The diagnosis should be suspected in patients who exhibit signs of impaired oxygen delivery despite adequate cardiac output and adequate arterial pO_2. Classically, methemoglobinemic blood is described as chocolate brown, without color change on exposure to air.

When methemoglobinemia is diagnosed, the treatment of choice is methylene blue, 1-2 mg/kg intravenously.

DOSAGE AND ADMINISTRATION

The suggested starting dose is between 0.2 mg/hr and 0.4 mg/hr. Doses between 0.4 mg/hr and 0.8 mg/hr have shown continued effectiveness for 10-12 hours daily for at least one month (the longest period studied) of intermittent administration. Although the minimum nitrate-free interval has not been defined, data show that a nitrate-free interval of 10-12 hours is sufficient (see **Clinical Pharmacology**). Thus, an appropriate dosing schedule for nitroglycerin patches would include a daily patch-on period of 12-14 hours and a daily patch-off period of 10-12 hours.

Although some well controlled clinical trials using exercise tolerance testing have shown maintenance of effectiveness when patches are worn continuously, the large majority of such controlled trials have shown the development of tolerance (i.e., complete loss of effect) within the first 24 hours after therapy was initiated. Dose adjustment, even to levels much higher than generally used, did not restore efficacy.

HOW SUPPLIED

Nitroglycerin Transdermal Therapeutic System.

Nitroglycerin transdermal Rated Release in vivo	Total Nitroglycerin in system	System Size	Carton Size
0.2 mg/hour	62.5 mg	10 cm^2	30 units
0.4 mg/hour	125.0 mg	20 cm^2	30 units
0.6 mg/hour	187.5 mg	30 cm^2	30 units

STORAGE CONDITIONS:

Store at controlled room temperature 15°-30°C (59°-86°F).

Do not refrigerate.

CAUTION:

Federal law prohibits dispensing without prescription.

REVISION DATE: July 1993

HCS-075 (7/93)

HERCON LABORATORIES CORPORATION

EMIGSVILLE, PA 17318

Figure 2.10 (*continued*) *A typical drug package insert*

The categories of information usually listed on a package insert are described in Table 2.3.

Notes/Workspace

Table 2.3 *Types of Information on Drug Package Inserts*

Information	Comments
Name of pharmaceutical company	
Name of the drug (trade/generic)	
Strength of drug and clinical formulation	
Clinical pharmacology	How the drug acts in the body.
Indications for using the drug	The conditions the drug is approved to treat.
Contraindications	Conditions under which the drug must not be given.
Warning information	Relative to the safety of the patient. For example, a potent diuretic drug that can deplete the body of electrolytes and fluid can cause a state of dehydration. Therefore, *close* medical supervision would be required for the patient.
Precautions	Indicate the assessments that must be done by a nurse to identify untoward results that could occur when a patient is given a medication. Serum diagnostic tests also identify changes in the patient's overall condition.
Adverse reactions	Drug reactions that could affect patient comfort and safety but that don't necessarily deter the prescriber from prescribing the drug.

Example 2.3

Read the excerpts provided from the package inserts in Figures 2.11 through 2.14 and fill in the requested information.

1. What is the name of the drug (Figure 2.11)?

Nitroglycerin Transdermal System

NITROGLYCERIN TRANSDERMAL SYSTEM

Prescribing Information

DESCRIPTION

Nitroglycerin is 1,2,3-propanetriol trinitrate, an organic nitrate whose structural formula is:

$$H_2CONO_2 \\ HCONO_2 \\ H_2CONO_2$$

Figure 2.11 *Description for Nitroglycerin Transdermal System*

Notes/Workspace

2. What is the most commonly reported side effect of this drug (Figure 2.12)?

Headache

ADVERSE REACTIONS
Adverse reactions to nitroglycerin are generally dose-related, and almost all of these reactions are the result of nitroglycerin's activity as a vasodilator. Headache, which may be severe, is the most commonly reported side effect. Headache may be recurrent with each daily dose, especially at higher doses. Transient episodes of lightheadedness, occasionally related to blood pressure changes, may also occur. Hypotension occurs infrequently, but in some patients it may be severe enough to warrant discontinuation of therapy. Syncope, crescendo angina, and rebound hypertension have been reported but are uncommon.

Figure 2.12 *Adverse reactions for Nitroglycerin Transdermal System*

3. According to the information in Figure 2.13, how is this drug administered?

cutaneously

The Nitroglycerin Transdermal System is a flat unit designed to provide continuous controlled release of nitroglycerin through intact skin. The rate of release of nitroglycerin is linearly dependent upon the area of the applied system; each cm^2 of applied system delivers approximately 0.02 mg of nitroglycerin per hour. Thus, the 10-, 20-, and 30-cm^2 systems deliver approximately 0.2, 0.4 and 0.6 mg of nitroglycerin per hour, respectively. The remainder of the nitroglycerin in each system serves as a reservoir and is not delivered in normal use. After 12 hours, for example, each system has delivered 4% of its original content of nitroglycerin.

Figure 2.13 *Administration for Nitroglycerin Transdermal System*

4. According to Figure 2.14, would this drug be ordered for a patient who is allergic to the adhesives used in nitroglycerin patches?

no

CONTRAINDICATIONS
Allergic reactions to organic nitrates are extremely rare, but they do occur. Nitroglycerin is contraindicated in patients who are allergic to it. Allergy to the adhesives used in nitroglycerin patches has also been reported, and it similarly constitutes a contraindication to the use of this product.

Figure 2.14 *Contraindications for Nitroglycerin Transdermal System*

5. According to Figure 2.15, what is an appropriate dosing schedule for Nitroglycerin Transdermal System?

patch on 10-12 hrs + off 10-12 hours

DOSAGE AND ADMINISTRATION
The suggested starting dose is between 0.2 mg/hr and 0.4 mg/hr. Doses between 0.4 mg/hr and 0.8 mg/hr have shown continued effectiveness for 10-12 hours daily for at least one month (the longest period studied) of intermittent administration. Although the minimum nitrate-free interval has not been defined, data show that a nitrate-free interval of 10-12 hours is sufficient (see **Clinical Pharmacology**). Thus, an appropriate dosing schedule for nitroglycerin patches would include a daily patch-on period of 12-14 hours and a daily patch-off period of 10-12 hours.

Figure 2.15 *Dosage for Nitroglycerin Transdermal System*

Notes/Workspace

Here is what you should have found:

1. Nitroglycerin patch.
2. Headaches.
3. Through the skin surface.
4. No.
5. Daily patch-on period of 12–14 hours and a daily patch-off period of 10–12 hours.

Medication Administration Records

Medication administration records (MARs) are used to record information about the drugs a patient receives under a prescriber's orders. The following list indicates the kinds of information recorded on an MAR.

- Person receiving the medications:
  - Name
  - Date of birth
  - Patient registration number
- Medication:
  - Name
  - Dosage
  - Time of administration
  - Route of administration
  - Date started
  - Date discontinued
- Staff member administering medications:
  - Initials of those administering medications
  - Signatures of staff members administering medications

Although the type of information appearing on an MAR is fairly standard, the appearance of these records varies from one health-care provider to another. For example, some MARs record the time of drug administration using the military clock. This system of recording time does not use A.M. or P.M. after the hour designation. Instead, the hours continue to increment past 12 noon. For example, 2:00 P.M. according to the standard clock is written 14:00 (pronounced "fourteen hundred hours"). Figure 2.16, page 37, compares military and standard clock hours.

In some health-care facilities, the MAR is computerized. Hard copy of an MAR can be readily printed from the computerized patient data base. Each time a medication is administered to a patient, the MAR is updated at a computer terminal by the staff member who administered the drug.

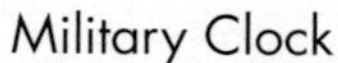

Notes/Workspace

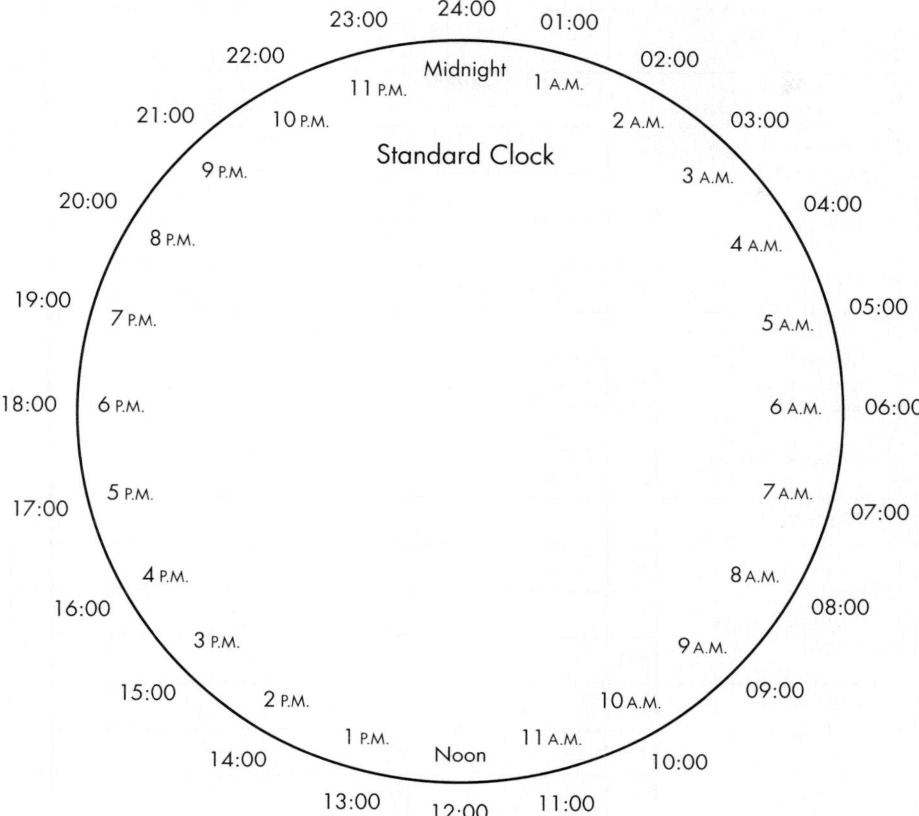

Figure 2.16 *A comparison of the military (outer) and standard (inner) clock. 10 P.M. on a standard clock is 22:00 (twenty-two hundred hours) on a military clock.*

Let's look at an MAR in greater detail (Figure 2.17, page 38). This MAR reveals the following information:

Drug administered at 5 P.M. (17:00) on 9/13/94: Inderal 40 mg

Drug administered at 6 A.M. (06:00) on 9/12/94: haloperidol 1 mg

Drugs administered between 12 noon and 11 P.M. (12:00–23:00): Inderal 40 mg, benztropine 1 mg, haloperidol 1 mg

Did Mr. Yates receive azithromycin 250 mg on 9/12/94, at 6 A.M. (06:00)? No, he received this medication at 9 A.M. (09:00)

When did Mr. Yates receive the last dose of haloperidol? 10 P.M. (22:00)

Notes/Workspace

⊕ GENERAL HOSPITAL ⊕

Year 19 *94* Month *September*	Day	*12*	*13*	*14*	*15*	*16*	*17*
Medication Dosage and Interval		Initials* and Hours	Initials and Hours	Initials and Hours	Initials and Hours	Initials and Hours	Initials and Hours
Date started: *9/12/94* *haloperidol 1 mg* *po tid* *0600, 1400, 2200*	I	*LA*	*LA*				
	AM	*0600*	*0600*				
	I	*MS SG*	*MS SG*				
Discontinued:	PM	*1400, 2200*	*1400, 2200*				
Date started: *9/12/94* *benztropine 1 mg* *po bid x 5 days* *0900, 1700*	I	*JO*	*JO*				
	AM	*0900*	*0900*				
	I	*MS*	*MS*				
Discontinued: *9/17/94*	PM	*1700*	*1700*				
Date started: *9/12/94* *azithromycin 500 mg* *po qd* *0600*	I	*JO*					
	AM	*0600*					
today only 9/12/94	I						
Discontinued: *9/12/94*	PM						
Date started: *9/13/94* *azithromycin 250 mg* *po qd x 5 days* *0900*	I	X	*JO*				
	AM	X	*0900*				
	I	X					
Discontinued: *9/17/94*	PM	X					
Date started: *9/13/94* *Inderal 40 mg* *po qid* *0900, 1300, 1700, 2100*	I	X	*JO*				
	AM	X	*0900*				
	I	X	*MS, MS, SG*				
Discontinued:	PM	X	*1300, 1700, 2100*				

Allergies: (Specify)
tomatoes, codeine, penicillin

Init*	Signature
MS	*Mary Smith*
SG	*Susan Green*
LA	*Louise Alvarez*
JO	*June Olsen*

MEDICATION ADMINISTRATION RECORD

PATIENT IDENTIFICATION

666244 9/11/94
John Yates 8/24/54
44 Chester Drive Christian
NY, NY 10003 Aetna
Dr. Leon Ablon

Figure 2.17 *Medication administration record*

Example 2.4

Study the MAR in Figure 2.18; then fill in the following chart and answer the questions.

Notes/Workspace

GENERAL HOSPITAL

Year 19 *94* Month *July* Day		*17*	*18*	*19*	*20*	*21*	*22*
Medication Dosage and Interval		Initials* and Hours	Initials and Hours	Initials and Hours	Initials and Hours	Initials and Hours	Initials and Hours
Date started: *7/17/94* *Interferon alpha-2a 3,000,000 u Sc 3 x 1 week (check CBC)* Discontinued: *7/23/94*	I	*LA*					
	AM	*0900*					
	I						
	PM						
Date started: *7/17/94* *amitriptyline 75 mg po hs* Discontinued: *7/23/94*	I						
	AM						
	I	*AG*					
	PM	*2100*					
Date started: *7/17/94* *zidovudine 200 mg po q4h (do not give during night)* Discontinued: *7/23/94*	I	*LA LA*					
	AM	*0600, 1000*					
	I	*LA SG AG*					
	PM	*1400, 1800, 2300*					
Date started: *7/17/94* *Ecotrin 650 mg po qd* Discontinued: *9/12/94*	I	*LA*					
	AM	*0900*					
	I						
	PM						

Allergies: (Specify) *penicillin*

Init*	Signature
LA	*Leon Ablon*
AG	*Anthony Giangrasso*
SG	*Susan Green*

PATIENT IDENTIFICATION

622326 7/3/94
David Smith 12/20/60
368-121 Brown Ave. RC
Stocie IL 63642 Medicaid

Dr. June Olsen

MEDICATION ADMINISTRATION RECORD

Figure 2.18 *Medication administration record*

Notes/Workspace

Name of Drug	Route of Administration	Time of Administration

1. Which drug was administered at 10 A.M.? ____________

2. Identify the drug administered po at 9 A.M. ____________

3. Which drug was administered subcutaneously? ____________

4. Who administered the Ecotrin? ____________

5. When was the amitriptyline given? ____________

Here is what you should have found:

Name of Drug	Route of Administration	Time of Administration
Interferon alpha-2a 3,000,000 u	sc	0900 (9 A.M.)
amitriptyline 75 mg	po	2100 hs (9 P.M.)
zidovudine 200 mg	po	q4h (6 A.M., 10 A.M., etc.)
Ecotrin 650 mg	po	0900 qd (9 A.M.)

1. zidovudine 200 mg
2. Ecotrin 650 mg
3. Interferon alpha-2a 3,000,000 u
4. Leon Ablon
5. 9:00 P.M.

x start here

Practice Sets

Notes/Workspace

You will find the answers to Try These for Practice and Exercises Practice Sets in Appendix A at the back of the book. Your instructor has the answers to the Additional Exercises.

Try These for Practice

Test your comprehension after reading the chapter. Study the drug labels in Figure 2.19, page 42, and supply the following information.

1. What is the route of administration for lidocaine hydrochloride?

intravenous

2. How many capsules are in a container of Zithromax?

50 capsules

3. What is the quantity of drug in each capsule of chlordiazepoxide hydrochloride?

10 mg

4. Write the trade name for the drug manufactured by Lilly.

Kefzol

5. What is the quantity of drug in each tablet of meclizine hydrochloride?

25mg.

Notes/Workspace

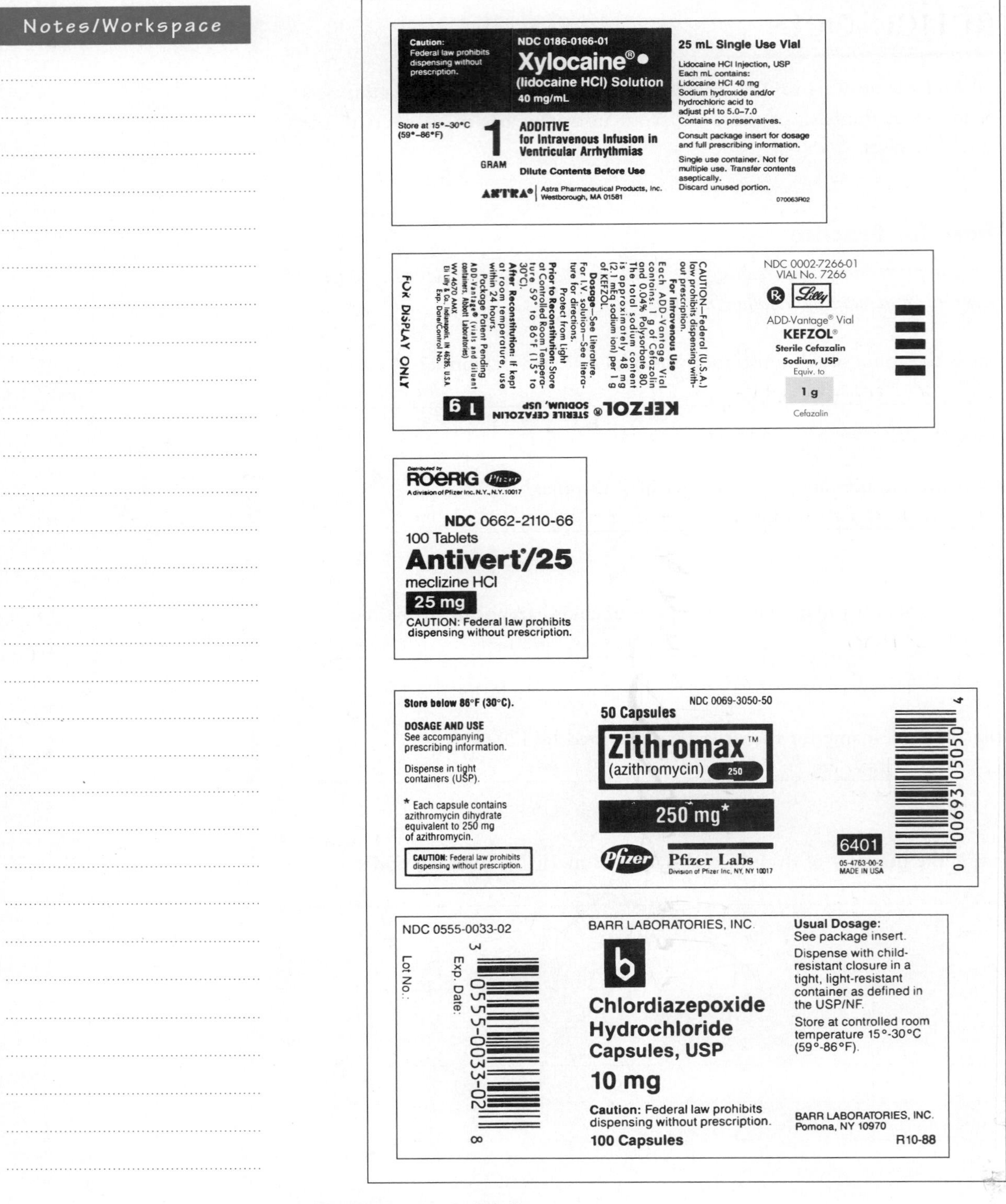

Figure 2.19 *Drug labels*

Exercises

Reinforce your understanding in class or at home. Study the drug labels shown in Figure 2.19, page 42, and supply the following information.

1. Write the generic name for Xylocaine.

(lidocaine HCl) Solution

2. Write the trade name for lidocaine HCl solution.

Xylocaine

3. What is the quantity of Xylocaine in each milliliter of prepared solution?

40 mg

4. What is the route of administration for Xylocaine?

Intravenous

5. Write the trade name for the drug distributed by Roerig.

Antivert/25

6. Study the MAR in Figure 2.20 on page 44. Fill in the following chart and answer the questions.

Name of Drug	Dose	Route of Administration	Time of Administration	Date Started	Date Discontinued
clofibrate	500mg tid	by mouth	10, 2, 6	7/18/94	7/25/94
Cardizem	60mg bid	by mouth	10am 6pm	7/18/94	7/25/95
Clinoril	200mg bid	by mouth	10am 6pm	7/19/94	7/26/94
digoxin	0.125mg bid	by mouth	10am	7/19/94	7/26/94
Lasix	20mg qd	by mouth	10am	7/19/94	7/26/94
Carafate	1g. qid	by mouth	before meals & at bedtime 7-12-5-10	7/20/94	7/27/94

a. Identify the drugs administered on July 18, 1994.

clofibrate & Cardizem

Notes/Workspace

⊕ GENERAL HOSPITAL ⊕

Year 19 *94* Month *July* Day		*18*	*19*	*20*	*21*	*22*	*23*
Medication Dosage and Interval		Initials* and Hours	Initials and Hours	Initials and Hours	Initials and Hours	Initials and Hours	Initials and Hours
Date started: *7/18/94*	I	*JO*	*JO*	*JO*			
clofibrate 500 mg po tid 10–2–6	AM	*10*	*10*	*10*			
	I		*LA LA*	*LA LA*			
Discontinued: *7/25/94*	PM		*2 6*	*2 6*			
Date started: *7/18/94*	I	*JO*	*JO*	*JO*			
Cardizem SR 60 mg po bid 10–6	AM	*10*	*10*	*10*			
	I		*LA*	*LA*			
Discontinued: *7/25/94*	PM		*6*	*6*			
Date started: *7/19/94*	I	X	*JO*	*JO*			
Clinoril 200 mg po bid 10–6	AM	X	*10*	*10*			
	I	X	*LA*	*LA*			
Discontinued: *7/26/94*	PM	X	*6*	*6*			
Date started: *7/19/94*	I	X	*JO*	*JO*			
digoxin 0.125 mg po bid 10 AM	AM	X	*10*	*10*			
	I	X					
Discontinued: *7/26/94*	PM	X					
Date started: *7/19/94*	I	X	*JO*	*JO*			
Lasix 20 mg po qd 10 AM	AM	X	*10*	*10*			
	I	X					
Discontinued: *7/26/94*	PM	X					
Date started: *7/20/94*	I	X	X	*JO*			
Carafate 1 g qid po ac + hs 7–12–5–10	AM	X	X	*7*			
	I	X	X	*JO SG LA*			
Discontinued: *7/27/94*	PM	X	X	*12–5–10*			

Allergies: (Specify)
NKA

Init*	Signature
JO	*June Olsen*
LA	*Leon Ablon*
SG	*Susan Green*

MEDICATION ADMINISTRATION RECORD

PATIENT IDENTIFICATION

177456 7/18/94

Mary Adams 3/12/34
755 Bay Bridge Ave Jewish
Brooklyn, NY 11209 Blue Cross

Dr. Anthony Giangrasso

Figure 2.20 *Medication administration record*

b. Identify the drugs administered po on July 20, 1994.

Clofibrate, cardizem, clinoril, digoxin, lasix carafate

c. How many drugs were administered at 10 P.M. on July 20, 1994?

1

7. Study the physician's order sheet in Figure 2.21; then answer the following questions.

a. What is the dose of Inderal?

120 mg (by mouth) once a day

b. How many times a day do you administer vitamin C to Mr. Sanchez?

twice a day

c. If the last dose of Declomycin was given at 12 noon, at what time would you administer the next dose?

6 p.m.

d. Which drug is administered once a day to Mr. Sanchez?

Inderal

GENERAL HOSPITAL

PRESS HARD WITH BALLPOINT PEN. WRITE DATE & TIME AND SIGN EACH ORDER

DATE	TIME	A.M. / P.M.
Oct 12, 1994	*6*	P.M. (circled)
Declomycin 300 mg po q6h		
vitamin C 11 g po bid		
Inderal 120 mg po qd		
SIGNATURE *L. Ablon* M.D.		

IMPRINT
731122 10/12/94
Jose Sanchez 3/2/45
24 Third Ave. RC
Chicago, IL 54312 Medicaid
Dr. Leon Ablon

ORDERS NOTED
DATE *10/12/94* TIME *6:30* A.M. / P.M. (P.M. circled)
❑ MEDEX ❑ KARDEX
NURSE'S SIG. *June Olsen*

FILLED BY DATE

PHYSICIAN'S ORDERS

Figure 2.21 *Physician's order sheet*

Notes/Workspace

Notes/Workspace

e. What was the patient's date of admission?

10/12/94.

8. Use the package insert excerpt shown in Figure 2.22 to answer the following questions.

a. What is the generic name of the drug?

Democlocycline Hydrochloride

b. What is the usual dose for an adult?

150mg qid or 300mg, bid

c. What is the initial oral dose of Declomycin for patients with gonorrhea?

600mg (+ 300mg q12h for 4 days)

d. How is this drug supplied?

gelatin capsules

8:12.24

DECLOMYCIN®

DEMECLOCYCLINE HYDROCHLORIDE

FOR ORAL USE

Adults: Usual daily dose - Four divided doses of 150 mg each or two divided doses of 300 mg each.

For children above eight years of age: Usual daily dose, 3-6 mg per pound body weight per day, depending upon the severity of the disease, divided into two to four doses.

Gonorrhea patients sensitive to penicillin may be treated with demeclocycline administered as an initial oral dose of 600 mg followed by 300 mg every 12 hours for four days to a total of 3 grams.

HOW SUPPLIED

DECLOMYCIN® demeclocycline hydrochloride Capsules, 150 mg are two-tone, coral colored, soft gelatin capsules, printed with LL followed by D9 on the light side in blue ink, are supplied as follows:

NDC 0005-9208-23 - Bottle of 100

Figure 2.22 *Package insert (excerpt) for Declomycin*

Additional Exercises

Now, on your own, test yourself! Ask your instructor to check your answers.

1. Study the MAR in Figure 2.23; then fill in the chart on page 48 and answer the questions.

⊕ GENERAL HOSPITAL ⊕							
Year 19 *94* Month *May*	Day	*3*	*4*	*5*	*6*	*7*	*8*
Medication Dosage and Interval		Initials* and Hours	Initials and Hours	Initials and Hours	Initials and Hours	Initials and Hours	Initials and Hours
Date started: *5/3/94* *allopurinol 100 mg po q12h*	I		*LA*				
	AM		*12*				
	I	*JO*	*JO*				
Discontinued: *5/9/94*	PM	*12*	*12*				
Date started: *5/3/94* *diphenhydramine 50 mg po hs*	I						
	AM						
	I	*CH*	*CH*				
Discontinued: *5/9/94*	PM	*10*	*10*				
Date started: *5/3/94* *Dilantin 100 mg po tid*	I	*JO*	*JO*				
	AM	*10*	*10*				
	I	*JO CH*	*JO CH*				
Discontinued: *5/9/94*	PM	*2 – 6*	*2 – 6*				
Date started: *5/3/94* *phenobarbital 30 mg po bid*	I	*JO*	*JO*				
	AM	*10*	*10*				
	I	*CH*	*CH*				
Discontinued: *5/9/94*	PM	*6*	*6*				
Date started: *5/3/94* *phenobarbital 60 mg po hs*	I						
	AM						
	I	*CH*	*CH*				
Discontinued: *5/9/94*	PM	*10*	*10*				

Figure 2.23 *Medication administration record*

Notes/Workspace

Notes/Workspace

Date started: *5/3/94* *heparin 5000 u sc q12h*	I		*LA*				
	AM		*12*				
	I	*JO*	*JO*				
Discontinued:	PM	*12*	*12*				
Date started: *5/4/94* *NPH insulin sc 44 u ac breakfast*	I		*MS*				
	AM		*7:30*				
	I						
Discontinued: *5/10/94*	PM						

Allergies: (Specify)

Init*	Signature
LA	*Leon Ablon*
JO	*June Olsen*
CH	*Claire Hill*
MS	*Mary Smith*

MEDICATION ADMINISTRATION RECORD

PATIENT IDENTIFICATION

455432 5/3/94

Sally Johnson 5/30/34
10-32 Fifth St. RC
Rutland VA 93071 BCBS

Anthony Giangrasso, M.D.

Figure 2.23 (*continued*) *Medication administration record*

	Name of Drug	Route of Administration	Time of Administration	Date Started	Date Discontinued
q12h	allopurinol	by mouth	q12h 12:00am 12:00pm	5/3/94	5/9/94
hs	diphenhydramine	by mouth	hour of sleep 10pm.	5/3/94	5/9/94
tid	Dilantin	by mouth	10am 2pm 6pm	5/3/94	5/9/94
bid	phenobarbital 30 mg	by mouth	twice a day bid 10am 6pm	5/3/94	5/9/94
hs	phenobarbital 60 mg	by mouth	hour of sleep 10 pm	5/3/94	5/9/94
	heparin	subcutaneous	every 12 hs. 12am 12pm	5/3/94	
	NPH insulin	subcutaneous	before meals 7:30	5/4/94	5/10/94

a. Which drug was administered at 12 noon on 5/4/94?

allopurinol + heparin

b. Name the drugs administered at 10 P.M. on 5/3/94.

diphenhydramine, phenobarbital 60mg

c. Which drugs are to be administered by mouth?

5

d. How many drugs were administered on May 4, 1994?

7 6 (phenobarbital dose contas 1 drug) for a total of 12 doses

Notes/Workspace

2. Study the physician's order sheet in Figure 2.24 and answer the following questions.

⊕ GENERAL HOSPITAL ⊕

PRESS HARD WITH BALLPOINT PEN. WRITE DATE & TIME AND SIGN EACH ORDER

DATE	TIME	A.M. / (P.M.)
5/3/94	*12 noon*	P.M. (circled)
Bumex 2 mg po qd		
digoxin 0.125 mg po bid for 3 days		
Spectrobid 400 mg po bid		
Quibron 300 mg po bid		
Reglan 5 mg po hs		
heparin 5000 u sc qd		
SIGNATURE *J. Olsen* M.D.		

IMPRINT
678123 5/3/94
Jennifer Dodson 6/6/60
333 West North Street Prot
Clearview, VT 05071 Aetna
Dr. June Olsen

ORDERS NOTED
DATE *5/3/94* TIME *12:15* A.M. (P.M.)
❑ MEDEX ❑ KARDEX
NURSE'S SIG. *Leon Ablon*

FILLED BY DATE

PHYSICIAN'S ORDERS

Figure 2.24 *Physician's order sheet*

a. What is the route of administration for Reglan?

by mouth

b. Which drugs should be administered at 10 P.M.?

Reglan

c. Identify the date digoxin is to be discontinued.

5/6/94

d. Identify the route of administration for heparin.

subcutaneously

Notes/Workspace

Study the drug labels in Figure 2.25 and supply the following information.

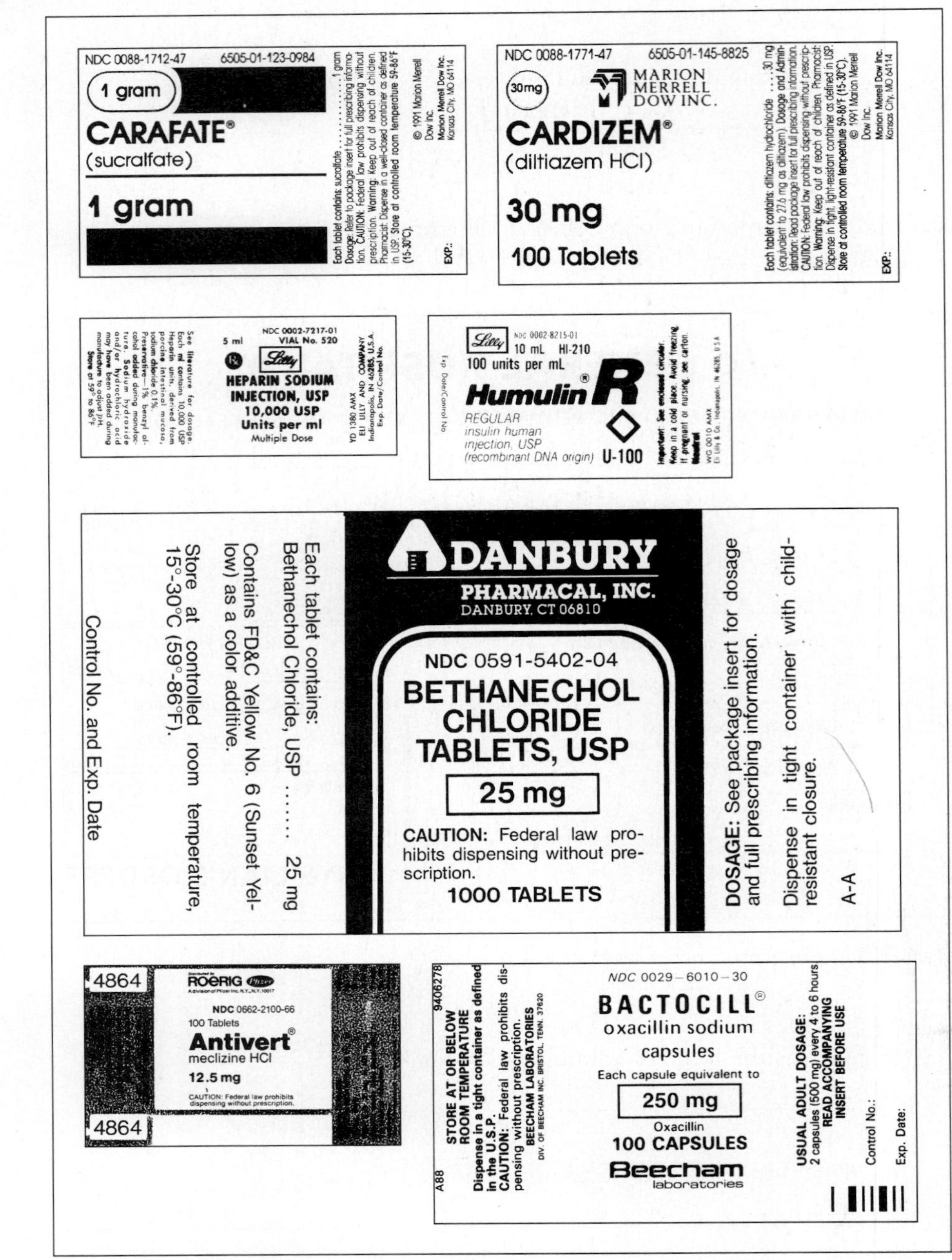

Figure 2.25 *Drug labels*

3. Write the generic name for Carafate.

sucralfate

4. What is the route of administration for regular Humulin insulin?

injection

5. What is the trade name of oxacillin?

Bactocill

6. What is the quantity of heparin in each milliliter of solution?

10,000 usp units per ml

7. What is the total quantity in the Humulin R vial?

10 mL

8. Write the trade name for meclizine HCl.

Antivert

9. What is the route of administration for bethanechol chloride?

by mouth

10. Write the generic name for Cardizem.

diltiazem HCL

11. What is the quantity of drug in each tablet of bethanechol chloride?

25 mg.

12. How many tablets are in the bottle of Antivert?

100 tablets

Notes/Workspace

chapter 3

Dimensional Analysis

Objectives

After completing this chapter, you will be able to

- *solve a calculation problem using dimensional analysis.*
- *identify some common units of measurement.*
- *recognize the abbreviations for these units.*
- *state the equivalents for these units of measurement.*
- *convert from one unit of measurement to another.*

In this chapter you will learn to use dimensional analysis to calculate drug dosages. Dimensional analysis is a common-sense approach to drug calculations that largely frees you from the need to memorize formulas. It is the method most commonly accepted in the physical sciences. Once you master this technique, you will be able to calculate drug dosages quickly and safely.

Table 3.1 *Abbreviations for Common Units*

Unit	Abbreviation
inch	in
foot	ft
yard	yd
ounce	oz
pound	lb
second	sec
minute	min
hour	h or hr or H
day	d
month	mon
year	yr

Notes/Workspace

Getting Started

One of the best ways to learn dimensional analysis is to convert some common units of measurement. Study the familiar units of measurement for length, weight, and time listed in Table 3.1. Some common equivalent measurements for these units are listed in Table 3.2.

Now, use this information and dimensional analysis to solve some problems.

If you have to wait 3 years until graduation, how many months is that? That is, you want to change 3 years into an equivalent number of months. The relationship is written as:

3 yr = ? mon

Table 3.2 *Equivalents for Common Units*

12 in = 1 ft
3 ft = 1 yd
16 oz = 1 lb
60 sec = 1 min
60 min = 1 h
24 h = 1 d
12 mon = 1 yr

Notes/Workspace

Whenever you divide something by itself, you get 1. Since 12 months is the same as 1 year, when you divide 12 months by 1 year, you get 1.

$$\frac{12\text{ mon}}{1\text{ yr}} = 1$$

Now see what happens when you multiply 3 years by $\frac{12\text{ mon}}{1\text{ yr}}$. The amount of time will not change, since you are really multiplying the time by 1.

$$3\text{ yr} = \frac{3\cancel{\text{ yr}}}{1} \times \frac{12\text{ mon}}{1\cancel{\text{ yr}}} = \frac{(3 \times 12)\text{ mon}}{1} = 36\text{ mon}$$

So 3 years is the same amount of time as 36 months.

Note

Cancel units just as you cancel numbers and letters in arithmetic and algebra.

Here is another problem. If a storm lasts for 72 hours, how many days does it last? You want to change 72 hours to days. The relationship is written as:

$$72\text{ h} = ?\text{ d}$$

Notice that $\frac{1\text{ d}}{24\text{ h}} = 1$, since 1 day is the same as 24 hours. Now you multiply 72 hours by $\frac{1\text{ d}}{24\text{ h}}$. The amount of time will not change, since you are really multiplying it by 1.

$$72\text{ h} \times \frac{1\text{ d}}{24\text{ h}} = ?$$

$$\frac{\overset{3}{\cancel{72\text{ h}}}}{1} \times \frac{1\text{ d}}{\underset{1}{\cancel{24\text{ h}}}} = \frac{(3 \times 1)\text{ d}}{1} = 3\text{ d}$$

So the 72-hour storm lasts for 3 days.

In both problems you canceled the original units and ended up with the desired units. You did this by multiplying a fraction that was equal to 1. The fraction had the old units on the bottom and the new units on the top.

Notes/Workspace

Example 3.1

Change 2 feet to an equivalent number of inches.

$$2 \text{ ft} = ? \text{ in}$$

You want to cancel the feet and get the answer in inches. Therefore, multiply 2 feet by a fraction that has feet on the bottom (in the denominator) and inches on the top (in the numerator).

$$2 \text{ ft} \times \frac{? \text{ in}}{? \text{ ft}} = ? \text{ in}$$

Next, put in numbers that will make the fraction $\frac{? \text{ in}}{? \text{ ft}}$ equal to 1. Since 12 in = 1 ft, the fraction you want is $\frac{12 \text{ in}}{1 \text{ ft}}$. Now, multiply 2 feet by $\frac{12 \text{ in}}{1 \text{ ft}}$.

$$\frac{2 \cancel{\text{ft}}}{1} \times \frac{12 \text{ in}}{1 \cancel{\text{ft}}} = \frac{(2 \times 12) \text{ in}}{1} = 24 \text{ in}$$

So 2 feet is the same as 24 inches.

Example 3.2

Change 36 inches to an equivalent number of feet.

$$36 \text{ in} = ? \text{ ft}$$

You want to cancel the inches and get the answer in feet. So you must multiply 36 inches by a fraction that has inches on the bottom (in the denominator) and feet on the top (in the numerator).

$$36 \text{ in} \times \frac{? \text{ ft}}{? \text{ in}} = ?$$

Note $\frac{1 \text{ ft}}{12 \text{ in}} = 1$, since 1 foot is the same as 12 inches. Now, multiply 36 inches by $\frac{1 \text{ ft}}{12 \text{ in}}$.

$$\overset{3}{\cancel{36}} \cancel{\text{in}} \times \frac{1 \text{ ft}}{\underset{1}{\cancel{12}} \cancel{\text{in}}} = \frac{3 \times 1 \text{ ft}}{1} = 3 \text{ ft}$$

So 36 inches is the same as 3 feet.

Notes/Workspace

Example 3.3

Change 15 yards to an equivalent length in feet.

$$15 \text{ yd} = ? \text{ ft}$$

You want to cancel the yards and get the answer in feet. So, multiply 15 yards by a fraction that has yards on the bottom (denominator). The answer must be in feet, so the fraction must have feet on the top (numerator).

$$15 \text{ yd} \times \frac{? \text{ ft}}{? \text{ yd}} = ? \text{ ft}$$

We must put in numbers that will make $\frac{? \text{ ft}}{? \text{ yd}}$ equal to 1. Since 3 ft = 1 yd, the fraction we want is $\frac{3 \text{ ft}}{1 \text{ yd}}$. Now, multiply 15 yards by $\frac{3 \text{ ft}}{1 \text{ yd}}$.

$$15 \cancel{\text{yd}} \times \frac{3 \text{ ft}}{1 \cancel{\text{yd}}} = \frac{15 \times 3 \text{ ft}}{1} = 45 \text{ ft}$$

So 15 yards is the same as 45 feet.

Example 3.4

Change 0.25 feet to an equivalent length in inches.

$$0.25 \text{ ft} = ? \text{ in}$$

You want to cancel feet and get the answer in inches. So, multiply 0.25 feet by a fraction that looks like $\frac{? \text{ in}}{? \text{ ft}}$.

$$0.25 \text{ ft} \times \frac{? \text{ in}}{? \text{ ft}} = ? \text{ in}$$

Since 12 in = 1 ft, the fraction we want is $\frac{12 \text{ in}}{1 \text{ ft}}$.

$$0.25 \cancel{\text{ft}} \times \frac{12 \text{ in}}{1 \cancel{\text{ft}}} = \frac{0.25 \times 12 \text{ in}}{1} = 3 \text{ in}$$

So 0.25 feet is the same as 3 inches.

Example 3.5

Change 64 ounces to pounds.

$$64 \text{ oz} = ? \text{ lb}$$

You want to cancel ounces and get the answer in pounds. So, multiply 64 ounces by a fraction that looks like $\frac{? \text{ lb}}{? \text{ oz}}$.

$$64 \text{ oz} \times \frac{? \text{ lb}}{? \text{ oz}} = ?$$

Since 16 oz = 1 lb, the fraction we want is $\frac{1 \text{ lb}}{16 \text{ oz}}$.

$$\overset{4}{\cancel{64}}\ \cancel{\text{oz}} \times \frac{1 \text{ lb}}{\cancel{16}\ \cancel{\text{oz}}} = 4 \text{ lb}$$

So 64 ounces is the same as 4 pounds.

Notes/Workspace

Notes/Workspace

Practice Sets

You will find the answers to Try These for Practice and Exercises Practice Sets in Appendix A at the back of the book. Your instructor has the answers to the Additional Exercises.

Try These for Practice

Test your compehension after reading the chapter.

1. An infant weighs 6 pounds. What is its weight in ounces? ________

2. A woman is 60 inches in height. How tall is she in feet? ________

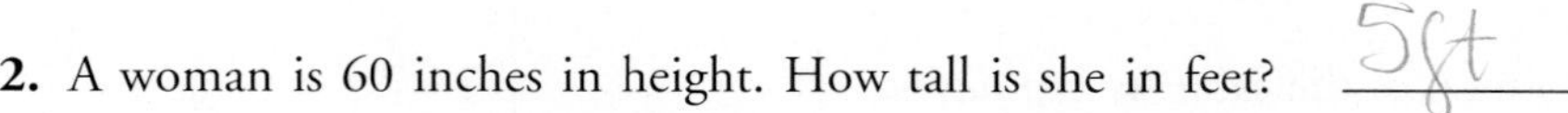

3. It takes 48 months to pay off an automobile loan. How many years is that? ________

4. How many seconds are in $2\frac{1}{2}$ minutes? ________

5. How many yards does 20 feet equal? ________

Exercises

Reinforce your understanding in class or at home.

> **Note**
>
> In several of the following problems, you will find decimal numbers used with units from the household system. As you will find in Chapter 5 where we discuss it in detail, this system uses only whole numbers and fractions. The following exercises are merely practice problems developed to increase your skills in dimensional analysis.

1. 1.5 yr = ________ mon

2. 3 d = ________ h

3. 2 lb = ________ oz

4. 120 sec = ________ min

5. 120 in = ________ ft

6. 18 ft = ________ yd

7. 8 oz = ________ lb

8. 0.5 yd = ________ ft

9. $1\frac{1}{2}$ yr = ________ mon

10. $\frac{1}{2}$ min = ________ sec

11. What is the height of a 6-foot-tall patient in inches? ________

12. An IV solution has been infusing for 10 minutes. How many seconds is that?

____

13. Change 2.75 hours to minutes. ________

14. How many years are there in 30 months? ________

15. What part of an hour is 45 minutes? ________

16. If your patient measures 66 inches in height, what would the patient measure in feet? ________

17. Convert 60 hours to days. ________

18. An infant weighs 7 pounds at birth. What is its weight in ounces?

____

19. A person is 5 feet 4 inches tall. Express this height in inches.

____

20. If an infant weighs $3\frac{1}{2}$ pounds, what would be the equivalent in ounces?

____

Notes/Workspace

Notes/Workspace

Additional Exercises

Now, on your own, test yourself! Ask your instructor to check your answers.

1. 720 mon = ________ yr

2. 36 h = ________ d

3. 32 oz = ________ lb

4. 6.5 min = ________ sec

5. $3\frac{1}{2}$ ft = ________ in

6. 4 yd = ________ ft

7. $6\frac{1}{4}$ lb = ________ oz

8. 1.25 ft = ________ in

9. 6 mon = ________ yr

10. 30 sec = ________ min

11. What is the height in feet of a child who is 36 inches tall? ________

12. Change 300 seconds to minutes. ________

13. What part of a pound is 4 ounces? ________

14. How many months are in 5 years? ________

15. Change $2\frac{1}{2}$ hours to minutes. ________

16. Convert 7 days to hours. ________

17. An infant weighs 88 ounces. What is its weight in pounds? ________

18. What is the weight in ounces of an infant who weighs 6 pounds 3 ounces? ________

19. What is the height in inches of a girl who is 5 feet 6 inches tall? ________

20. Change 150 seconds to minutes. ________

Unit Two

Systems of Measurement for Dosage Calculations

chapter 4

The Metric System

Objectives

After completing this chapter, you will be able to

- *identify metric system units of measurement.*
- *recognize the abbreviations for the metric units of measurement.*
- *state the metric equivalents for the units of volume for liquids.*
- *state the metric equivalents for the units of weight for solids.*
- *convert from one unit to another within the metric system.*

At present, there are three systems used to measure drugs: the *household* system, the *apothecary* system, and the *International System of Units* (SI). The SI, commonly known as the *metric system,* is replacing the other systems of measurement. However, the other systems are still in use, so you must understand all three systems and learn how to convert from one to another. In this chapter you will be introduced to the metric system.

Liquid Volume in the Metric System

Drugs in liquid form are measured by volume. The volume of a liquid is the amount of space it occupies. The units of measurement for liquid volume in the metric system are shown in Table 4.1 along with their abbreviations.

Table 4.1 *Metric Units of Volume*

Unit	Abbreviation
liter	L
milliliter	mL or ml
cubic centimeter	cc or cm^3

Note

The prefix "milli" means "$\frac{1}{1000}$". So a milliliter is $\frac{1}{1000}$ of a liter.

The milliliter (mL) and cubic centimeter (cc) are equivalent measurements. A 30 mL vial of meperidine hydrochloride (Demerol) is therefore the same as a 30 cc vial of meperidine hydrochloride. Table 4.2 lists some of the frequently used equivalent measurements for liquid volume in the metric system.

Table 4.2 *Metric Equivalents of Liquid Volume*

1 cc	=	1 mL
1000 mL	=	1 L
1000 cc	=	1 L

Using dimensional analysis and the information in Table 4.2, you can convert a quantity written in one unit of metric volume to another. The next examples show how to do this.

Example 4.1

If the prescriber ordered 2.5 liters of 5% dextrose in water (D/W), how many cubic centimeters were ordered?

2.5 L = ? cc

Notes/Workspace

Notes/Workspace

You want to cancel the liters and obtain the equivalent amount in cubic centimeters.

$$2.5 \text{ L} \times \frac{? \text{ cc}}{? \text{ L}} = ? \text{ cc}$$

Since 1000 cc = 1 L (see Table 4.2), the fraction you want is $\frac{1000 \text{ cc}}{1 \text{ L}}$.

$$2.5 \cancel{\text{L}} \times \frac{1000 \text{ cc}}{1 \cancel{\text{L}}} = 2500 \text{ cc}$$

So the prescriber ordered 2500 cubic centimeters of 5% D/W.

Note

Write 2.5 liters instead of $2\frac{1}{2}$ liters because, in the metric system, quantities are written as decimal numbers instead of fractions.

Example 4.2

Your patient is to receive 1750 milliliters of 10% dextrose (D) in 0.45% normal saline (NS). What is the same dose in liters?

$$1750 \text{ mL} = ? \text{ L}$$

You want to cancel the milliliters and obtain the equivalent amount in liters.

$$1750 \text{ mL} \times \frac{? \text{ L}}{? \text{ mL}} = ? \text{ L}$$

Since 1000 mL = 1 L, the fraction you want is $\frac{1 \text{ L}}{1000 \text{ mL}}$.

$$1750 \cancel{\text{mL}} \times \frac{1 \text{ L}}{1000 \cancel{\text{mL}}} = \frac{1750 \text{ L}}{1000} = 1.75 \text{ L}$$

So 1750 milliliters of 10% D/0.45% NS is the same dose as 1.75 liters of 10% D/0.45% NS.

Weight in the Metric System

Drugs in dry form are measured by weight in the metric system. Table 4.3 on page 65 lists common metric units of measurement for weight along with their abbreviations. Metric equivalents for weight are shown in Table 4.4, page 65.

Notes/Workspace

Table 4.3	*Metric Units of Weight*
Unit	**Abbreviation**
kilogram	kg
gram	g
milligram	mg
microgram	μg or mcg

Note

"Kilo" means "thousand" (1000). So a kilogram is 1000 grams.
"Milli" means "one thousandth" $\left(\frac{1}{1000}\right)$. So a milligram is $\frac{1}{1000}$ of a gram.
"Micro" means "one millionth" $\left(\frac{1}{1,000,000}\right)$. So a microgram is $\frac{1}{1,000,000}$ of a gram.

Table 4.4	*Metric Equivalents for Weight*	
1 kg	=	1000 g
1 g	=	1000 mg
1 mg	=	1000 μg or 1000 mcg

Using dimensional analysis and the information in Table 4.4, you can convert a quantity written in one unit of metric weight to an equivalent quantity in another unit of metric weight. The following examples show you how to do this.

Example 4.3

The prescriber has ordered 100 micrograms of cyanocobalomin (vitamin B_{12}). How many milligrams is this dose?

$$100\ \mu g = ?\ mg$$

You want to cancel the micrograms and obtain the equivalent amount in milligrams.

$$100\ \mu g \times \frac{?\ mg}{?\ \mu g} = ?\ mg$$

Notes/Workspace

Since 1000 μg = 1 mg, the fraction you want is $\frac{1\text{ mg}}{1000\ \mu g}$.

$$\overset{1}{\cancel{100}\ \cancel{\mu g}} \times \frac{1\text{ mg}}{\underset{10}{\cancel{1000}\ \cancel{\mu g}}} = \frac{1\text{ mg}}{10} = 0.1\text{ mg}$$

So 100 micrograms is the same as 0.1 milligram.

Example 4.4

The order reads 250 micrograms of digoxin (Lanoxin). How many milligrams of this anti-arrythmic drug would you administer to the patient?

$$250\text{ mcg} = ?\text{ mg}$$

You want to cancel the micrograms and obtain the equivalent amount in milligrams.

$$250\text{ mcg} \times \frac{?\text{ mg}}{?\text{ mcg}} = ?\text{ mg}$$

Since 1000 mcg = 1 mg, you have:

$$250\ \cancel{\text{mcg}} \times \frac{1\text{ mg}}{1000\ \cancel{\text{mcg}}} = 0.25\text{ mg}$$

So 250 micrograms is the same as 0.25 milligram, and you would administer 0.25 milligram of digoxin.

Example 4.5

The order reads 0.016 gram of the analgesic morphine sulfate. How many milligrams would you administer?

$$0.016\text{ g} = ?\text{ mg}$$

You want to cancel the grams and obtain the equivalent amount in milligrams.

$$0.016\text{ g} \times \frac{?\text{ mg}}{?\text{ g}} = ?\text{ mg}$$

$$0.016\ \cancel{\text{g}} \times \frac{1000\text{ mg}}{1\ \cancel{\text{g}}} = 16\text{ mg}$$

So 0.016 gram is the same as 16 milligrams, and you would administer 16 milligrams of morphine sulfate.

By the way

A dose is always expressed in the form of a number and a unit. Both are important. For example:

15 cc	2 capsules
2.5 mg	1.5 mL
3 tablets	0.5 L

When you write your answer, be sure to include the appropriate unit.

Notes/Workspace

Prerequisite Equivalents

In order to do the exercises at the end of this chapter, you need to memorize the metric equivalents for volume and weight. To test yourself, fill in the missing numbers in the following chart and check your answers on page A-4 before you start the exercises.

Volume

1 mL = 1 cc = 1 cm^3

1 L = 1000 cc

1000 mL = 1 L

Weight

1 kg = 1000 g

1 g = 1000 mg

1 mg = 1000 µg

1 mg = 1000 mcg

1 µg = 1 mcg

Notes/Workspace

Practice Sets

You will find the answers to Try These for Practice and Exercises Practice Sets in Appendix A at the back of the book. Your instructor has the answers to the Additional Exercises.

Try These for Practice

Test your comprehension after reading the chapter.

1. The prescriber ordered:

Premarin 1.25 mg po qd

Convert this dose to grams. _________

2. According to the label in Figure 4.1, each tablet of furosemide contains 40 milligrams. Convert 40 milligrams to grams. _________

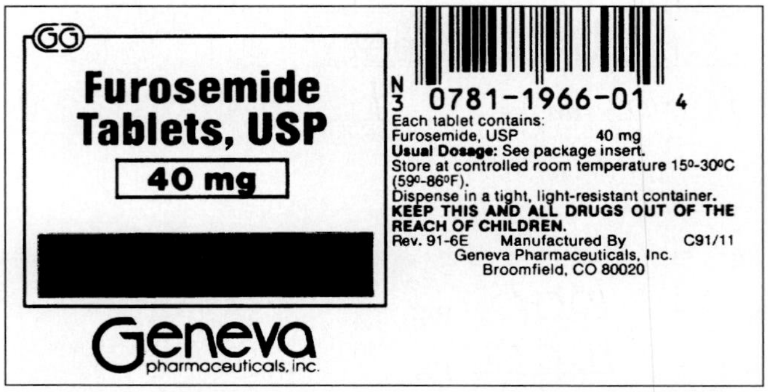

Furosemide Tablets, USP
40 mg
N 3 0781-1966-01 4
Each tablet contains:
Furosemide, USP 40 mg
Usual Dosage: See package insert.
Store at controlled room temperature 15°-30°C (59°-86°F).
Dispense in a tight, light-resistant container.
KEEP THIS AND ALL DRUGS OUT OF THE REACH OF CHILDREN.
Rev. 91-6E Manufactured By C91/11
Geneva Pharmaceuticals, Inc.
Broomfield, CO 80020
Geneva
pharmaceuticals, inc.

Figure 4.1 *Drug label for furosemide*

3. The prescriber ordered:

methimazole 0.005 g po tid

Convert this dose to milligrams. _________

4. An order of 2000 milliliters of 5% D/W has been placed for a patient. What is the same dose in liters? _________

5. A prescriber has ordered 1500 micrograms of cyanocobalamin (vitamin B_{12}). How many milligrams is this dose? _________

Exercises

Reinforce your understanding in class or at home.

Notes/Workspace

1. 7500 g = ________ kg
2. 1.5 L = ________ cc
3. 2 L = ________ mL
4. 750 mg = ________ g
5. 0.005 g ________ mg
6. 0.372 g = ________ mg
7. 0.4 kg = ________ g
8. 3000 cc = ________ L
9. 1.75 mg = ________ g
10. 0.0004 g = ________ mg
11. 15,000 mcg = ________ mg
12. 200 μg = ________ mg
13. The prescriber orders 30 milligrams of the narcotic morphine sulfate (Roxanol). What is the equivalent dose in grams? ________
14. How many milligrams would you administer to the patient if the order for the sedative triazolam (Halcion) was 0.025 gram? ________
15. The order reads 0.6 gram of clindamycin (Cleocin). What is the equivalent dose in milligrams? ________
16. The prescriber ordered: 5% D/W 0.8 L IV q8h. How many milliliters is contained in this amount of solution? ________
17. A prescriber ordered: methocarbamol 2000 mg po bid. What is the equivalent amount in grams for this skeletal muscle relaxant? ________
18. The patient must receive 0.3 milligram of digoxin (Lanoxin) po immediately. What is the equivalent dose in micrograms? ________
19. The prescriber ordered: butorphanol 500 μg IV q4h prn. What is the equivalent dose in milligrams of this narcotic analgesic drug? ________

Notes/Workspace

20. The label in Figure 4.2 indicates that each capsule contains 25 milligrams of chlordiazepoxide hydrochloride. Convert 25 milligrams to grams.

____

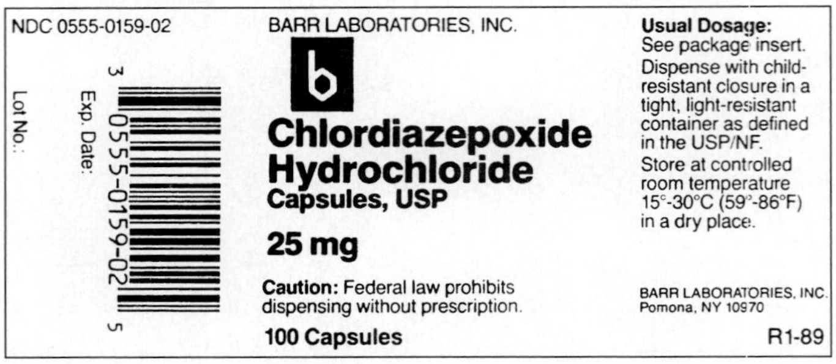

NDC 0555-0159-02
Lot No.:
Exp. Date:
3 0555-0159-02 5
BARR LABORATORIES, INC.
b
Chlordiazepoxide Hydrochloride
Capsules, USP
25 mg
Caution: Federal law prohibits dispensing without prescription.
100 Capsules
Usual Dosage:
See package insert.
Dispense with child-resistant closure in a tight, light-resistant container as defined in the USP/NF.
Store at controlled room temperature 15°-30°C (59°-86°F) in a dry place.
BARR LABORATORIES, INC.
Pomona, NY 10970
R1-89

Figure 4.2 *Drug label for chlordiazepoxide hydrochloride*

Additional Exercises

Now, on your own, test yourself! Ask your instructor to check your answers.

1. 35 kg = ________ g

2. 400 mcg = ________ mg

3. 250 mcg = ________ mg

4. 2.25 L = ________ mL

5. 16 kg = ________ g

6. 0.007 g = ________ mg

7. 0.6 mg = ________ g

8. 0.75 g = ________ mg

9. 0.001 L = ________ cc

10. 250 mg = ________ g

11. The prescriber ordered: zalcitabine 375 μg po bid. How many milligrams of this antiviral drug would you administer to the patient? ________

12. How many milliliters are contained in 3.75 liters of Ringer's lactate?

____

13. The order reads: Inderal 60 mg po bid. How many grams of this beta-adrenergic blocker would you administer? ________

14. The bronchodilator terbutaline sulfate (Bricanyl) has been prescribed for a patient po. The amount ordered is 250 micrograms. What is the equivalent quantity in milligrams? _________

15. The physician ordered 40 milligrams of the anti-anginal drug, nifedipine (Procardia). How many micrograms equal 40 milligrams? _________

16. If an infant weighs 3.5 kilograms, what would be its weight in grams?

____

17. An order for a cardiac glycoside is as follows: digoxin 0.00025 g po qd. How many milligrams would you prepare? _________

18. How many milligrams are contained in the order written in Figure 4.3 for azithromycin? _________

GENERAL HOSPITAL

PRESS HARD WITH BALLPOINT PEN. WRITE DATE & TIME AND SIGN EACH ORDER

DATE	TIME	A.M. / P.M.
1/29/94	*1*	P.M. (circled)
azithromycin 0.5 g po bid		
D/C ampicillin 500 mg po tid		
Sustagen po 60 mL per 12 h		
soft diet		
OOB		
SIGNATURE	*L. Ablon*	M.D.

IMPRINT
129941 01/29/94
John Peters 03/14/65
23 Jones Court Prot
San Diego, CA 09774 Prud
Dr. Leon Ablon

ORDERS NOTED
DATE *1/29/94* TIME *1:15* A.M. P.M. (circled)
❑ MEDEX ❑ KARDEX
NURSE'S SIG. *C. Hill*

FILLED BY DATE

PHYSICIAN'S ORDERS

Figure 4.3 *Physician's order sheet*

19. Calculate the amount of fluid in milliliters a patient must receive each hour if the order is 0.1 liter per hour. _________

Notes/Workspace

Notes/Workspace

20. In Figure 4.4, each tablet of hydroxyzine HCl (Atarax) contains 25 milligrams. Convert this quantity to micrograms. ________

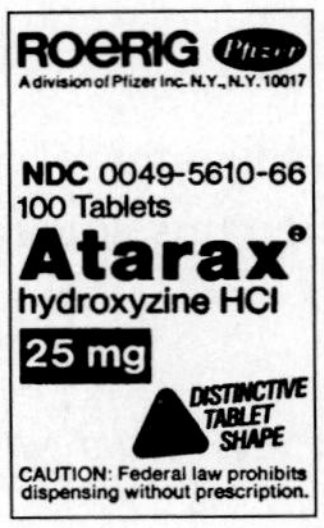

ROERIG Pfizer
A division of Pfizer Inc. N.Y., N.Y. 10017
NDC 0049-5610-66
100 Tablets
Atarax®
hydroxyzine HCl
25 mg
DISTINCTIVE TABLET SHAPE
CAUTION: Federal law prohibits dispensing without prescription.

Figure 4.4 *Drug label for Atarax*

chapter 5

The Apothecary and Household Systems

Objectives

After completing this chapter, you will be able to

- *identify units of measurement in the apothecary system.*
- *recognize the abbreviations for apothecary units.*
- *state the apothecary equivalents for units of liquid volume.*
- *convert from one unit to an equivalent unit within the apothecary system.*
- *understand the commonly used Roman numerals.*
- *identify units of measurement in the household system.*
- *recognize the abbreviations for household units.*
- *state the household equivalents for units of liquid volume.*
- *convert from one unit to an equivalent unit within the household system.*

The apothecary system is one of the oldest systems of drug measurement. Although infrequently used, the apothecary system must still be understood in order to safely administer medications. Unlike the metric system, which expresses quantities in decimal numbers such as 0.5 and 3.75, the apothecary system uses fractions such as $\frac{1}{2}$ and $3\frac{3}{4}$.

Notes/Workspace

1 gtt= ml = minum

1m

Liquid Volume in the Apothecary System

The units of measurement for liquid volume in the apothecary system are shown in Table 5.1 along with their abbreviations.

Table 5.1 *Apothecary Units of Measurement for Liquid Volumes*

Unit	Abbreviation
quart	qt
pint	pt
ounce	℥ or oz
dram	ʒ or dr
minim	♍

You may already be familiar with quarts, pints, and ounces since these liquid measurements are commonly used outside the health-care field. Table 5.2 lists the equivalents for these units.

Table 5.2 *Common Equivalents for Apothecary Liquid Volume Units*

qt 1	=	pt 2
qt 1	=	℥ 32
pt 1	=	℥ 16
℥ 1	=	ʒ 8
ʒ 1	=	♍ 60

Note

In the apothecary system, the abbreviation or symbol for the unit is placed before the quantity (as in pt 2). However, it is sometimes written the other way (2 pt) as well.

You can use dimensional analysis to convert from one unit to an equivalent unit within the apothecary system the same way you converted units within the metric system. You multiply the old measurement by a fraction that is equal to 1; the fraction has the old units on the bottom (the denominator) and the new units on top (the numerator) as the following examples show.

Notes/Workspace

Example 5.1

The order reads minims 120 of guaifenesin (Robitussin). How many drams of this expectorant would you administer?

$$♍ 120 = \text{dr } ?$$

You want to cancel the minims and obtain the equivalent amount in drams.

$$♍ 120 \times \frac{\text{dr } ?}{♍ ?} = \text{dr } ?$$

Since ♍ 60 = dr 1, the fraction you want is $\frac{\text{dr } 1}{♍ 60}$.

$$\overset{2}{\cancel{♍ 120}} \times \frac{\text{dr } 1}{\underset{1}{\cancel{♍ 60}}} = \text{dr } 2$$

So minims 120 is the same as drams 2, and you would administer drams 2 of guaifenesin.

Example 5.2

The prescriber has ordered drams 2 of theophylline (Elixophyllin). How many minims would you administer of this drug?

$$ʒ 2 = ♍ ?$$

You want to cancel the drams and obtain the equivalent amount in minims.

$$ʒ 2 \times \frac{♍ ?}{ʒ ?} = ♍ ?$$

Since ♍ 60 = ʒ 1, the fraction you want is $\frac{♍ 60}{ʒ 1}$.

$$\cancel{ʒ} 2 \times \frac{♍ 60}{\cancel{ʒ} 1} = ♍ 120$$

So drams 2 is the same as minims 120, and you would administer minims 120 of theophylline.

Notes/Workspace

Example 5.3

The patient is to receive drams 6 of magaldrate (Riopan). How many ounces of this antacid would you administer?

$$\text{ʒ}\ 6 = \text{℥}\ ?$$

You want to cancel the drams and get the answer in ounces.

$$\text{ʒ}\ 6 \times \frac{\text{℥}\ ?}{\text{ʒ}\ ?} = \text{℥}\ ?$$

Since ʒ 8 = ℥ 1, the fraction you want is $\frac{\text{℥}\ 1}{\text{ʒ}\ 8}$.

$$\text{ʒ}\ \overset{3}{\cancel{6}} \times \frac{\text{℥}\ 1}{\cancel{\text{ʒ}\ 8}_{4}} = \text{℥}\ \frac{3}{4}$$

So drams 6 is the same as ounce $\frac{3}{4}$, and you would administer ounce $\frac{3}{4}$ of Riopan.

Weight in the Apothecary System

The grain (gr) is the only unit of weight in the apothecary system that is used in administering medication. You will be converting this unit to its equivalent in other systems of measurement in Chapter 6.

Roman Numerals

Dosages in the apothecary system are sometimes written using Roman numerals. Roman numeral values above 30 are seldom encountered in the apothecary system. Table 5.3 shows four different ways medication orders can be written using Roman numerals. In addition, you may sometimes see dots over the i's.

The symbol **ss** written after a Roman numeral indicates $\frac{1}{2}$. Table 5.4 illustrates the uses of ss; it should only be used in these instances.

Table 5.3 *Values of Roman Numerals*

Arabic Number	Roman Numeral Equivalent[†]			
1	$\overline{\underline{\text{I}}}$	$\overline{\text{I}}$	I	$\overline{\text{i}}$
2	$\overline{\underline{\text{II}}}$	$\overline{\text{II}}$	II	$\overline{\text{ii}}$
3	$\overline{\underline{\text{III}}}$	$\overline{\text{III}}$	III	$\overline{\text{iii}}$
4	$\overline{\underline{\text{IV}}}$	$\overline{\text{IV}}$	IV	$\overline{\text{iv}}$
5	$\overline{\underline{\text{V}}}$	$\overline{\text{V}}$	V	$\overline{\text{v}}$
6	$\overline{\underline{\text{VI}}}$	$\overline{\text{VI}}$	VI	$\overline{\text{vi}}$
7	$\overline{\underline{\text{VII}}}$	$\overline{\text{VII}}$	VII	$\overline{\text{vii}}$
8	$\overline{\underline{\text{VIII}}}$	$\overline{\text{VIII}}$	VIII	$\overline{\text{viii}}$
9	$\overline{\underline{\text{IX}}}$	$\overline{\text{IX}}$	IX	$\overline{\text{ix}}$
10	$\overline{\underline{\text{X}}}$	$\overline{\text{X}}$	X	$\overline{\text{x}}$
15	$\overline{\underline{\text{XV}}}$	$\overline{\text{XV}}$	XV	$\overline{\text{xv}}$
20	$\overline{\underline{\text{XX}}}$	$\overline{\text{XX}}$	XX	$\overline{\text{xx}}$
25	$\overline{\underline{\text{XXV}}}$	$\overline{\text{XXV}}$	XXV	$\overline{\text{xxv}}$
30	$\overline{\underline{\text{XXX}}}$	$\overline{\text{XXX}}$	XXX	$\overline{\text{xxx}}$

[†] The Roman numerals may appear in any of these styles.

Table 5.4 *The Symbol* ss $\left(\frac{1}{2}\right)$ *with Roman Numerals*

Arabic Number	Roman Numeral Equivalent[†]		
$\frac{1}{2}$	$\overline{\text{SS}}$	SS	ss
$1\frac{1}{2}$	$\overline{\text{ISS}}$	ISS	iss
$7\frac{1}{2}$	$\overline{\text{VIISS}}$	VIISS	viiss

[†]The symbol may appear in any of these styles.

Notes/Workspace

Example 5.4

The dose is ounce ss of Kaopectate. How many drams of this antidiarrheal agent would you administer?

$$\text{℥}\,\frac{1}{2} = \text{ʒ}\,?$$

You want to cancel the ounces and obtain an equivalent amount in drams.

$$\text{℥}\,\frac{1}{2} \times \frac{\text{ʒ}\,?}{\text{℥}\,?} = \text{ʒ}?$$

Since ʒ 8 = ℥ 1, the fraction you want is $\frac{\text{ʒ}\,8}{\text{℥}\,1}$.

$$\cancel{\text{℥}}\,\frac{1}{\cancel{2}_{1}} \times \frac{\text{ʒ}\,\cancel{8}^{4}}{\cancel{\text{℥}}\,1} = \text{ʒ}\,4$$

So ounce ss is the same as drams 4, and you would administer drams 4 of Kaopectate.

Example 5.5

Change drams $\overline{\text{III}}$ to minims.

$$\text{ʒ}\,3 = \text{♏}\,?$$

You want to cancel the drams and obtain the equivalent amount in minims.

$$\text{ʒ}\,3 \times \frac{\text{♏}\,?}{\text{ʒ}\,?} = \text{♏}\,?$$

Since ♏ 60 = ʒ 1, the fraction is $\frac{\text{♏}\,60}{\text{ʒ}\,1}$.

$$\cancel{\text{ʒ}}\,3 \times \frac{\text{♏}\,60}{\cancel{\text{ʒ}}\,1} = \text{♏}\,180$$

So drams $\overline{\text{III}}$ is the same as minims 180.

Liquid Volume in the Household System

Notes/Workspace

Occasionally household measurements are used in prescribing liquid medication. It may be your responsibility to convert metric or apothecary units to household measurements when explaining a prescribed dosage to a patient who will be taking medication at home. The household units of measurement for liquid volumes are shown in Table 5.5 along with their abbreviations. Table 5.6 lists equivalent values for units of liquid measurement in the household system.

Table 5.5 ***Household Units***

Unit	Abbreviation
glass	—
measuring cup	—
teacup	—
tablespoon	T or tbs
teaspoon	t or tsp
ounce (fluid)	℥ or oz
drop	gtt

Since these units are measured using household utensils, which are not necessarily accurate, the equivalents listed in Table 5.6 are only *approximate.* Unlike the metric system, which uses decimal numbers such as 0.5 and 3.75, the household system uses fractions such as $\frac{1}{2}$ and $3\frac{3}{4}$.

Table 5.6 ***Equivalent Measurements in the Household System***

1 glass (usually)	=	℥ 8 or 8 oz
1 measuring cup	=	℥ 8 or 8 oz
1 teacup	=	℥ 6 or 6 oz
1 oz	=	2 T
1 T	=	3 t
1 t	=	60 gtt

Notes/Workspace

Example 5.6

The patient is to receive 15 drops of the gastrointestinal antispasmodic paregoric. How many teaspoons would the patient receive?

$$15 \text{ gtt} = ? \text{ t}$$

You want to cancel drops and obtain the equivalent amount in teaspoons.

$$15 \text{ gtt} \times \frac{? \text{ t}}{? \text{ gtt}} = ? \text{ t}$$

Since 60 gtt = 1 t, the fraction is $\frac{1 \text{ t}}{60 \text{ gtt}}$.

$$\overset{1}{\cancel{15}}\ \cancel{\text{gtt}} \times \frac{1 \text{ t}}{\underset{4}{\cancel{60}}\ \cancel{\text{gtt}}} = \frac{1}{4} \text{ t}$$

So 15 drops is approximately the same as $\frac{1}{4}$ teaspoon, and the patient would receive $\frac{1}{4}$ teaspoon of paregoric.

Example 5.7

The prescriber directs the patient to take 2 ounces of a cathartic, citrate of magnesia, at home whenever necessary. How many tablespoons would the patient take?

$$2 \text{ oz} = ? \text{ T}$$

You want to cancel the ounces and obtain the equivalent amount in tablespoons.

$$2 \text{ oz} \times \frac{? \text{ T}}{? \text{ oz}} = ? \text{ T}$$

Since 2 T = 1 oz, the fraction is $\frac{2 \text{ T}}{1 \text{ oz}}$.

$$2\ \cancel{\text{oz}} \times \frac{2 \text{ T}}{1\ \cancel{\text{oz}}} = 4 \text{ T}$$

So 2 ounces is approximately the same as 4 tablespoons, and the patient would take 4 tablespoons of citrate of magnesia whenever necessary.

Example 5.8

If the patient asks you how many drops are in $1\frac{1}{2}$ teaspoons, what would you tell him?

$$1\frac{1}{2} \text{ t} = ? \text{ gtt}$$

You want to cancel the teaspoons and obtain the equivalent amount in drops.

$$1\frac{1}{2}\text{ t} \times \frac{?\text{ gtt}}{?\text{ t}} = ?\text{ gtt}$$

Since 60 gtt = 1 t, the fraction is $\frac{60\text{ gtt}}{1\text{ t}}$.

$$\frac{3\cancel{\text{t}}}{\cancel{2}} \times \frac{\overset{30}{\cancel{60}}\text{ gtt}}{1\cancel{\text{t}}} = 90\text{ gtt}$$

So you would tell the patient that there are 90 drops in $1\frac{1}{2}$ teaspoons.

Weight in the Household System

The only units of weight used in the household system are ounces (oz) and pounds (lb), as shown in Table 5.7.

Table 5.7 *Weight in the Household System*

16 oz = 1 lb

Example 5.9

An infant weighs 7 pounds 11 ounces. What is the weight of the infant in ounces?

First you change the 7 pounds to ounces.

$$7\text{ lb} = ?\text{ oz}$$

You want to cancel the pounds and obtain the equivalent amount in ounces.

$$7\text{ lb} = \frac{?\text{ oz}}{?\text{ lb}} = ?\text{ oz}$$

Since 16 oz = 1 lb, the fraction is $\frac{16\text{ oz}}{1\text{ lb}}$.

$$7\cancel{\text{lb}} \times \frac{16\text{ oz}}{1\cancel{\text{lb}}} = 112\text{ oz}$$

Now you add the extra 11 ounces.

$$112\text{ oz} + 11\text{ oz} = 123\text{ oz}$$

So the 7-pound, 11-ounce infant weighs 123 ounces.

Notes/Workspace

Notes/Workspace

Practice Sets

You will find the answers to Try These for Practice, Exercises, and Cumulative Review Practice Sets in Appendix A at the back of the book. Your instructor has the answers to the Additional Exercises.

Try These for Practice

Test your comprehension after reading the chapter.

1. The prescriber has ordered 8 ounces of the food supplement Ensure. How many drams will you administer to the patient? ________

2. If a patient has an order for 12 ounces of the cathartic citrate of magnesia, how many teacups do you give to the patient? ________

3. Convert 2 tablespoons to teaspoons. ________

4. The prescriber ordered:

   cranberry juice ℥ 12 q A.M. po

   Convert ounces 12 to pints. ________

5. In order to do the exercises at the end of this chapter, you need to memorize all the apothecary, household, and metric equivalents. To test yourself, fill in the missing numbers in the following chart and check your answers on page A-5 before you start the exercises.

   Apothecary System

qt 1	=	pt 2
pt 1	=	℥ 16
fl. oz. ℥ 1	=	ʒ 8
ʒ 1	=	♏ 60

Prescribed amount

Household System

1 glass = ℥ 8

1 measuring cup = ℥ 8

1 teacup = ℥ 6

1 oz = 2 T

1 T = 3 t

1 t = 60 gtt

1 lb = 16 oz

Metric System

1 mL = 1 cc

1 g = 1000 mg

1 kg = 1000 g

1000 μg = 1 mg

Exercises

Reinforce your understanding in class or at home.

1. ♏ 120 = dr ________

2. qt 4 = pt ________

3. pt 10 = qt ________

4. 3 t = ________ gtt

5. ʒ 30 = ♏ ________

6. ℥ $\frac{1}{8}$ = ʒ ________

7. ʒ 32 = ℥ ________

8. 4 T = ________ t

9. ℥ 24 = ʒ ________

10. ♏ 90 = ʒ ________

Notes/Workspace

Notes/Workspace

11. The label in Figure 5.1 indicates the quantity of colchicine in 1 tablet using both the metric and apothecary system. Indicate the quantity of colchicine in 1 tablet using:

a. the apothecary system ________

b. the metric system ________

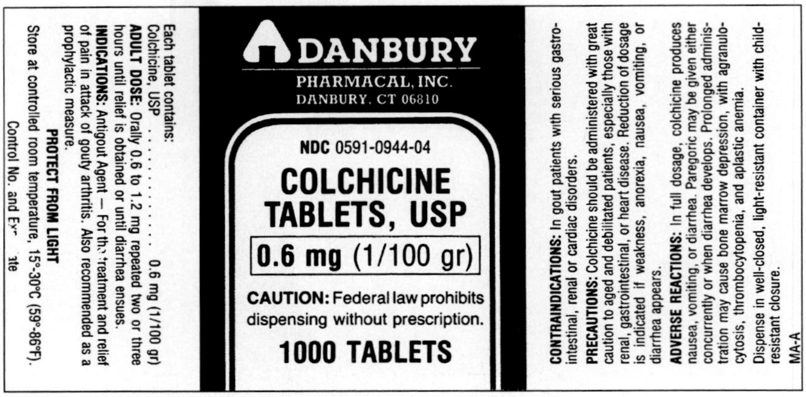

Figure 5.1 *Drug label for colchicine*

12. The order reads 3 teaspoons of the antidiarrheal medication bismuth subsalicylate (Pepto-Bismol). Change to the equivalent in tablespoons. ________

13. The patient is to receive ounces $\overline{\text{ISS}}$ of castor oil for bowel preparation before surgery. What is the equivalent quantity in drams? ________

14. The order reads $2\frac{1}{2}$ quarts of H_2O. What is the equivalent quantity in pints?
____

15. According to the physician's order sheet in Figure 5.2, what is the dose of guaifenesin (Robitussin) in ounces? ________

Notes/Workspace

GENERAL HOSPITAL

PRESS HARD WITH BALLPOINT PEN. WRITE DATE & TIME AND SIGN EACH ORDER

DATE	TIME	(A.M.) P.M.
3/8/94	11	
Robitussin oz 4 po q6h		

SIGNATURE A. Giangrasso M.D.

IMPRINT
273189 3/7/94
Jane Campbell 2/1/75
2 Elm St. Buddhist
Silver Springs, CO Aetna
43612
Anthony Giangrasso, M.D.

ORDERS NOTED
DATE 3/8/94 TIME 11:20 (A.M.) P.M.
❑ MEDEX ❑ KARDEX
NURSE'S SIG. J. Olsen

FILLED BY DATE

PHYSICIAN'S ORDERS

Figure 5.2 *Physician's order sheet*

16. The prescriber ordered drams 2 of elixir of potassium gluconate (Kaon Liquid). How many minims of this electrolyte are contained in this dose?

____

17. The prescriber ordered: tincture of belladonna 15 gtt po prn. Convert the drops of this antidiarrheal drug to teaspoons. ________

18. A patient has been prescribed: docusate sodium dr 3 po qd. How many ounces of this stool softener will you administer? ________

19. The order reads: milk 2 qt po qd. What is the equivalent in ounces?

____

20. The prescriber ordered: H_2O $\frac{1}{4}$ pt po q1h. How many ounces should be given every hour? ________

Notes/Workspace

Additional Exercises

Now, on your own, test yourself! Ask your instructor to check your answers.

1. $\frac{1}{3}$ t = ________ gtt

2. 9 t = ________ T

3. 18 oz = ________ teacups

4. $\frac{3}{4}$ qt = ________ pt

5. ℥ 12 = ʒ ________

6. 30 gtt = ________ t

7. ʒ 6 = ♏ ________

8. ʒ 3 = ℥ ________

9. ʒ 4 = ♏ ________

10. 2 t = ________ gtt

11. Change 5 ounces to drams. ________

12. How many ounces are contained in 5 tablespoons? ________

13. The prescriber ordered $\frac{1}{2}$ teaspoon of tincture of opium (paregoric) as an antidiarrheal agent. How many drops are contained in $\frac{1}{2}$ teaspoon?

____

14. The prescriber ordered 2 cups (teacups) of magnesium citrate. What would be the equivalent in ounces of this cathartic? ________

15. The order reads 2 teaspoons of mineral oil, a laxative. How many drops are contained in 2 teaspoons? ________

16. How many drops are contained in 3 teaspoons of cimetidine (Tagamet), an anti-ulcer agent? ________

17. The prescriber ordered:

castor oil dr 8 po 9 P.M.

Convert this amount to ounces. ________

18. If the patient must receive ounces 4 of sodium phosphate (Phospho-Soda) po, how many drams of this laxative will you prepare? ________

19. The patient is to receive:

$$\text{syrup of prochlorperazine } 1\frac{1}{2} \text{ tsp po q4h prn}$$

What is the equivalent in drops of this anti-emetic drug? ________

20. Read the physician's order sheet in Figure 5.3. How many teaspoons are equivalent to this dose of magnesium hydroxide and aluminum hydroxide (Mylanta)? ________

GENERAL HOSPITAL

PRESS HARD WITH BALLPOINT PEN. WRITE DATE & TIME AND SIGN EACH ORDER

DATE	TIME	A.M. / P.M.
7/2/94	2	P.M. (circled)
Mylanta 2 T po q4h		
SIGNATURE J. Olsen		M.D.

IMPRINT
721492 7/21/94
Robert Jones 12/2/60
32 Broadway RC
Irvine, CA Blue Cross
77461
June Olsen, M.D.

ORDERS NOTED
DATE 7/21/94 TIME 2:30 A.M. P.M. (P.M. circled)
❑ MEDEX ❑ KARDEX
NURSE'S SIG. A. Giangrasso

FILLED BY DATE

PHYSICIAN'S ORDERS

Figure 5.3 *Physician's order sheet*

Notes/Workspace

Notes/Workspace

Cumulative Review Exercises

Review your mastery of earlier chapters.

1. 2.5 g = ________ mg

2. 200 mcg = ________ mg

3. ♏ 180 = ʒ ________

4. ℥ 4 = ʒ ________

5. 25 mg = ________ μg

6. 6 t = ________ T

7. 1200 cc = ________ L

8. 6000 mg = ________ g

9. 2.35 kg = ________ g

10. 2.5 g = ________ mg

11. How many teaspoons are contained in $\frac{1}{2}$ tablespoon? ________

12. How many milliliters are contained in 3.25 liters? ________

13. The prescriber ordered drams 6 of magnesium hydroxide and aluminum hydroxide (Mylanta), an antacid. How many ounces would you administer to the patient? ________

14. If the prescriber ordered 30 drops of a drug, how many teaspoons would you administer to the patient? ________

15. The order reads:

orange juice 240 mL po qd

Convert 240 milliliters to liters. ________

chapter 6

Converting from One System of Measurement to Another

Objectives

After completing this chapter, you will be able to

- *state the equivalent units of weight for the metric, apothecary, and household systems.*
- *state the equivalent units of volume for the metric, apothecary, and household systems.*
- *state the equivalent units of length for the metric and household systems.*
- *convert from one unit to its equivalent among the three systems.*

When calculating drug dosages, you will sometimes need to convert a quantity expressed in one unit of measurement to an equivalent quantity expressed in another. For example, you might need to convert a quantity measured in drams to the same quantity measured in milliliters. This chapter will show you how to use dimensional analysis to accomplish this conversion.

Notes/Workspace

Equivalents of Common Units of Measurement

To get started, you will need to learn some basic equivalent values of the various units in the different systems. Tables 6.1 through 6.3 list some common equivalent values for weight, volume, and length in the metric, apothecary, and household systems of measurement. Although these equivalents are considered standards, many of them are still only approximations.

Table 6.1 *Equivalent Values for Units of Weight*

Metric		Apothecary		Household
60 milligrams (mg)	=	grain (gr) 1		
1 gram (g)	=	grains (gr) 15		
1 kilogram (kg)			=	2.2 pounds (lb)
0.45 kilogram (kg)			=	1 pound (lb)

Table 6.2 *Equivalent Values for Units of Volume*

Metric		Apothecary		Household
		minim (♏) 1	=	1 drop (gtt)
1 milliliter (mL)	=	minims (♏) 15 or 16	=	15 or 16 drops (gtt)
4 or 5 milliliters (mL)	=	dram (ʒ) 1	=	1 teaspoon (t)
		minims (♏) 60	=	1 teaspoon (t)
		minims (♏) 60	=	60 drops (gtt)
30 milliliters (mL)	=	ounce (℥) 1	=	1 ounce (℥) or 2 T
500 milliliters (mL)	=	ounces (℥) 16	=	1 pt (pt)
1000 milliliters (mL)	=	ounces (℥) 32	=	1 quart (qt)

Note

Here are some useful equivalents:

1 t = 60 gtt = ♏ 60 = ʒ 1 = 4 or 5 mL

2 T = ℥ 1 = ʒ 8 = 30 or 32 mL

Table 6.3 *Equivalent Values for Units of Length*

Metric		Household
1 centimeter (cm)	=	0.4 inch (in)
		or $\frac{2}{5}$ inch
2.5 centimeters (cm)	=	1 inch (in)

Notes/Workspace

Note

Equivalent values for units of weight, volume, and length can also be found on the inside front cover.

You can use dimensional analysis to convert from one system to another in exactly the same way you converted from one unit to another within the same system. Multiply the original measurement by a fraction that is equal to 1. This fraction will have the original units on the bottom and the new units on the top.

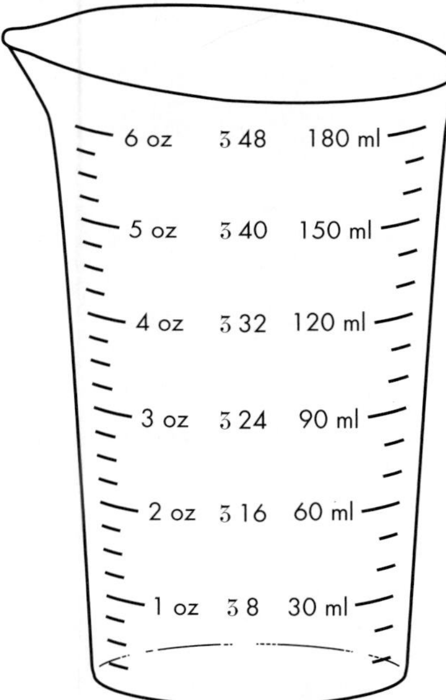

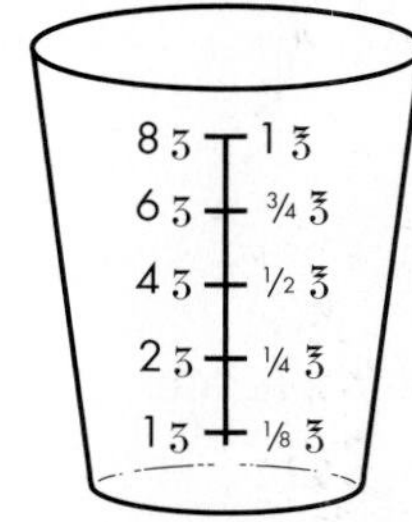

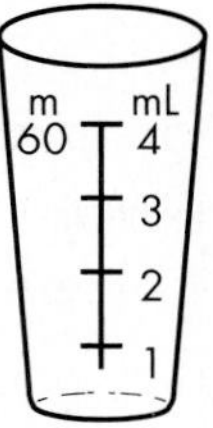

Figure 6.1 *Units of volume in the apothecary, household, and metric systems*

Notes/Workspace

Metric-to-Apothecary Conversions

Example 6.1

Convert 300 milligrams to grains.

$$300 \text{ mg} = \text{gr } ?$$

You want to cancel the milligrams and obtain the equivalent amount in grains.

$$300 \text{ mg} \times \frac{\text{gr } ?}{? \text{ mg}} = \text{gr } ?$$

Since 60 mg = gr 1, the fraction is $\frac{\text{gr } 1}{60 \text{ mg}}$.

$$300 \cancel{\text{mg}} \times \frac{\text{gr } 1}{60 \cancel{\text{mg}}} = \frac{\text{gr } 300}{60} = \text{gr } 5$$

So 300 milligrams is equivalent to grains 5.

Example 6.2

Convert 10 milligrams to grains.

$$10 \text{ mg} = \text{gr } ?$$

You want to cancel the milligrams and obtain the equivalent amount in grains.

$$10 \text{ mg} \times \frac{\text{gr } ?}{? \text{ mg}} = \text{gr } ?$$

Since 60 mg = gr 1, the fraction is $\frac{\text{gr } 1}{60 \text{ mg}}$.

$$\overset{1}{\cancel{10}} \cancel{\text{mg}} \times \frac{\text{gr } 1}{\underset{6}{\cancel{60}} \cancel{\text{mg}}} = \text{gr } \frac{1}{6}$$

So 10 milligrams is equivalent to grain $\frac{1}{6}$.

Example 6.3

Convert 0.1 milligram to grains.

$$0.1 \text{ mg} = \text{gr } ?$$

You want to cancel the milligram and obtain the equivalent amount in grains.

$$0.1 \text{ mg} \times \frac{\text{gr } ?}{? \text{ mg}} = \text{gr } ?$$

Since 60 mg = gr 1, the fraction is $\frac{\text{gr } 1}{60 \text{ mg}}$.

$$0.1 \cancel{\text{mg}} \times \frac{\text{gr } 1}{60 \cancel{\text{mg}}} = \frac{\text{gr } 0.1}{60} \times \frac{10}{10} = \text{gr } \frac{1}{600}$$

So 0.1 milligram is equivalent to grain $\frac{1}{600}$.

In Example 6.3, we multiplied both the numerator and the denominator of the fraction $\frac{\text{gr } 0.1}{60}$ by 10 to eliminate the decimal number.

Example 6.4

Convert 4 grams to grains.

$$4 \text{ g} = \text{gr } ?$$

You want to cancel the grams and obtain the equivalent amount in grains.

$$4 \text{ g} \times \frac{\text{gr } ?}{? \text{ g}} = \text{gr } ?$$

Since 1 g = gr 15, the fraction is $\frac{\text{gr } 15}{1 \text{ g}}$.

$$4 \cancel{\text{g}} \times \frac{\text{gr } 15}{1 \cancel{\text{g}}} = \text{gr } 60$$

So 4 grams is equivalent to grains 60.

Example 6.5

Convert 0.25 gram to grains.

$$0.25 \text{ g} = \text{gr } ?$$

You want to cancel the gram and obtain the equivalent amount in grains.

$$0.25 \text{ g} \times \frac{\text{gr } ?}{? \text{ g}} = \text{gr } ?$$

Since 1 g = gr 15, the fraction is $\frac{\text{gr } 15}{1 \text{ g}}$.

$$0.25 \cancel{\text{g}} \times \frac{\text{gr } 15}{1 \cancel{\text{g}}} = \text{gr } 3.75 = \text{gr } 3\frac{3}{4}$$

So 0.25 gram is equivalent to grains $3\frac{3}{4}$.

Notes/Workspace

Notes/Workspace

Note

Grains are expressed in fractions and whole numbers. Therefore, grains 3.75 is changed to grains $3\frac{3}{4}$.

Apothecary-to-Metric Conversions

Example 6.6

Convert grain $\frac{1}{2}$ to milligrams.

$$\text{gr } \frac{1}{2} = ?\text{ mg}$$

You want to cancel the grain and obtain the equivalent amount in milligrams.

$$\text{gr } \frac{1}{2} \times \frac{?\text{ mg}}{\text{gr } ?} = ?\text{ mg}$$

Since 60 mg = gr 1, the fraction is $\frac{60\text{ mg}}{\text{gr } 1}$.

$$\cancel{\text{gr}}\ \frac{1}{\cancel{2}_{1}} \times \frac{\overset{30}{\cancel{60}}\text{ mg}}{\cancel{\text{gr}}\ 1} = 30\text{ mg}$$

So grain $\frac{1}{2}$ is equivalent to 30 milligrams.

Example 6.7

Convert grains 5 to milligrams.

$$\text{gr } 5 = ?\text{ mg}$$

You want to cancel the grains and obtain the equivalent amount in milligrams.

$$\text{gr } 5 \times \frac{?\text{ mg}}{\text{gr } ?} = ?\text{ mg}$$

Since 60 mg = gr 1, the fraction is $\frac{60\text{ mg}}{\text{gr } 1}$.

$$\cancel{\text{gr}}\ 5 \times \frac{60\text{ mg}}{\cancel{\text{gr}}\ 1} = 300\text{ mg}$$

So grains 5 is equivalent to 300 milligrams.

Example 6.8

Convert grains $7\frac{1}{2}$ to grams.

$$\text{gr } 7\frac{1}{2} = ?\text{ g}$$

You want to cancel the grains and obtain the equivalent amount in grams.

$$\text{gr } \frac{15}{2} \times \frac{?\text{ g}}{\text{gr } ?} = ?\text{ g}$$

Since 1 g = gr 15, the fraction is $\frac{1\text{ g}}{\text{gr } 15}$.

$$\cancel{\text{gr}}\ \frac{\overset{1}{\cancel{15}}}{2} \times \frac{1\text{ g}}{\cancel{\text{gr}}\ \underset{1}{\cancel{15}}} = \frac{1}{2}\text{ g} = 0.5\text{ g}$$

So grains $7\frac{1}{2}$ is equivalent to 0.5 gram.

Note

Grams are expressed in decimals or whole numbers. Therefore, $\frac{1}{2}$ gram is changed to 0.5 gram.

Example 6.9

Convert grains $1\frac{1}{2}$ to grams.

$$\text{gr } 1\frac{1}{2} = ?\text{ g}$$

You want to cancel the grains and obtain the equivalent amount in grams.

$$\text{gr } \frac{3}{2} \times \frac{?\text{ g}}{\text{gr } ?} = ?\text{ g}$$

Since 1 g = gr 15, the fraction is $\frac{1\text{ g}}{\text{gr } 15}$.

$$\cancel{\text{gr}}\ \frac{\overset{1}{\cancel{3}}}{2} \times \frac{1\text{ g}}{\cancel{\text{gr}}\ \underset{5}{\cancel{15}}} = \frac{1\text{ g}}{10} = 0.1\text{ g}$$

So grains $1\frac{1}{2}$ is equivalent to 0.1 gram.

Notes/Workspace

Notes/Workspace

Household to Apothecary or Metric Conversions

Example 6.10

Convert 6 teaspoons to milliliters.

$$6 \text{ t} = ? \text{ mL}$$

You want to cancel the teaspoons and obtain the equivalent in milliliters.

$$6 \text{ t} \times \frac{? \text{ mL}}{? \text{ t}} = ? \text{ mL}$$

You can either use 4 mL = 1 t or 5 mL = 1 t. For this calculation, use 5 mL = 1 t; the fraction is therefore $\frac{5 \text{ mL}}{1 \text{ t}}$.

$$6 \cancel{\text{t}} \times \frac{5 \text{ mL}}{1 \cancel{\text{t}}} = 30 \text{ mL}$$

So 6 teaspoons is equivalent to 30 milliliters.

By the way

If you used the equivalent 4 mL = 1 t in this example, the answer would be 24 milliliters instead of 30 milliliters. This illustrates the approximate nature of the equivalents between systems.

Example 6.11

Change $\frac{1}{4}$ teaspoon to drops.

$$\frac{1}{4} \text{ t} = ? \text{ gtt}$$

You want to cancel the teaspoon and obtain the equivalent amount in drops.

$$\frac{1}{4} \text{ t} \times \frac{? \text{ gtt}}{? \text{ t}} = ? \text{ gtt}$$

Since 60 gtt = 1 t, the fraction is $\frac{60 \text{ gtt}}{1 \text{ t}}$.

$$\frac{1}{\cancelto{1}{4}} \cancel{\text{t}} \times \frac{\cancelto{15}{60} \text{ gtt}}{1 \cancel{\text{t}}} = 15 \text{ gtt}$$

So $\frac{1}{4}$ teaspoon is equivalent to 15 drops.

Example 6.12

Dixie is 5 feet 9 inches tall. What is her height in centimeters?

$$5 \text{ ft } 9 \text{ in} \quad \text{means} \quad 5 \text{ ft} + 9 \text{ in}$$

First determine Dixie's height in inches. To do this, convert 5 feet to inches.

$$5 \text{ ft} = ? \text{ in}$$

You want to cancel feet and obtain the equivalent height in inches.

$$5 \text{ ft} \times \frac{? \text{ in}}{? \text{ ft}} = ? \text{ in}$$

Since 1 ft = 12 in, the fraction is $\frac{12 \text{ in}}{1 \text{ ft}}$.

$$5 \cancel{\text{ft}} \times \frac{12 \text{ in}}{1 \cancel{\text{ft}}} = 60 \text{ in}$$

Second, add the extra 9 inches.

$$60 \text{ in} + 9 \text{ in} = 69 \text{ in}$$

Now convert 69 inches to centimeters.

$$69 \text{ in} = ? \text{ cm}$$

You want to cancel inches and obtain the equivalent length in centimeters.

$$69 \text{ in} \times \frac{? \text{ cm}}{? \text{ in}} = ? \text{ cm}$$

Since 1 in = 2.5 cm, the fraction is $\frac{2.5 \text{ cm}}{1 \text{ in}}$.

$$69 \cancel{\text{in}} \times \frac{2.5 \text{ cm}}{1 \cancel{\text{in}}} = 172.5 \text{ cm}$$

So Dixie is 172.5 centimeters tall.

Notes/Workspace

Notes/Workspace

Example 6.13

Jennifer weighs 103 pounds 8 ounces. What is her weight in kilograms?

$$103 \text{ lb } 8 \text{ oz} \quad \text{means} \quad 103 \text{ lb} + 8 \text{ oz}$$

First determine Jennifer's weight in pounds. To do this, convert 8 ounces to pounds.

$$8 \text{ oz} = ? \text{ lb}$$

You want to cancel ounces and obtain the equivalent amount in pounds.

$$8 \text{ oz} \times \frac{? \text{ lb}}{? \text{ oz}} = ? \text{ lb}$$

Since 1 lb = 16 oz, the fraction is $\frac{1 \text{ lb}}{16 \text{ oz}}$.

$$\overset{1}{\cancel{8 \text{ oz}}} \times \frac{1 \text{ lb}}{\underset{2}{\cancel{16 \text{ oz}}}} = \frac{1}{2} \text{ lb}$$

So Jennifer weighs 103 lb + $\frac{1}{2}$ lb or 103.5 pounds.

Second, convert 103.5 pounds to kilograms.

$$103.5 \text{ lb} = ? \text{ kg}$$

You want to cancel pounds and obtain the equivalent amount in kilograms.

$$103.5 \text{ lb} \times \frac{? \text{ kg}}{? \text{ lb}} = ? \text{ kg}$$

Since 1 kg = 2.2 lb, the fraction is $\frac{1 \text{ kg}}{2.2 \text{ lb}}$.

$$103.5 \cancel{\text{lb}} \times \frac{1 \text{ kg}}{2.2 \cancel{\text{lb}}} = 47.0 \text{ kg}$$

So Jennifer weighs 47 kilograms.

Prerequisite Equivalents

Notes/Workspace

In order to do the exercises at the end of this chapter, you need to memorize all the equivalents presented so far. To test yourself, fill in the missing numbers in the following chart. Check your answers on page A-6 before you start the exercises.

Metric System

1 mL = 1 cc = 1 cm^3

1 L = 1000 mL

1 kg = 1000 g

1000 mg = 1 g

1000 μg = 1 mg

101 μg = 1 mcg

Apothecary System

1 qt = 2 pt

1 pt = ℥ 16

℥ 1 = ʒ 8

ʒ 1 = ♏ 60

Household System

1 glass = ℥ 8

1 teacup = ℥ 6

℥ 1 = 2 T

1 T = 3 t

1 t = 60 gtt

1 lb = 16 oz

1 ft = 12 in

Mixed Systems

ʒ 1 = 1 t = ♏ 60 = 60 gtt = 5 mL

℥ 1 = 2 T = ʒ 8 = 30 mL

1 measuring cup = 1 glass = ℥ 8 = ½ pt

gr 1 = 60 mg

1 g = gr 15

1 mL = 15-16 gtt

1 kg = 2.2 lb

1 lb = 0.45 kg

1 in = 2.5 cm

Household + apothecary are written in fraction - metric is written as decimal

Notes/Workspace

Practice Sets

You will find the answers to Try These for Practice, Exercises, and Cumulative Review Practice Sets in Appendix A at the back of the book. Your instructor has the answers to the Additional Exercises.

Try These for Practice

Test your comprehension after reading the chapter.

1. The prescriber has ordered grains 20 of acetylsalicylic acid (aspirin). Convert this quantity to milligrams. ________

2. If a patient has an order for 0.25 milligram of cosyntropin (Cortrosyn) IM, how many grains will you administer to the patient? ________

3. The prescriber ordered: atropine sulfate gr $\frac{1}{500}$ sc stat. Convert this quantity to milligrams. ________

4. A child weighs 62 pounds. Convert this weight to kilograms. ________

5. The patient is to receive 4 milliliters of diphenhydramine (Benylin). How many minims will you administer to the patient? ________

Exercises

Reinforce your understanding in class or at home.

1. Convert 25 micrograms to milligrams. ________

2. How many grams does 1.5 kilograms equal? ________

3. 0.0001 g = ________ mg

4. 0.008 mg = ________ mcg

5. gr $\frac{1}{6}$ = ________ mg

6. 0.6 mg = gr ________

7. 0.1 mg = ________ g

8. 0.2 mg = ________ mcg

9. gr $\frac{1}{240}$ = ________ g

10. gr $3\frac{3}{4}$ = ________ mg

11. 0.75 g = gr ________

12. gr $\frac{1}{600}$ = ________ mg

Notes/Workspace

13. The prescriber ordered: atropine sulfate gr $\frac{1}{300}$ sc q6h prn. What is the equivalent dose in milligrams? ________

14. The order reads grains 4 of a drug. Change this order to grams.

____

15. A prescriber has ordered 12.5 milligrams of captopril (Capoten). What is the equivalent quantity in micrograms? ________

16. According to the medication administration record in Figure 6.2, how many milligrams of glipizide will you give the patient each day? ________

17. The prescriber has ordered 0.75 gram of cefuroxime (Ceftin) for a patient. What is the equivalent quantity of this antibiotic in milligrams?

____

GENERAL HOSPITAL

Year 19 *94* Month *February* Day		*12*	*13*	*14*	*15*	*16*	
Medication Dosage and Interval		Initials* and Hours	Initials and Hours	Initials and Hours	Initials and Hours	Initials and Hours	Initials and Hours
Date started: *2/12/94* *glipizide gr $\frac{1}{3}$ po qd*	I	*JO*					
	AM	*10*					
	I						
Discontinued:	PM						

Allergies: (Specify) *none*

Init*	Signature
JO	*June Olsen*

PATIENT IDENTIFICATION

789102 2/12/94

Susan Walters 6/16/60
40 Water Street Prot
Merrymount, NY 10301 BCBS

L. Ablon, M.D.

MEDICATION ADMINISTRATION RECORD

Figure 6.2 *Medication administration record*

Notes/Workspace

18. Read the information on the label in Figure 6.3 and change the milligrams to grains. ________

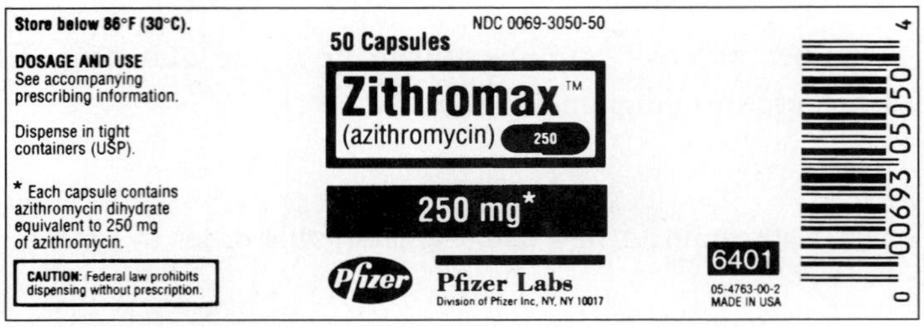

Figure 6.3 *Drug label for Zithromax*

19. Using the information in Figure 6.4, calculate the amount of grains in 1 tablet. ________

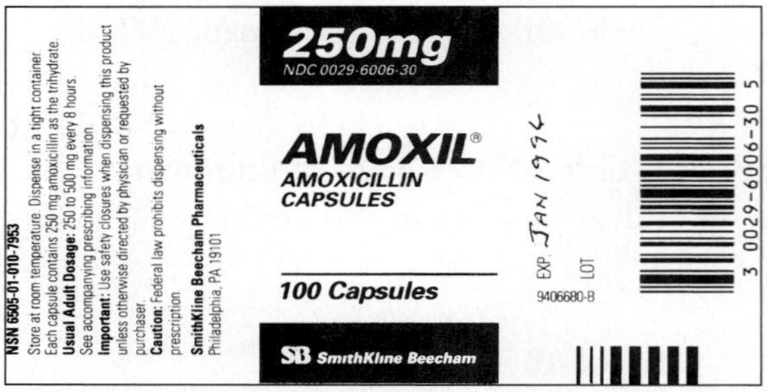

Figure 6.4 *Drug label for Amoxil*

20. The prescriber ordered: diphenhydramine hydrochloride 50 mg po tid. Calculate the amount of grains in 1 capsule from the label in Figure 6.5.

____

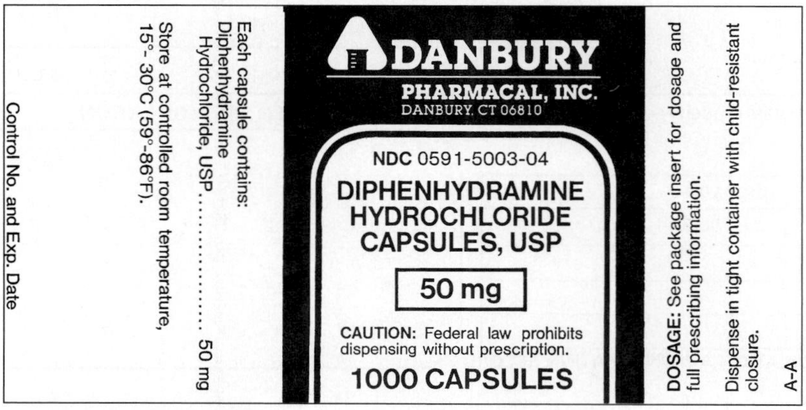

Figure 6.5 *Drug label for diphenhydramine hydrochloride*

Additional Exercises

Now, on your own, test yourself! Ask your instructor to check your answers.

1. From the medication administration record in Figure 6.6, calculate the amount of grains of digoxin (Lanoxin) you would prepare. _________

GENERAL HOSPITAL

Year 19 94 · Month February · Day	13					
Medication Dosage and Interval	Initials* and Hours	Initials and Hours	Initials and Hours	Initials and Hours	Initials and Hours	Initials and Hours
Date started: 2/13/94 digoxin 0.25 mg po qd — I	JO					
AM	10					
I						
Discontinued: — PM						

Allergies: (Specify)
none

Init*	Signature
JO	June Olsen

MEDICATION ADMINISTRATION RECORD

PATIENT IDENTIFICATION

789102 2/12/94
John Walters 5/31/47
140 Waiter Street Prot
Barrie, NY 10301 BCBS
L. Ablon, M.D.

Figure 6.6 *Medication administration record*

2. If a physician orders grain $\frac{1}{200}$ of atropine sulfate, how many milligrams would you administer of this anti-arrhythmic drug? _________

3. The order is 0.5 milligram of digoxin (Lanoxin). Change this quantity to grains. _________

4. The prescriber ordered: neostigmine gr $\frac{1}{200}$ IM q4h prn. What is the dose of this cholinergic drug in grams? _________

5. An order reads 0.0003 gram. Change this quantity to milligrams.

____

Notes/Workspace

Notes/Workspace

6. gr 20 = ________ mg

7. A capsule of acetaminophen (Tylenol), an antipyretic, contains 0.5 gram. How much is this in milligrams? ________

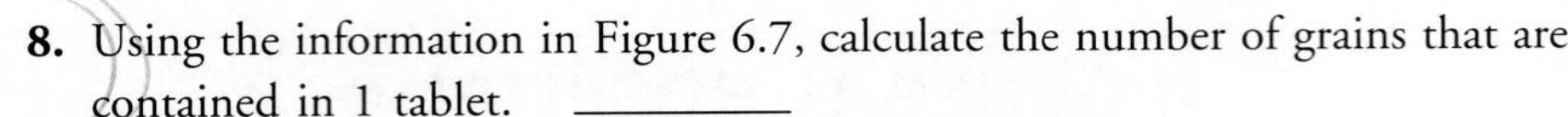

8. Using the information in Figure 6.7, calculate the number of grains that are contained in 1 tablet. ________

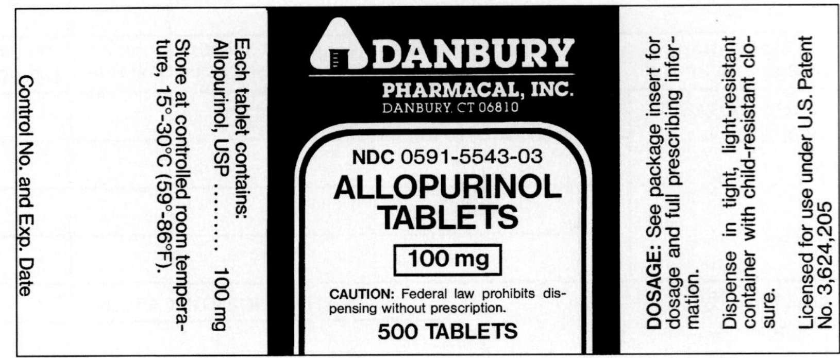

DANBURY
PHARMACAL, INC.
DANBURY, CT 06810
NDC 0591-5543-03
ALLOPURINOL
TABLETS
100 mg
CAUTION: Federal law prohibits dispensing without prescription.
500 TABLETS
Each tablet contains:
Allopurinol, USP .... 100 mg
Store at controlled room temperature, 15°-30°C (59°-86°F).
Control No. and Exp. Date
DOSAGE: See package insert for dosage and full prescribing information.
Dispense in tight, light-resistant container with child-resistant closure.
Licensed for use under U.S. Patent No. 3,624,205

Figure 6.7 *Drug label for allopurinol*

9. 5000 μg = ________ mg

10. Convert 2700 grams to kilograms. ________

11. Change 15,000 micrograms to milligrams. ________

12. gr $\frac{1}{150}$ = ________ g

13. gr $\frac{1}{60}$ = ________ mg

14. 0.012 g = ________ mg

15. gr 45 = ________ g

16. The order reads: quinidine gluconate 200 mg po q12h. How many grains of this anti-arrhythmic drug are contained in 200 milligrams? ________

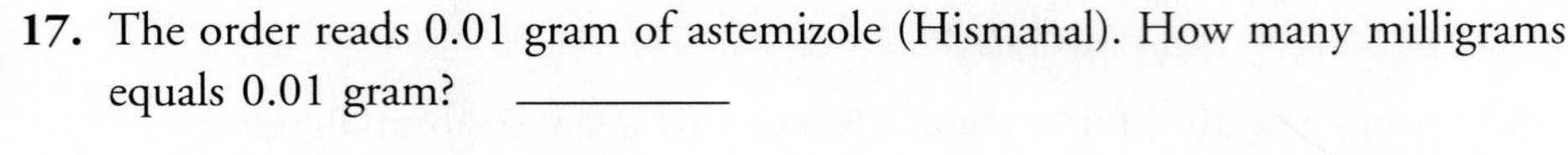

17. The order reads 0.01 gram of astemizole (Hismanal). How many milligrams equals 0.01 gram? ________

18. Read the information on the label in Figure 6.8. Change the milligrams to grains. ________

ROERIG Pfizer
A division of Pfizer Inc., N.Y., N.Y. 10017
NDC 0049-5710-66
100 Capsules
Navane®
thiothixene
1 mg
CAUTION: Federal law prohibits dispensing without prescription.
ROERIG Pfizer
A division of Pfizer Inc., N.Y., N.Y. 10017

Figure 6.8 *Drug label for Navane*

19. The label in Figure 6.9 is for Procardia. How many milligrams are contained in 100 capsules? ________

RECOMMENDED STORAGE
STORE BETWEEN 59°F-77°F (15°C-25°C)
DO NOT PERMIT TO FREEZE
PROTECT CAPSULES FROM LIGHT AT ALL TIMES
PROTECT FROM MOISTURE AND HUMIDITY
REPLACE CAP TIGHTLY AFTER EACH OPENING
Each capsule contains 10 mg nifedipine.
Manufactured by Pfizer Inc.
Encapsulated by Banner Gelatin Products Corp.
Chatsworth, California 91311
MADE IN U.S.A. 3
1473
6505-01 126-3842
NDC 0069-2600-66
100 Capsules
Procardia®
nifedipine
10 mg
CAUTION: Federal law prohibits dispensing without prescription.
READ ACCOMPANYING PROFESSIONAL INFORMATION
DOSAGE: See accompanying prescribing information.
Dispense in tight, light resistant containers (USP)

Figure 6.9 *Drug label for Procardia*

20. The drug in Figure 6.10 is hydrochlorothiazide. Convert the milligrams to grams. ________

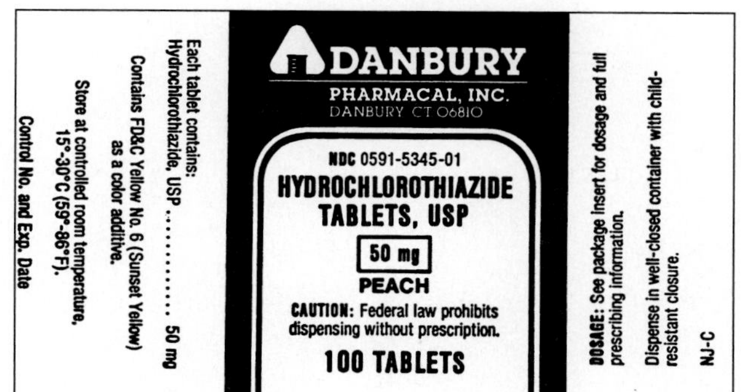

Each tablet contains:
Hydrochlorothiazide, USP .... 50 mg
Contains FD&C Yellow No. 6 (Sunset Yellow) as a color additive.
Store at controlled room temperature, 15°-30°C (59°-86°F).
Control No. and Exp. Date
DANBURY
PHARMACAL, INC.
DANBURY CT 06810
NDC 0591-5345-01
HYDROCHLOROTHIAZIDE
TABLETS, USP
50 mg
PEACH
CAUTION: Federal law prohibits dispensing without prescription.
100 TABLETS
DOSAGE: See package insert for dosage and full prescribing information.
Dispense in well-closed container with child-resistant closure.
NJ-C

Figure 6.10 *Drug label for hydrochlorothiazide*

Notes/Workspace

Notes/Workspace

Cumulative Review Exercises

Review your mastery of earlier chapters.

1. 9 mg = gr ________

2. 4 t = ʒ ________

3. 0.25 g = gr ________

4. 45 mg = gr ________

5. gr $\frac{1}{3}$ = ________ mg

6. 180 mg = gr ________

7. 0.003 g = gr ________

8. 1.5 mg = gr ________

9. ʒ 16 = ℥ ________

10. 15 gtt = ________ mL

11. The order reads 1.25 mg of reserpine (Serpasil), an antihypertensive drug. What would be the equivalent amount in grams? ________

12. The prescriber ordered 15 milligrams of the sedative flurazepam (Dalmane). Convert this quantity to grains. ________

13. Read the information on the label in Figure 6.11. Calculate the number of grains in each tablet. ________

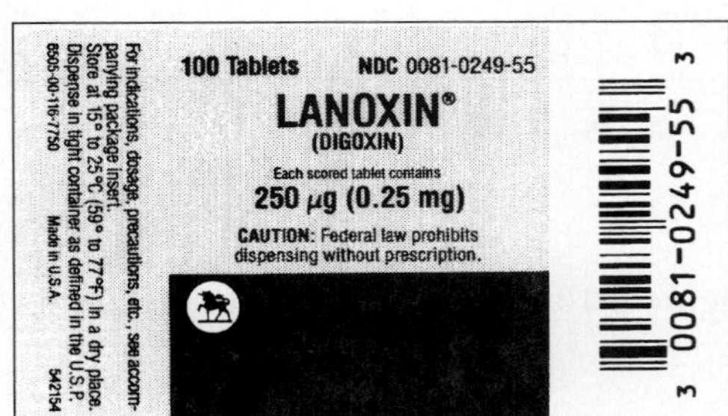

100 Tablets
NDC 0081-0249-55
LANOXIN®
(DIGOXIN)
Each scored tablet contains
250 μg (0.25 mg)
CAUTION: Federal law prohibits dispensing without prescription.
For indications, dosage, precautions, etc., see accompanying package insert.
Store at 15° to 25°C (59° to 77°F) in a dry place.
Dispense in tight container as defined in the U.S.P.
Made in U.S.A.
3 0081-0249-55 3

Figure 6.11 *Drug label for Lanoxin*

14. How many grains are equal to the number of milligrams contained in 1 tablet of the drug Cardilate shown in Figure 6.12? ________

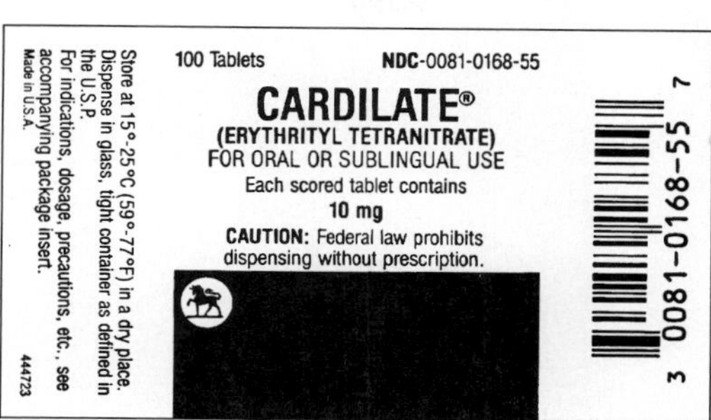
100 Tablets
NDC-0081-0168-55
CARDILATE®
(ERYTHRITYL TETRANITRATE)
FOR ORAL OR SUBLINGUAL USE
Each scored tablet contains
10 mg
CAUTION: Federal law prohibits dispensing without prescription.
Store at 15°-25°C (59°-77°F) in a dry place.
Dispense in glass, tight container as defined in the U.S.P.
For indications, dosage, precautions, etc., see accompanying package insert.
Made in U.S.A.
44723
3 0081-0168-55 7

Figure 6.12 *Drug label for Cardilate*

15. The label for furosemide is shown in Figure 6.13. Convert the milligrams to grams. ________

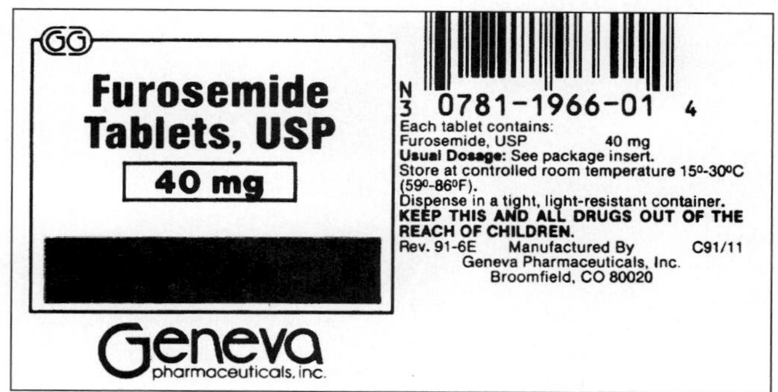
Furosemide Tablets, USP
40 mg
Geneva
pharmaceuticals, inc.
N 3 0781-1966-01 4
Each tablet contains:
Furosemide, USP 40 mg
Usual Dosage: See package insert.
Store at controlled room temperature 15°-30°C (59°-86°F).
Dispense in a tight, light-resistant container.
KEEP THIS AND ALL DRUGS OUT OF THE REACH OF CHILDREN.
Rev. 91-6E Manufactured By C91/11
Geneva Pharmaceuticals, Inc.
Broomfield, CO 80020

Figure 6.13 *Drug label for furosemide*

Notes/Workspace

Unit Three

Common Medication Preparations

chapter 7

Calculating Oral Medication Doses

Objectives

After completing this chapter, you will be able to

- *use dimensional analysis to calculate drug doses when the dose is dependent on the strength of the medication.*
- *calculate doses by body weight.*
- *do multistep conversion problems.*
- *calculate doses for oral medications in liquid form.*
- *calculate doses for oral medications in tablet, capsule, and caplet form.*
- *calculate doses for oral medications from the information given on drug labels.*

In this chapter you will learn the computations necessary to calculate doses of oral medication in liquid, tablet (tab), capsule (cap), or caplet (cap) form.

One-Step Conversions

In the calculations you have done in previous chapters, all the equivalents have come from standard tables. For example, 60 mg = gr 1. In this section the equivalent used will depend on the strength of the drug that is available. The equivalent used is found on the label of the drug container.

Notes/Workspace

Example 7.1

The order reads 2 milligrams po of haloperidol, an antipsychotic drug. Read the drug label in Figure 7.1 and determine how many tablets you would administer to the patient.

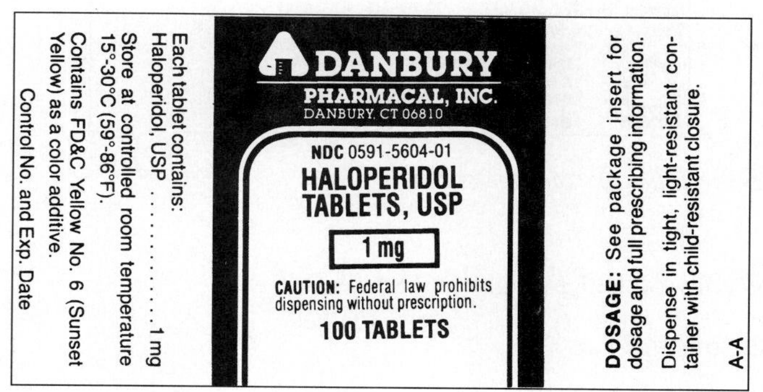
Each tablet contains:
Haloperidol, USP .... 1 mg
Store at controlled room temperature 15°-30°C (59°-86°F).
Contains FD&C Yellow No. 6 (Sunset Yellow) as a color additive.
Control No. and Exp. Date
DANBURY
PHARMACAL, INC.
DANBURY, CT 06810
NDC 0591-5604-01
HALOPERIDOL
TABLETS, USP
1 mg
CAUTION: Federal law prohibits dispensing without prescription.
100 TABLETS
DOSAGE: See package insert for dosage and full prescribing information.
Dispense in tight, light-resistant container with child-resistant closure.
A-A

Figure 7.1 *Drug label for haloperidol*

You want to convert the order, 2 milligrams, to tablets.

$$2 \text{ mg} = ? \text{ tab}$$

You want to cancel the milligrams and obtain the equivalent amount in tablets.

$$2 \text{ mg} \times \frac{? \text{ tab}}{? \text{ mg}} = ? \text{ tab}$$

Since the label states that 1 tab = 1 mg, the fraction is $\frac{1 \text{ tab}}{1 \text{ mg}}$.

$$2 \cancel{\text{mg}} \times \frac{1 \text{ tab}}{1 \cancel{\text{mg}}} = 2 \text{ tab}$$

So, 2 milligrams is equivalent to 2 tablets, and you would give 2 tablets of haloperidol to the patient.

Notes/Workspace

Example 7.2

The order reads:

codeine sulfate 120 mg po qd

The label is shown in Figure 7.2. How many tablets will you administer to the patient?

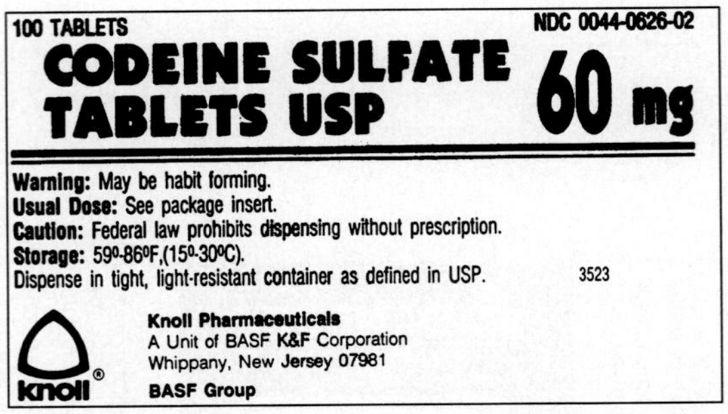

Figure 7.2 *Drug label for codeine sulfate*

You want to convert 120 milligrams to tablets.

$$120 \text{ mg} = ? \text{ tab}$$

You want to cancel the milligrams and calculate the equivalent amount in tablets.

$$120 \text{ mg} \times \frac{? \text{ tab}}{? \text{ mg}} = ? \text{ tab}$$

Since the label indicates that each tablet contains 60 milligrams, you use the equivalent $\frac{1 \text{ tab}}{60 \text{ mg}}$.

$$\overset{2}{\cancel{120 \text{ mg}}} \times \frac{1 \text{ tab}}{\cancel{60 \text{ mg}}} = 2 \text{ tab}$$

So you would administer 2 tablets of codeine sulfate to the patient.

Notes/Workspace

Example 7.3

How many tablets should you give a patient if the order is for grain $\frac{1}{2}$ of codeine sulfate and each tablet contains grain $\frac{1}{4}$?

In this problem you want to convert the order grain $\frac{1}{2}$ to tablets.

$$\text{gr}\ \frac{1}{2} = ?\ \text{tab}$$

You want to cancel the grain and determine the equivalent amount in tablets.

$$\text{gr}\ \frac{1}{2} \times \frac{?\ \text{tab}}{?\ \text{gr}} = ?\ \text{tab}$$

Since 1 tab = gr $\frac{1}{4}$, the fraction is $\frac{1\ \text{tab}}{\text{gr}\ \frac{1}{4}}$.

$$\cancel{\text{gr}}\ \frac{1}{2} \times \frac{1\ \text{tab}}{\cancel{\text{gr}}\ \frac{1}{4}} = \frac{1\ \text{tab}}{\frac{2}{4}} = 1\ \text{tab} \div \frac{2}{4} = 1\ \text{tab} \times \frac{4}{2} = 2\ \text{tab}$$

So grain $\frac{1}{2}$ is equivalent to 2 tablets, and you should give the patient 2 tablets of codeine sulfate.

Example 7.4

The order reads 100 milligrams of the anti-infective drug nitrofurantoin (Macrodantin). The label indicates that each capsule contains 50 milligrams of nitrofurantoin. How many capsules should be given to the patient po?

You want to convert the order, 100 milligrams, to capsules.

$$100\ \text{mg} = ?\ \text{cap}$$

You want to cancel the milligrams and obtain the equivalent amount in capsules.

$$100\ \text{mg} \times \frac{?\ \text{cap}}{?\ \text{mg}} = ?\ \text{cap}$$

Since each capsule contains 50 milligrams, the equivalent fraction is $\frac{1\ \text{cap}}{50\ \text{mg}}$.

$$\overset{2}{\cancel{100\ \text{mg}}} \times \frac{1\ \text{cap}}{\underset{1}{\cancel{50\ \text{mg}}}} = 2\ \text{cap}$$

So, 100 milligrams is equivalent to 2 capsules, and the patient should be given 2 capsules of nitrofurantoin.

Example 7.5

The prescriber orders 15 milligrams of the anticoagulant warfarin sodium (Coumadin). This is a loading dose. Examine the drug label shown in Figure 7.3 and determine how many of these scored tablets you would give the patient.

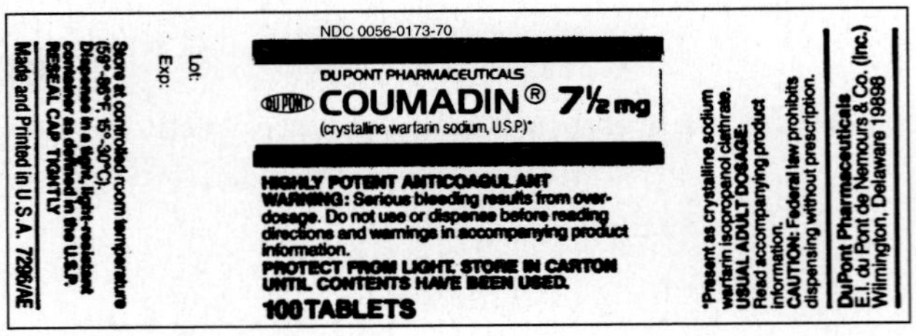

Figure 7.3 *Drug label for Coumadin*

You want to convert 15 milligrams to tablets.

$$15 \text{ mg} = ? \text{ tab}$$

You want to cancel the milligrams and obtain the equivalent amount in tablets.

$$15 \text{ mg} \times \frac{? \text{ tab}}{? \text{ mg}} = ? \text{ tab}$$

Since 1 tab = 10 mg, the equivalent fraction is $\frac{1 \text{ tab}}{10 \text{ mg}}$.

$$15 \cancel{\text{mg}} \times \frac{1 \text{ tab}}{7\frac{1}{2} \cancel{\text{mg}}} = \frac{15}{7\frac{1}{2}} \text{ tab} = 2 \text{ tab}$$

So 15 milligrams is equivalent to 2 tablets, and you would give 2 tablets of Coumadin to the patient.

Note

The loading dose of a drug is the amount necessary to allow the drug to become therapeutic in its action.

Dosage by Body Weight

Sometimes the amount of medication prescribed depends on the patient's body weight. So a patient who weighs more will receive more of the drug, and a patient who weighs less will receive less of the drug.

Notes/Workspace

Example 7.6

The prescriber orders 10 milligrams per kilogram of aminophylline (Phyllocontin) for a patient who weighs 50 kilograms. How much of this bronchodilating drug should the patient receive?

Note

The expression 10 mg/kg means that the patient is to receive 10 milligrams of the drug for each kilogram of body weight. So you will use the equivalent 10 mg (of drug) = 1 kg (of body weight).

You want to convert body weight to dosage.

$$50 \text{ kg (of body weight)} = ? \text{ mg (of drug)}$$

$$50 \text{ kg (of body weight)} \times \frac{? \text{ mg (of drug)}}{? \text{ kg (of body weight)}} = \text{mg (of drug)}$$

So you use the fraction $\frac{10 \text{ mg}}{1 \text{ kg}}$, which relates dosage to body weight.

$$50 \cancel{\text{kg}} \times \frac{10 \text{ mg}}{1 \cancel{\text{kg}}} = 500 \text{ mg}$$

So the patient should receive 500 milligrams of aminophylline.

Example 7.7

The order is 10 milligrams per kilogram of the antitubercular drug, isoniazid (Laniazid). How many milligrams would you administer to a patient who weighs 75 kilograms?

You want to convert body weight to dosage.

$$75 \text{ kg} = ? \text{ mg}$$

$$75 \text{ kg} \times \frac{? \text{ mg}}{? \text{ kg}} = ? \text{ mg}$$

You use the equivalent 10 mg = 1 kg. So the fraction you use is $\frac{10 \text{ mg}}{1 \text{ kg}}$.

$$75 \cancel{\text{kg}} \times \frac{10 \text{ mg}}{1 \cancel{\text{kg}}} = 750 \text{ mg}$$

So the patient should receive 750 milligrams of isoniazid.

Notes/Workspace

When doing conversions of

$\frac{1 \text{ lb}}{2.2 \text{ kg}} = \frac{10}{22}$

makes the math easier

mL per kg is

same logic as miles per gallon

Notes/Workspace

Multistep Conversions

Sometimes drug dosage calculations involve more than one step. For example, suppose you want to find out how many seconds are in 2 hours. You can do this conversion in two steps.

Step 1 Change hours to minutes. Since 60 minutes is 1 hour, the fraction to change hours to minutes is $\frac{60 \text{ min}}{1 \text{ hr}}$.

$$2 \text{ hr} \times \frac{60 \text{ min}}{1 \text{ hr}}$$

Step 2 Change minutes to seconds. Since 60 seconds is 1 minute, the fraction to change minutes to seconds is $\frac{60 \text{ sec}}{1 \text{ min}}$.

$$2 \text{ hr} \times \frac{60 \text{ min}}{1 \text{ hr}} \times \frac{60 \text{ sec}}{1 \text{ min}}$$

Cancel hours and minutes.

$$2 \cancel{\text{hr}} \times \frac{60 \cancel{\text{min}}}{1 \cancel{\text{hr}}} \times \frac{60 \text{ sec}}{1 \cancel{\text{min}}} = \frac{2 \times 60 \times 60}{1} \text{ sec} = 7200 \text{ sec}$$

This is the general method you will use in the following examples. When you do this kind of calculation, you must make sure that each equivalent fraction you use is equal to 1 and that it gives the units needed.

Example 7.8

The order is 600 milligrams of acetylsalicylic acid (aspirin); grains 5 caplets are available. How many caplets of this antipyretic should be given to the patient?

In this problem you need to convert 600 milligrams to grains and then convert grains to caplets.

$$600 \text{ mg} \rightarrow \text{gr ?} \rightarrow \text{? cap}$$

This is done in two steps as follows.

Step 1 Change milligrams to grains.

$$600 \text{ mg} \times \frac{\text{gr ?}}{\text{? mg}}$$

Step 2 Change grains to caplets.

$$600 \text{ mg} \times \frac{\text{gr ?}}{\text{? mg}} \times \frac{\text{? cap}}{\text{gr ?}} = \text{? cap}$$

Since gr 1 = 60 mg, the first fraction is $\frac{\text{gr } 1}{60 \text{ mg}}$. Since 1 cap = gr 5, the second fraction is $\frac{1 \text{ cap}}{\text{gr } 5}$.

$$\overset{10}{\cancel{600}\,\cancel{\text{mg}}} \times \frac{\cancel{\text{gr}}\ 1}{\underset{1}{\cancel{60}\,\cancel{\text{mg}}}} \times \frac{1\ \text{cap}}{\cancel{\text{gr}}\ 5} = 2\ \text{cap}$$

So 600 milligrams is equivalent to 2 caplets, and 2 caplets of Aspirin should be given to the patient.

Note

Equivalent values for units of weight are given in Table 6.1. At this point in the text, however, all the equivalent values should be memorized.

Example 7.9

The order is 0.2 milligram per kilogram qid of nifedipine (Procardia) for a patient who weighs 50 kilograms. Read the drug label in Figure 7.4 and determine the number of capsules of this calcium antagonist you would give to the patient.

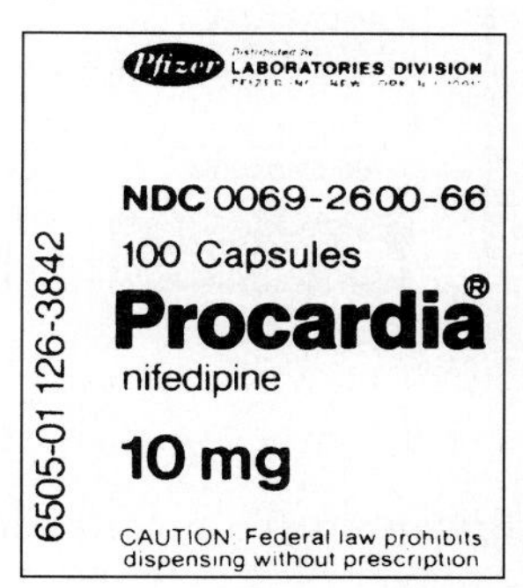

Figure 7.4 *Drug label for Procardia*

In this problem you want to convert 50 kilograms to milligrams and then convert milligrams to capsules.

$$50\ \text{kg} \rightarrow ?\ \text{mg} \rightarrow ?\ \text{cap}$$

This is done in two steps.

Step 1 Change body weight in kilograms to dosage in milligrams.

$$50\ \text{kg} \times \frac{?\ \text{mg}}{?\ \text{kg}}$$

Step 2 Change milligrams to capsules.

$$50\ \text{kg} \times \frac{?\ \text{mg}}{?\ \text{kg}} \times \frac{?\ \text{cap}}{?\ \text{mg}} = ?\ \text{cap}$$

Notes/Workspace

Notes/Workspace

Since the patient is to receive 0.2 milligram of nifedipine per kilogram of body weight, the first equivalent fraction is $\frac{0.2 \text{ mg}}{1 \text{ kg}}$. Since the label indicates that 1 cap = 10 mg, the second equivalent fraction is $\frac{1 \text{ cap}}{10 \text{ mg}}$.

$$\overset{5}{\cancel{50}} \cancel{\text{kg}} \times \frac{0.2 \cancel{\text{mg}}}{1 \cancel{\text{kg}}} \times \frac{1 \text{ cap}}{\underset{1}{\cancel{10}} \cancel{\text{mg}}} = 1 \text{ cap}$$

So the patient should receive 1 capsule of nifedipine.

Example 7.10

The order is 0.5 gram of the antibiotic, amoxicillin (Amoxil). Read the label shown in Figure 7.5 and calculate how many capsules should be given.

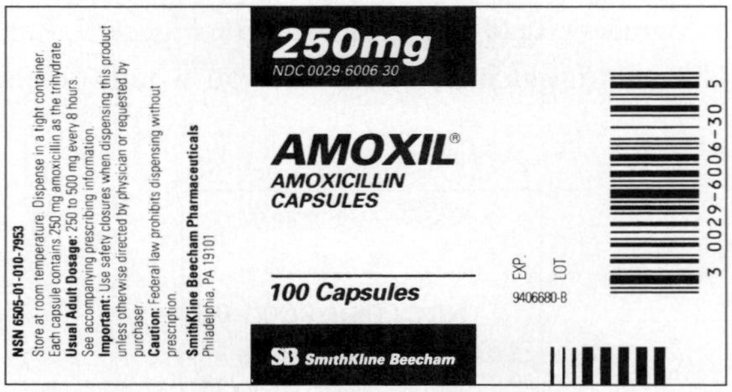

Figure 7.5 *Drug label for Amoxil*

In this problem you want to convert 0.5 gram to milligrams and then convert milligrams to capsules.

$$0.5 \text{ g} \rightarrow ? \text{ mg} \rightarrow ? \text{ cap}$$

Do the two steps on one line as follows:

$$0.5 \text{ g} \times \frac{? \text{ mg}}{? \text{ g}} \times \frac{? \text{ cap}}{? \text{ mg}} = ? \text{ cap}$$

Since 1000 mg = 1 g, the first equivalent fraction is $\frac{1000 \text{ mg}}{1 \text{ g}}$. Since 250 mg = 1 cap, the second equivalent fraction is $\frac{1 \text{ cap}}{250 \text{ mg}}$.

$$0.5 \cancel{\text{g}} \times \frac{1000 \cancel{\text{mg}}}{1 \cancel{\text{g}}} \times \frac{1 \text{ cap}}{250 \cancel{\text{mg}}} = \frac{500}{250} \text{ cap} = 2 \text{ cap}$$

So 0.5 gram is equivalent to 2 capsules, and 2 capsules of amoxicillin should be given to the patient.

Sometimes prescribed oral medications are in liquid form. The calculations for these drugs follow the same format you have been using. The label will always state how much drug is contained in a certain amount of liquid.

Example 7.11

The prescriber orders 0.5 gram of the antibiotic amoxillicin/clavulanate potassium (Augmentin). Study the label shown in Figure 7.6 and calculate how many milliliters you will administer.

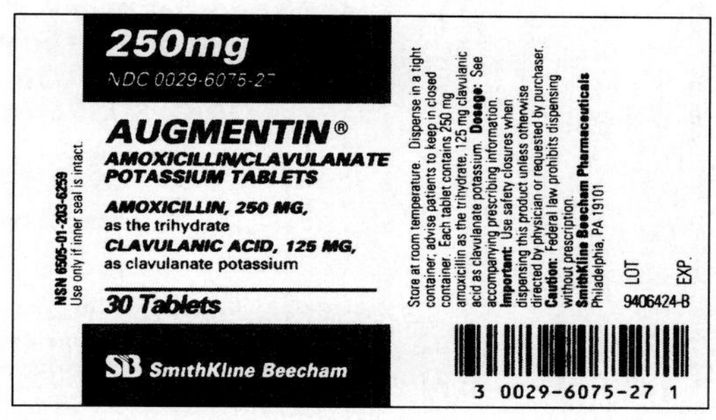

250mg
NDC 0029-6075-27
AUGMENTIN®
AMOXICILLIN/CLAVULANATE POTASSIUM TABLETS
AMOXICILLIN, 250 MG,
as the trihydrate
CLAVULANIC ACID, 125 MG,
as clavulanate potassium
30 Tablets
SB SmithKline Beecham
NSN 6505-01-203-6259
Use only if inner seal is intact.
Store at room temperature. Dispense in a tight container; advise patients to keep in closed container. Each tablet contains 250 mg amoxicillin as the trihydrate, 125 mg clavulanic acid as clavulanate potassium. Dosage: See accompanying prescribing information.
Important: Use safety closures when dispensing this product unless otherwise directed by physician or requested by purchaser.
Caution: Federal law prohibits dispensing without prescription.
SmithKline Beecham Pharmaceuticals
Philadelphia, PA 19101
LOT
9406424-B
EXP.
3 0029-6075-27 1

Figure 7.6 *Drug label for Augmentin*

In this problem you want to convert 0.5 gram to milligrams and then convert milligrams to tablets.

$$0.5 \text{ g} \rightarrow \text{? mg} \rightarrow \text{? tab}$$

You do the two steps on one line as follows:

$$0.5 \text{ g} \times \frac{\text{? mg}}{\text{? g}} \times \frac{1 \text{ tab}}{\text{? mg}} = \text{? tab}$$

Since 1000 mg = 1 g, the first equivalent fraction is $\frac{1000 \text{ mg}}{1 \text{ g}}$. The label on the bottle indicates that each tablet contains 250 milligrams of Augmentin. So the second equivalent fraction is $\frac{1 \text{ tab}}{250 \text{ mg}}$.

$$0.5 \cancel{\text{g}} \times \frac{\overset{4}{\cancel{1000 \text{ mg}}}}{1 \cancel{\text{g}}} \times \frac{1 \text{ tab}}{\underset{1}{\cancel{250 \text{ mg}}}} = 2 \text{ tab}$$

So you would administer 2 tablets of Augmentin.

Notes/Workspace

Notes/Workspace

Example 7.12

The patient is to receive 0.375 gram of the antibiotic cefaclor (Ceclor). Read the information on the drug label in Figure 7.7 and determine how many milliliters you would administer.

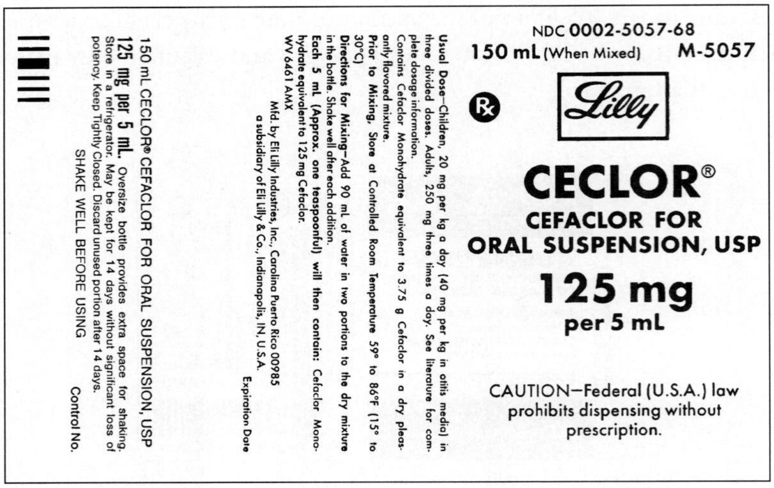

Figure 7.7 *Drug label for Ceclor*

The label on the bottle reads 125 milligrams per 5 milliliters. This means that each 5 milliliters of liquid contains 125 milligrams of cefaclor. In this problem you want to convert 0.375 gram to milligrams and then get its equivalent in milliliters.

$$0.375 \text{ g} \rightarrow ? \text{ mg} \rightarrow ? \text{ mL}$$

Do this on one line as follows:

$$0.375 \text{ g} \times \frac{? \text{ mg}}{? \text{ g}} \times \frac{? \text{ mL}}{? \text{ mg}} = ? \text{ mL}$$

Since 1000 mg = 1 g, the first equivalent fraction is $\frac{1000 \text{ mg}}{1 \text{ g}}$. Since 5 mL = 125 mg, the second equivalent fraction is $\frac{5 \text{ mL}}{125 \text{ mg}}$.

$$0.375 \cancel{\text{g}} \times \frac{\overset{8}{\cancel{1000 \text{ mg}}}}{1 \cancel{\text{g}}} \times \frac{5 \text{ mL}}{\underset{1}{\cancel{125 \text{ mg}}}} = 15 \text{ mL}$$

So you would administer 15 milliliters of cefaclor.

Example 7.13

The prescriber orders 0.00025 gram po of digoxin (Lanoxin), an anti-arrhythmic drug. Study the information on the label shown in Figure 7.8 and calculate the number of tablets of this drug you would administer.

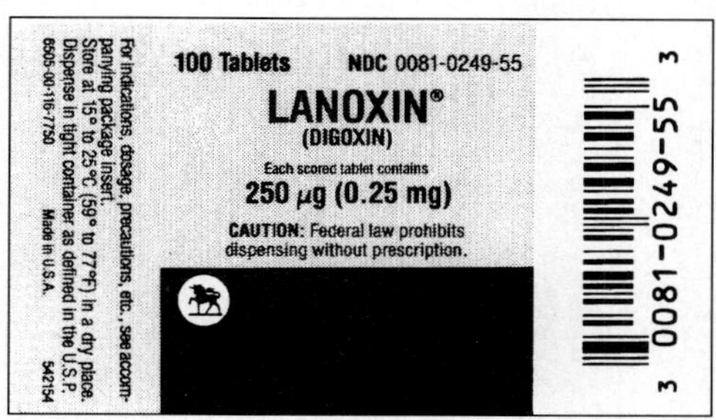
100 Tablets
NDC 0081-0249-55
LANOXIN®
(DIGOXIN)
Each scored tablet contains
250 μg (0.25 mg)
CAUTION: Federal law prohibits dispensing without prescription.
For indications, dosage, precautions, etc., see accompanying package insert.
Store at 15° to 25°C (59° to 77°F) in a dry place.
Dispense in tight container as defined in the U.S.P.
6505-00-116-7750
Made in U.S.A.
542154
3 0081-0249-55 3

Figure 7.8 *Drug label for Lanoxin*

The label on the bottle reads 0.25 milligrams per tablet. In this problem you want to convert 0.00025 gram to milligrams and then get its equivalent in tablets.

$$0.00025 \text{ g} \rightarrow \text{? mg} \rightarrow \text{? tab}$$

Do this on one line as follows:

$$0.00025 \text{ g} \times \frac{\text{? mg}}{\text{? g}} \times \frac{\text{? tab}}{\text{? mg}} = \text{? tab}$$

Since 1000 mg = 1 g, the first equivalent fraction is $\frac{1000 \text{ mg}}{1 \text{ g}}$. Since 1 tab = 0.25 mg, the second equivalent fraction is $\frac{1 \text{ tab}}{0.25 \text{ mg}}$.

$$0.00025 \cancel{\text{g}} \times \frac{1000 \cancel{\text{mg}}}{1 \cancel{\text{g}}} \times \frac{1 \text{ tab}}{0.25 \cancel{\text{mg}}} = 1 \text{ tab}$$

So you would administer 1 tablet of Lanoxin.

Note

In Example 7.14, the unit value is milliequivalents. Electrolytes are usually measured in milliequivalents, which is abbreviated mEq.

Notes/Workspace

Notes/Workspace

Example 7.14

The order for Mr. Jones is 15 milliequivalents of potassium chloride (K-Lor, Kay Ciel). The label on the bottle reads 10 milliequivalents in 5 cubic centimeters. How many drams of this electrolyte would you administer?

In this problem you want to change 15 milliequivalents to drams. You must first convert 15 milliequivalents to cubic centimeters and then convert cubic centimeters to drams.

$$15\text{ mEq} \rightarrow ?\text{ cc} \rightarrow ʒ\ ?$$

Do this on one line as follows:

$$15\text{ mEq} \times \frac{?\text{ cc}}{?\text{ mEq}} \times \frac{ʒ\ ?}{?\text{ cc}} = ʒ\ ?$$

The label on the bottle indicates that every 5 cubic centimeters of liquid contains 10 milliequivalents of potassium chloride. So the first fraction is $\frac{5\text{ cc}}{10\text{ mEq}}$. Since ʒ 1 = 5 cc, the second fraction is $\frac{ʒ\ 1}{5\text{ cc}}$.

$$15\ \cancel{\text{mEq}} \times \frac{\cancel{5\text{ cc}}}{10\ \cancel{\text{mEq}}} \times \frac{ʒ\ 1}{\cancel{5\text{ cc}}} = ʒ\ \frac{15}{10} \text{ or } ʒ\ 1\frac{1}{2}$$

So you would administer drams $1\frac{1}{2}$ of potassium chloride to the patient.

Practice Reading Labels

Calculate the following doses using the labels shown. (You will find the answers to Practice Reading Labels in Appendix A at the back of the book.)

1. Cephalexin 0.75 g = ____3____ cap

Lederle NDC 0005-3413-23

Cephalexin Capsules, USP

250 mg

CAUTION: Federal law prohibits dispensing without prescription. This package not for household dispensing.

100 CAPSULES BC1 18120

Each capsule contains cephalexin monohydrate equivalent to 250 mg cephalexin. Usual Adult Dose: One capsule every 6 hours. For more severe infections, dose may be increased, not to exceed 4 g a day. See accompanying literature.

Store at Controlled Room Temperature 15-30°C (59-86°F). Keep Tightly Closed.

Dispense in tight containers as defined in the USP.

Control No. Exp. Date 7-7-98

Manufactured for LEDERLE LABORATORIES DIVISION American Cyanamid Company Pearl River, NY 10965 by BIOCRAFT LABORATORIES, INC., Elmwood Park, NJ 07407

Notes/Workspace

2. Moderil 0.0005 g = ______ tab

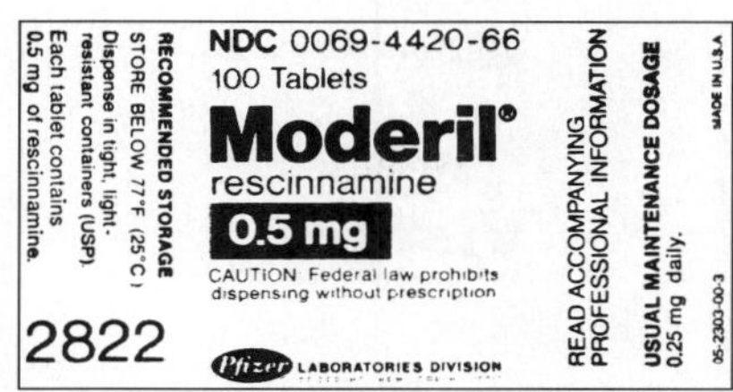

3. Feldene 0.02 g = ______ cap

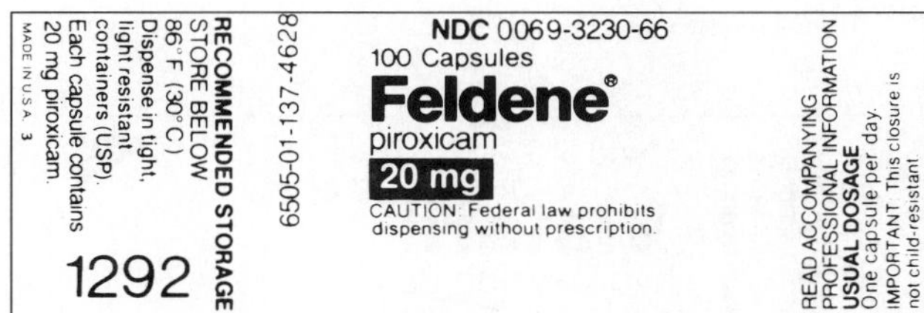

4. Vibramycin 200 mg = ______ cap

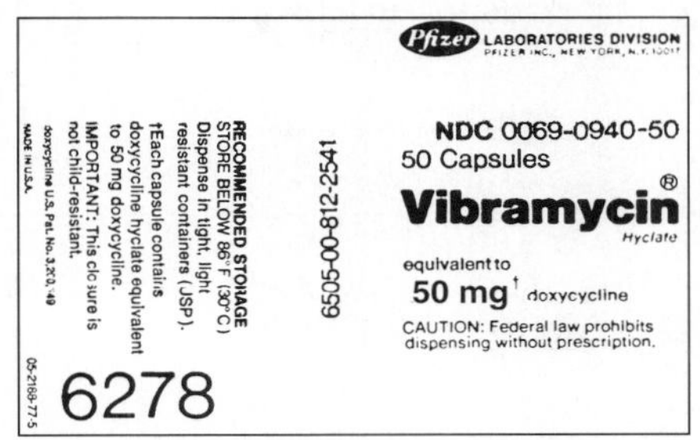

5. Procardia 0.02 g = ______ cap

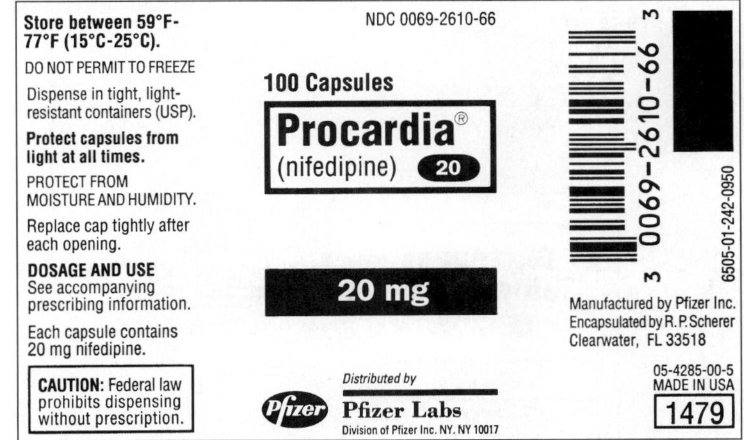

Notes/Workspace

6. Vistaril 100 mg = ___4___ cap

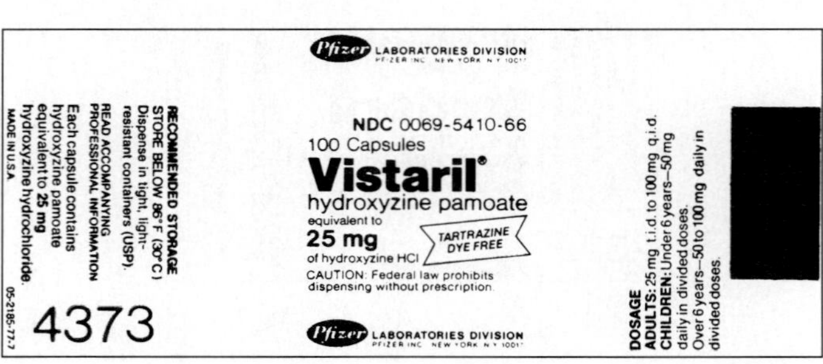

7. Vistaril 50 mg = ___10___ mL

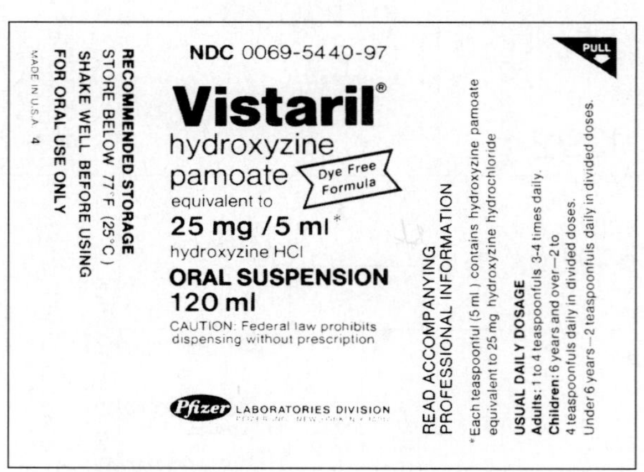

8. Platinol 25 mg = ___25___ mL

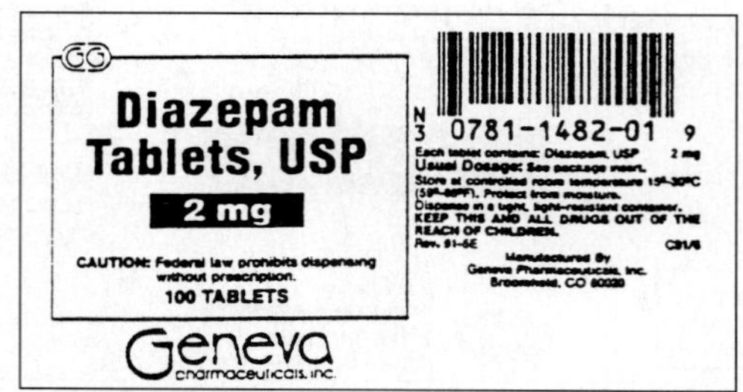

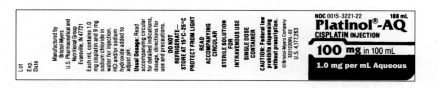

9. Diazepam gr $\frac{1}{15}$ = ___2___ tab

Diazepam Tablets, USP
2 mg
CAUTION: Federal law prohibits dispensing without prescription.
100 TABLETS
Geneva pharmaceuticals, inc.
N 3 0781-1482-01 9

Notes/Workspace

10. Minipress 5000 mcg = ________ cap

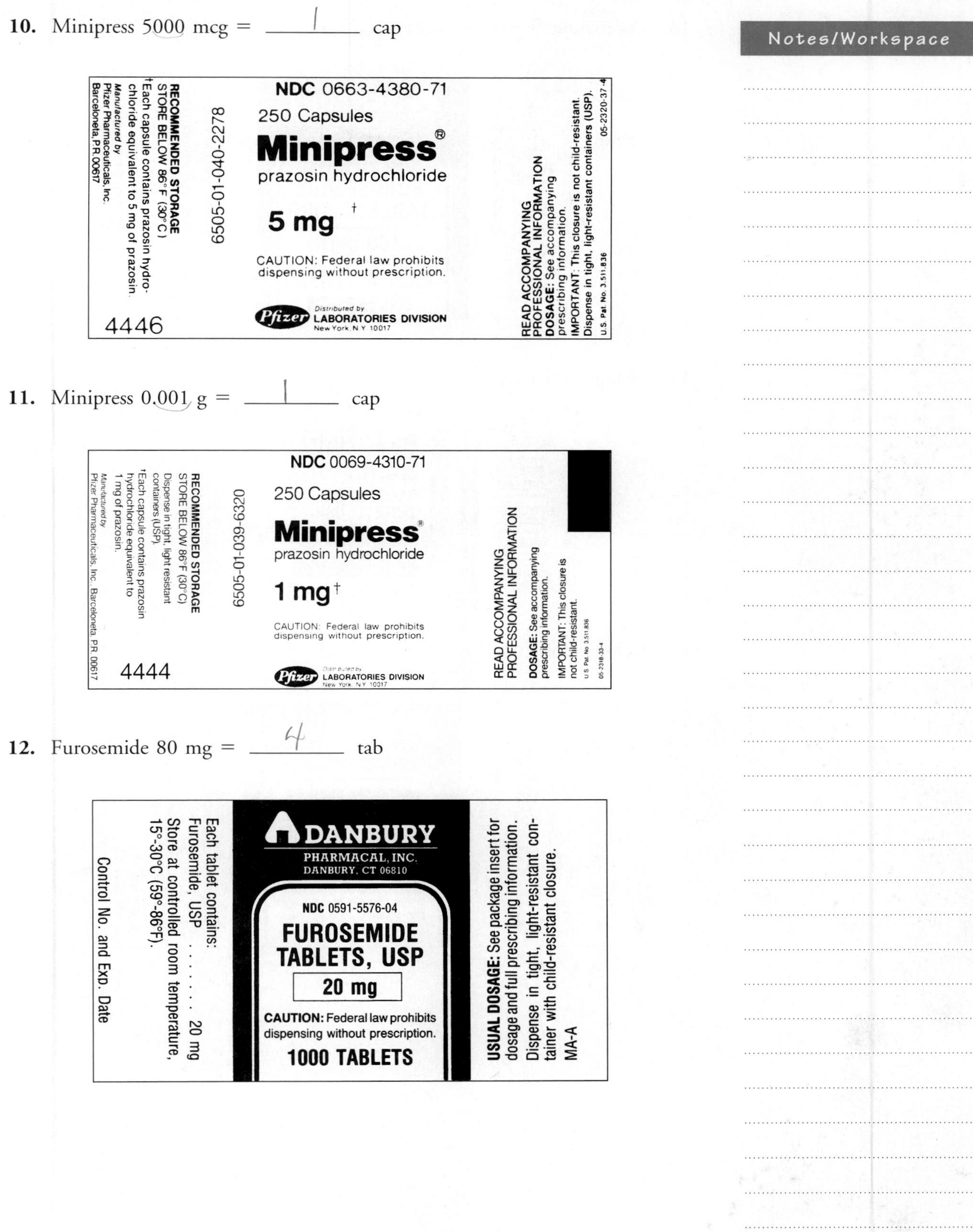
NDC 0663-4380-71
250 Capsules
Minipress®
prazosin hydrochloride
5 mg†
CAUTION: Federal law prohibits dispensing without prescription.
Pfizer Distributed by LABORATORIES DIVISION New York, N.Y. 10017
6505-01-040-2278
RECOMMENDED STORAGE
STORE BELOW 86°F (30°C)
†Each capsule contains prazosin hydrochloride equivalent to 5 mg of prazosin.
Manufactured by Pfizer Pharmaceuticals, Inc. Barceloneta, P.R. 00617
4446
READ ACCOMPANYING PROFESSIONAL INFORMATION
DOSAGE: See accompanying prescribing information.
IMPORTANT: This closure is not child-resistant.
Dispense in tight, light-resistant containers (USP).
U.S. Pat. No. 3,511,836
05-2320-37-4
NDC 0069-4310-71
250 Capsules
Minipress®
prazosin hydrochloride
1 mg†
CAUTION: Federal law prohibits dispensing without prescription.
Pfizer Distributed by LABORATORIES DIVISION New York, N.Y. 10017
6505-01-039-6320
RECOMMENDED STORAGE
STORE BELOW 86°F (30°C)
Dispense in tight, light resistant containers (USP).
†Each capsule contains prazosin hydrochloride equivalent to 1 mg of prazosin.
Manufactured by Pfizer Pharmaceuticals, Inc. Barceloneta, P.R. 00617
4444
READ ACCOMPANYING PROFESSIONAL INFORMATION
DOSAGE: See accompanying prescribing information.
IMPORTANT: This closure is not child-resistant.
U.S. Pat. No. 3,511,836
05-2318-33-4
DANBURY PHARMACAL, INC.
DANBURY, CT 06810
NDC 0591-5576-04
FUROSEMIDE TABLETS, USP
20 mg
CAUTION: Federal law prohibits dispensing without prescription.
1000 TABLETS
Each tablet contains:
Furosemide, USP .... 20 mg
Store at controlled room temperature, 15°-30°C (59°-86°F).
Control No. and Exp. Date
USUAL DOSAGE: See package insert for dosage and full prescribing information.
Dispense in tight, light-resistant container with child-resistant closure.
MA-A

11. Minipress 0.001 g = ________ cap

12. Furosemide 80 mg = ________ tab

Notes/Workspace

13. Furosemide 0.16 g = __2__ tab

DANBURY
PHARMACAL INC
DANBURY CT 06810
NDC 0591-5659-01
FUROSEMIDE TABLETS, USP
80 mg
CAUTION: Federal law prohibits dispensing without prescription.
100 TABLETS
Each tablet contains: Furosemide, USP .... 80 mg
Store at controlled room temperature, 15°-30°C (59°-86°F).
Control No. and Exp. Date
USUAL DOSAGE: See package insert for dosage and full prescribing information.
Dispense in tight, light-resistant container with child-resistant closure.

14. Haloperidol 1 mg = __2__ tab

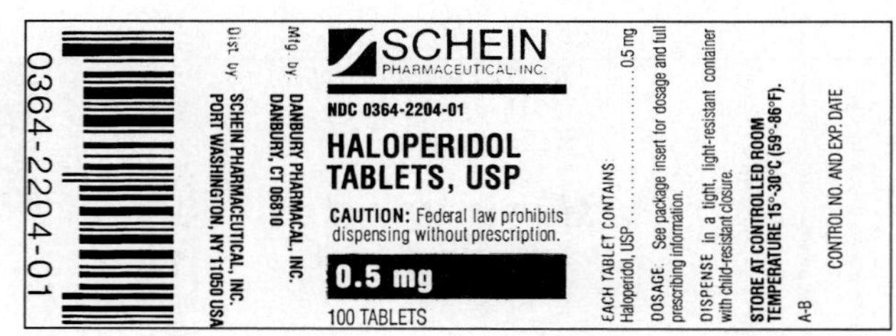

SCHEIN
PHARMACEUTICAL, INC.
NDC 0364-2204-01
HALOPERIDOL TABLETS, USP
CAUTION: Federal law prohibits dispensing without prescription.
0.5 mg
100 TABLETS
Mfg. by: DANBURY PHARMACAL, INC. DANBURY, CT 06810
Dist. by: SCHEIN PHARMACEUTICAL, INC. PORT WASHINGTON, NY 11050 USA
0364-2204-01
EACH TABLET CONTAINS Haloperidol, USP .... 0.5 mg
DOSAGE: See package insert for dosage and full prescribing information.
DISPENSE in a tight, light-resistant container with child-resistant closure.
STORE AT CONTROLLED ROOM TEMPERATURE 15°-30°C (59°-86°F).
A-B
CONTROL NO. AND EXP. DATE

15. Haloperidol 0.01 g = __1__ tab

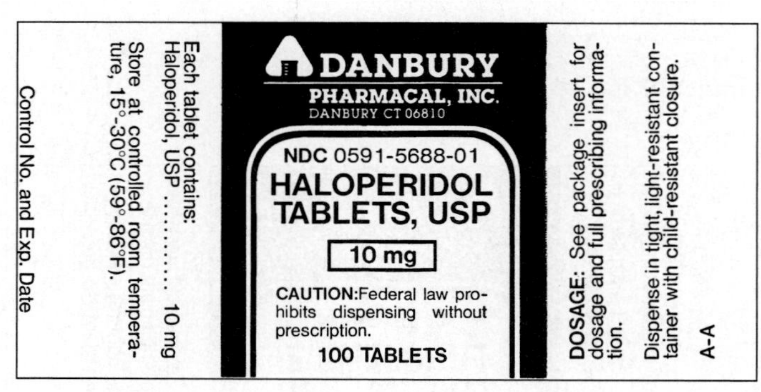

DANBURY
PHARMACAL, INC.
DANBURY CT 06810
NDC 0591-5688-01
HALOPERIDOL TABLETS, USP
10 mg
CAUTION:Federal law prohibits dispensing without prescription.
100 TABLETS
Each tablet contains: Haloperidol, USP .... 10 mg
Store at controlled room temperature, 15°-30°C (59°-86°F).
Control No. and Exp. Date
DOSAGE: See package insert for dosage and full prescribing information.
Dispense in tight, light-resistant container with child-resistant closure.
A-A

16. Vibramycin 0.2 g = ____4____ cap

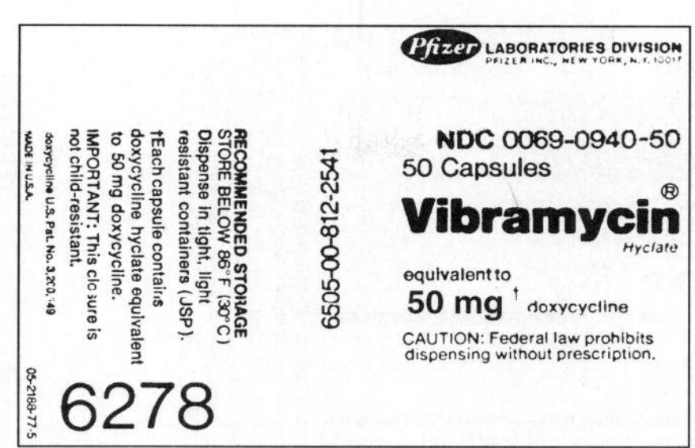

17. Moderil 1 mg = ____2____ tab

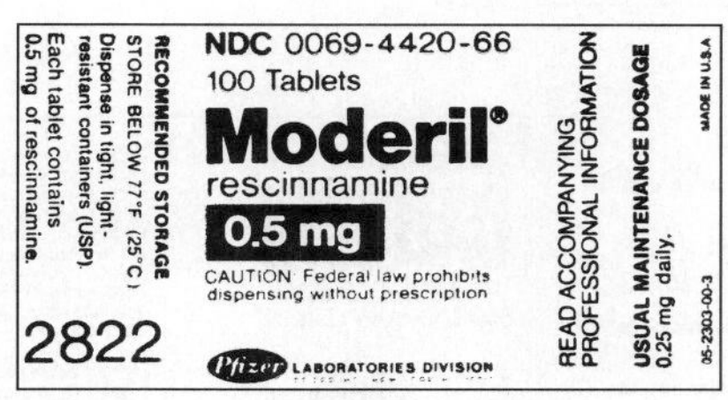

18. Carafate 1000 mg = ____1____ tab

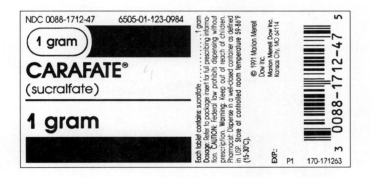

19. Cardizem 60 mg = ____2____ tab

NDC 0088-1771-47 6505-01-145-8825

30mg MARION MERRELL DOW INC.

CARDIZEM®
(diltiazem HCl)
30 mg
100 Tablets

Each tablet contains: diltiazem hydrochloride . . . . 30 mg (equivalent to 27.6 mg as diltiazem). Dosage and Administration: Read package insert for full prescribing information. CAUTION: Federal law prohibits dispensing without prescription. Warning: Keep out of reach of children. Pharmacist: Dispense in tight, light-resistant container as defined in USP. Store at controlled room temperature 59-86°F (15-30°C).

© 1991 Marion Merrell Dow Inc.
Marion Merrell Dow Inc.
Kansas City, MO 64114

EXP.: C1 170-177164

3 0088-1771-47 2

Notes/Workspace

Notes/Workspace

20. Cardizem 0.09 g = ________ tab

NDC 0088-1791-47
6505-01-259-8459
MARION LABORATORIES INC
90 mg
CARDIZEM®
(diltiazem HCl)
90 mg
100 Tablets
CAUTION: Federal law prohibits dispensing without prescription.
Each tablet contains: diltiazem hydrochloride .....90 mg
Dosage and Administration: Read package insert for full prescribing information. Warning: Keep out of reach of children. Pharmacist: Dispense in tight, light-resistant container as defined in USP. Store at controlled room temperature 59-86°F (15-30°C). © 1989 Marion Laboratories, Inc.
Marion Laboratories, Inc.
Kansas City, MO 64137
EXP:
0088-1791-47
P9 3
1170-177161

21. Calcium 1 g = ________ tab

OS-CAL®500
ADEQUATE DAILY CALCIUM CAN HELP KEEP YOUR BONES HEALTHY
EACH TABLET CONTAINS:
1250 mg of calcium carbonate from oyster shell, an organic calcium source.
Elemental calcium .... 500 mg
DIRECTIONS:
One tablet 2 to 3 times a day with meals, or as recommended by your physician.
TWO TABLETS PROVIDE:
1000 mg calcium, 100% of U.S. RDA for adults and children 12 or more years of age.
THREE TABLETS PROVIDE:
1500 mg calcium, 115% of U.S. RDA for pregnant and lactating women.
STORE AT ROOM TEMPERATURE.
KEEP OUT OF REACH OF CHILDREN.
IMPORTANT: Do not use if foil inner seal printed M in white is disturbed or missing.
R7

NDC 0088-1651-41
CALCIUM
HIGH POTENCY
500 MG SUPPLEMENT
OS-CAL® 500
60 TABLETS

INGREDIENTS:
Oyster shell powder, corn syrup solids, talc, hydroxypropyl methylcellulose, cornstarch, sodium starch glycolate, calcium stearate, polysorbate 80, pharmaceutical glaze, titanium dioxide, methyl propyl paraben, polyethylene glycol, polyvinylpyrrolidone, carnauba wax, D&C yellow #10, acetylated monoglyceride, edetate disodium, FD&C blue #1, simethicone emulsion.
PHARMACEUTICAL DIVISION
MARION LABORATORIES, INC.
KANSAS CITY, MISSOURI 64137
Control No.
Exp. Date

22. Terramycin 0.25 g = ________ cap

6720
Pfizer LABORATORIES DIVISION
PFIZER INC., NEW YORK, N.Y. 10017
NDC 0069-0730-73
500 Capsules
Terramycin®
oxytetracycline hydrochloride
250 mg†
CAUTION: Federal law prohibits dispensing without prescription.
RECOMMENDED STORAGE
STORE BELOW 86°F (30°C.)
Dispense in tight, light resistant containers (USP).
†Each capsule contains oxytetracycline hydrochloride equivalent to 250 mg of oxytetracycline with glucosamine hydrochloride.

23. Clonidine hydrochloride 0.2 mg = 2 tab

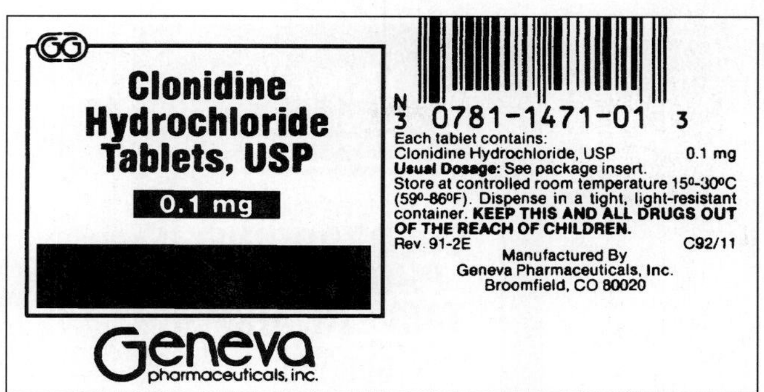
Clonidine Hydrochloride Tablets, USP
0.1 mg
N 3 0781-1471-01 3
Each tablet contains:
Clonidine Hydrochloride, USP 0.1 mg
Usual Dosage: See package insert.
Store at controlled room temperature 15°-30°C (59°-86°F). Dispense in a tight, light-resistant container. KEEP THIS AND ALL DRUGS OUT OF THE REACH OF CHILDREN.
Rev. 91-2E C92/11
Manufactured By
Geneva Pharmaceuticals, Inc.
Broomfield, CO 80020
Geneva
pharmaceuticals, inc.

24. Clonidine hydrochloride 0.4 mg = 2 tab

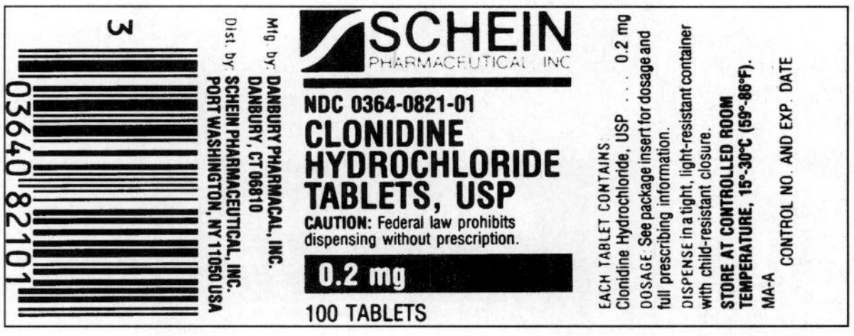
3
03640 82101
Mfg by: DANBURY PHARMACAL, INC.
DANBURY, CT 06810
Dist. by: SCHEIN PHARMACEUTICAL, INC.
PORT WASHINGTON, NY 11050 USA
SCHEIN
PHARMACEUTICAL INC
NDC 0364-0821-01
CLONIDINE HYDROCHLORIDE TABLETS, USP
CAUTION: Federal law prohibits dispensing without prescription.
0.2 mg
100 TABLETS
EACH TABLET CONTAINS
Clonidine Hydrochloride, USP . . . 0.2 mg
DOSAGE See package insert for dosage and full prescribing information.
DISPENSE in a tight, light-resistant container with child-resistant closure.
STORE AT CONTROLLED ROOM TEMPERATURE, 15°-30°C (59°-86°F).
MA-A
CONTROL NO. AND EXP. DATE

25. Chlorpropamide 0.1 g = 1 tab

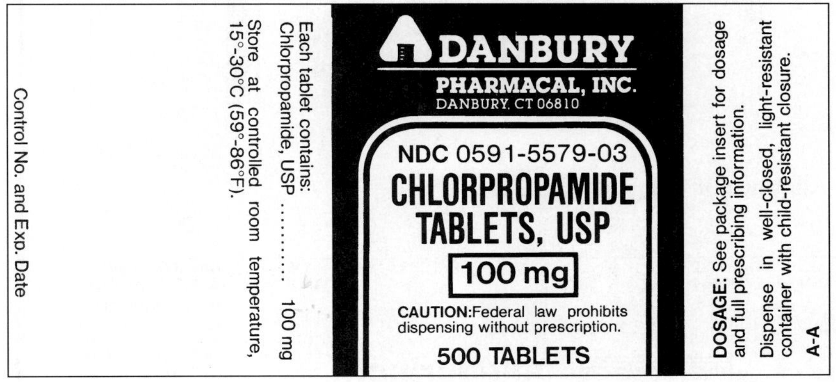
Control No. and Exp. Date
Each tablet contains:
Chlorpropamide, USP .... 100 mg
Store at controlled room temperature, 15°-30°C (59°-86°F).
DANBURY
PHARMACAL, INC.
DANBURY, CT 06810
NDC 0591-5579-03
CHLORPROPAMIDE TABLETS, USP
100 mg
CAUTION: Federal law prohibits dispensing without prescription.
500 TABLETS
DOSAGE: See package insert for dosage and full prescribing information.
Dispense in well-closed, light-resistant container with child-resistant closure.
A-A

Notes/Workspace

Notes/Workspace

26. Chloroquine phosphate 1 g = ___2___ tab

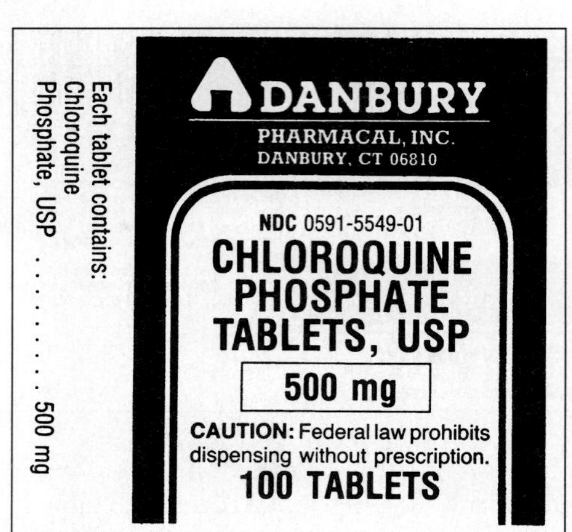
DANBURY
PHARMACAL, INC.
DANBURY, CT 06810
NDC 0591-5549-01
CHLOROQUINE PHOSPHATE TABLETS, USP
500 mg
CAUTION: Federal law prohibits dispensing without prescription.
100 TABLETS
Each tablet contains: Chloroquine Phosphate, USP .... 500 mg

27. Bethanechol chloride 0.025 g = ___1___ tab

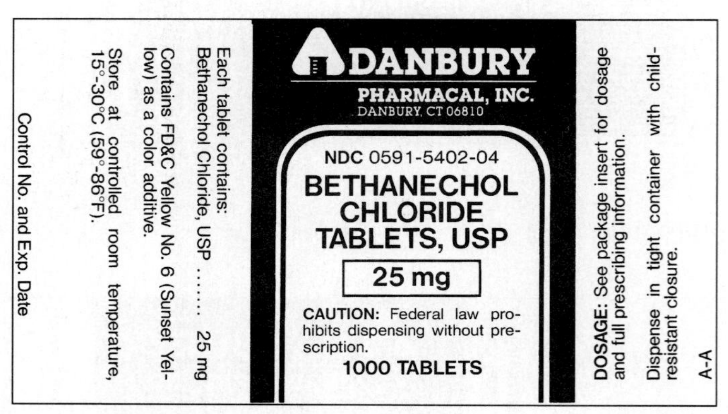
DANBURY
PHARMACAL, INC.
DANBURY, CT 06810
NDC 0591-5402-04
BETHANECHOL CHLORIDE TABLETS, USP
25 mg
CAUTION: Federal law prohibits dispensing without prescription.
1000 TABLETS
Each tablet contains: Bethanechol Chloride, USP ...... 25 mg
Contains FD&C Yellow No. 6 (Sunset Yellow) as a color additive.
Store at controlled room temperature, 15°-30°C (59°-86°F).
Control No. and Exp. Date
DOSAGE: See package insert for dosage and full prescribing information.
Dispense in tight container with child-resistant closure.
A-A

28. Allopurinol 0.3 g = ___1___ tab

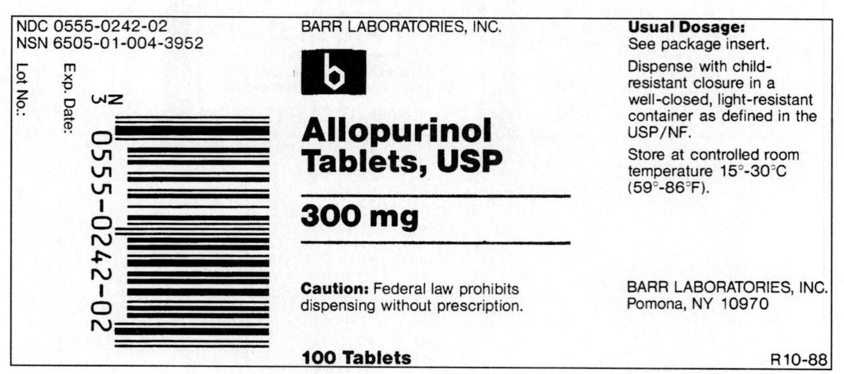
NDC 0555-0242-02
NSN 6505-01-004-3952
Lot No.:
Exp. Date:
N 3 0555-0242-02
BARR LABORATORIES, INC.
b
Allopurinol Tablets, USP
300 mg
Caution: Federal law prohibits dispensing without prescription.
100 Tablets
Usual Dosage:
See package insert.
Dispense with child-resistant closure in a well-closed, light-resistant container as defined in the USP/NF.
Store at controlled room temperature 15°-30°C (59°-86°F).
BARR LABORATORIES, INC.
Pomona, NY 10970
R10-88

29. Acetazolamide 0.5 g = __________ tab

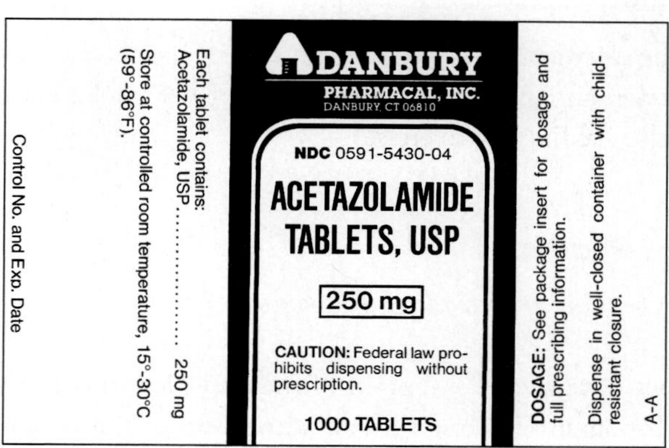

DANBURY
PHARMACAL, INC.
DANBURY, CT 06810
NDC 0591-5430-04
ACETAZOLAMIDE TABLETS, USP
250 mg
CAUTION: Federal law prohibits dispensing without prescription.
1000 TABLETS
Each tablet contains:
Acetazolamide, USP.............. 250 mg
Store at controlled room temperature, 15°-30°C (59°-86°F).
Control No. and Exp. Date
DOSAGE: See package insert for dosage and full prescribing information.
Dispense in well-closed container with child-resistant closure.
A-A

30. Platinol 0.010 g = __________ mL

NDC 0015-3070-20 6505-01-074-7590

Platinol®

CISPLATIN FOR INJECTION

10 mg

Lot
Exp. Date

U.S. Patent No. 4,177,263
Manufactured by Bristol-Myers
U.S. Pharmaceutical and Nutritional Group
Evansville, IN 47721

When reconstituted with 10 mL Sterile Water for Injection, USP, each mL will contain 1 mg of cisplatin, 10 mg mannitol and 9 mg of sodium chloride. HCl added to adjust pH.
DO NOT REFRIGERATE RECONSTITUTED SOLUTION—USE WITHIN 20 HOURS OF RECONSTITUTION.
Usual Dosage: Read accompanying circular for detailed indications, dosage, directions for use, and precautions.
PRIOR TO RECONSTITUTION PROTECT FROM LIGHT.
READ ACCOMPANYING CIRCULAR

BRISTOL LABORATORIES
ONCOLOGY PRODUCTS
A Bristol-Myers Company
Evansville, Indiana 47721

307020DRL-09

Notes/Workspace

Notes/Workspace

Practice Sets

You will find the answers to Try These for Practice, Exercises, and Cumulative Review Practice Sets in Appendix A at the back of the book. Your instructor has the answers to the Additional Exercises.

Try These for Practice

Test your comprehension after reading the chapter.

1. The prescriber has ordered 0.2 gram of the anti-ulcer medication misoprostol (Cytotec). How many tablets will you administer to the patient if each tablet contains 200 micrograms? ________

2. The patient is to receive grain $\frac{1}{120}$ of the antigout medication colchicine (ColBENEMID). Each tablet contains 0.5 milligram. How many tablets will you administer? ________

3. The order reads:

   zalpidine 10 mg po q12h

   Tablets are grain $\frac{1}{6}$ each. How many tablets will you administer to the patient?

   ____

4. The prescriber has ordered 0.04 gram of the anti-ulcer drug famotidine (Pepcid). Each 5 mL = 40 mg. How many milliliters must you administer?

   ____

5. The antivertigo drug meclizine HCl (Antivert) has been prescribed for a patient. The dose ordered is 0.65 milligram per kilogram, and the patient weighs 38 kilograms. Read the label in Figure 7.9 and calculate the number of tablets you will administer to the patient. ________

Distributed by
ROERIG (Pfizer)
A division of Pfizer Inc. N.Y., N.Y. 10017
NDC 0662-2100-66
100 Tablets
Antivert®
meclizine HCl
12.5 mg
CAUTION: Federal law prohibits dispensing without prescription.

Figure 7.9 *Drug label for Antivert*

Exercises

Reinforce your understanding in class or at home.

Notes/Workspace

1. Amantadine hydrochloride (Symmetrel) is an antiviral drug, and 0.2 gram has been ordered for a patient. Each capsule contains 100 milligrams. How many capsules will you administer to the patient? ________

2. If a patient is unable to swallow Symmetrel capsules, the patient must receive the oral suspension labeled 50 milligrams per 5 milliliters. How many milliliters equals 200 milligrams? ________

3. The order reads 0.15 gram of disopyramide phosphate (Norpace). If each tablet contains 150 milligrams, how many tablets of this anti-arrhythmic drug equals the prescribed dose? ________

4. The patient has been prescribed 0.3 gram po of the uricosuric drug allopurinol (Zyloprim), an antigout medication. Each scored tablet contains 300 milligrams. How many tablets will you administer? ________

5. The order reads:

   phenytoin 0.1 g po bid

   If each capsule of this anti-arrhythmic drug contains 100 milligrams, how many capsules will yield the prescribed dose? ________

6. Ten milligrams po of the antihypertensive drug amlodipine (Norvasc) is ordered for your patient. If each tablet contains 0.005 gram, how many tablets will you give your patient? ________

7. The order in Problem 6 has been reduced to 5 milligrams po. How many tablets equal this dose? ________

8. Read the first order on the medication administration record in Figure 7.10. How many capsules will you administer to the patient if the label reads 250 milligrams per capsule? ________

Notes/Workspace

⊕ GENERAL HOSPITAL ⊕

Year 19 *94* Month *December* Day		*17*	*18*				
Medication Dosage and Interval		Initials* and Hours	Initials and Hours	Initials and Hours	Initials and Hours	Initials and Hours	Initials and Hours
Date started: *12/17/94* *ciprofloxacin 0.75 g po qd*	I	*LA*					
	AM	*10*					
	I						
Discontinued:	PM						
Date started: *12/18/94* *Norvane 0.002 g po hs*	I	/					
	AM	/					
	I	/	*JO*				
Discontinued:	PM	/	*10*				

Allergies: (Specify)
penicillin, codeine

Init*	Signature
LA	*Leon Ablon*
JO	*June Olsen*

MEDICATION ADMINISTRATION RECORD

PATIENT IDENTIFICATION

226310 12/17/94

Susan Jackson 1/30/63
80 Martin Ave. Epis
Little Rock, AR HIP
76412

Dr. Anthony Giangrasso

Figure 7.10 *Medication administration record*

9. Read the second order from the MAR in Figure 7.10. How many tablets will you administer if each tablet contains 2 milligrams of this antipsychotic drug? ________

10. Your patient is to receive 0.25 milligram of the cardiac glycoside digoxin (Lanoxin) po. Each scored tablet contains 0.5 milligram. How many tablets will you administer to the patient? ________

11. The order reads: metoclopramide 0.01 g q4h prn. Each tablet contains 10 milligrams. How many tablets equals 0.01 gram? ________

12. A patient with tuberculosis has an order for the antitubercular drug ethambutol hydrochloride (Myambutol). Each tablet contains 400 milligrams. If the order is 1.6 grams po, how many tablets will you administer to the patient?

____

Notes/Workspace

13. The prescriber has ordered 20 milligrams of piroxicam (Feldene), and each capsule contains 0.01 gram. How many capsules of this nonsteroidal anti-inflammatory drug (NSAID) will you give the patient? ________

14. If the order in Problem 13 was changed to 0.375 gram po of the NSAID naproxen (Naprosyn) and each scored tablet contained 250 milligrams, how many tablets would you administer to the patient? ________

15. The order reads: clonazepam 0.03 mg/kg po qd. The patient weighs 67 kilograms. Each tablet contains 0.5 milligram. How many tablets of this anticonvulsant drug will equal the prescribed dose? ________

16. The prescriber has ordered 0.01 gram tid sublingual (under the tongue) of the anti-anginal medication erythrityl tetranitrate (Cardilate) for a patient. If each tablet contains 5 milligrams, how many tablets equal this dosage?

____

17. If a patient has an order for 100 milligrams po q6h of the antibiotic doxycycline (Vibramycin) and the oral suspension is labeled 25 milligrams per 5 milliliters, how many milliliters would equal the prescribed dosage?

____

18. The patient has been prescribed 0.45 mg of clonidine hydrochloride (Catapres), an antihypertensive drug. The drug is available in 0.3 mg scored tablets. How many tablets equals the prescribed dose? ________

19. A patient has been prescribed 0.001 gram of the estrogen estradiol (Estrace). If the tablets are labeled 1 milligram each, how many tablets equal this dose?

____

20. The order reads: azithromycin 7.2 mg/kg po qd. Each capsule contains 250 milligrams. How many capsules will you prepare of this antiviral drug for a patient weighing 154 pounds? ________

Notes/Workspace

Additional Exercises

Now, on your own, test yourself! Ask your instructor to check your answers.

1. The order is 2.5 milligrams per kilogram of a drug for a patient weighing 60 kilograms. Each capsule contains 50 milligrams. How many capsules would you administer to the patient? ________

2. Calculate the number of tablets a patient would be given if the order is 0.5 milligram and each tablet contains grain $\frac{1}{120}$. ________

3. The order reads:

   methyldopa 0.25 g po tid

   How many tablets of this antihypertensive drug will you administer each day if each tablet is labeled 125 milligrams? ________

4. A patient has been prescribed 0.01 gram bid of a central nervous system (CNS) stimulant, methylphenidate hydrochloride (Ritalin). If each tablet contains 10 milligrams, how many tablets equal 0.01 gram? ________

5. Aminophylline (Phyllocontin) is frequently ordered for patients with chronic obstructive disease—specifically, bronchial asthma. The usual dosage is 600 milligrams po qid. Your patient's order is 0.6 gram po qid. Is this an appropriate dosage for this patient? ________

6. The prescriber has ordered 0.5 gram po q8h of the antibiotic doxycycline hyclate (Vibramycin) for the treatment of Lyme disease. Is this an appropriate dosage for a patient weighing 74 kilograms when the usual dosage is 4.4 milligrams per kilogram? ________

7. The prescriber ordered:

   elixir of digoxin 250 mcg po qd

   The label reads 0.05 milligram per milliliter. How many milliliters would you administer to the patient? ________

Notes/Workspace

8. A patient has been prescribed 0.4 milligram sl (sublingual) of nitroglycerin (Nitrostat). Each tablet contains grain $\frac{1}{150}$. How many tablets will you administer to this patient of this anti-anginal drug? _________

9. The order reads:

   ascorbic acid 0.5 g po qd

   If each tablet contains 250 milligrams, how many tablets will you administer? _________

10. An order has been placed for 4 milligrams per kilogram of theophylline (Theo-Dur). Each capsule is labeled 300 milligrams. How many capsules of this bronchodilating drug will you prepare for a patient weighing 75 kilograms? _________

11. Your patient must receive 1.4 milligrams per kilogram of the antihypertensive drug metoprolol tartrate (Lopressor). The drug is available in the form of 50 mg tablets. If your patient weighs 72 kilograms, how many tablets will you administer? _________

12. Read the first order on the MAR in Figure 7.11 on page 138. How many milliliters will you prepare of the anticonvulsant drug if the label reads 100 milligrams per 4 milliliters? _________

13. The second order on the MAR in Figure 7.11 reads:

   amoxicillin 0.25 g po q6h

   The amoxicillin label reads 50 milligrams per milliliter. How many milliliters of this antibiotic will you prepare for Mr. Thompson? _________

14. Read the third order on the MAR in Figure 7.11. If the drug carteolol hydrochloride (Cartrol) is available in 2.5 mg scored tablets, how many tablets will you administer? _________

Notes/Workspace

⊕ GENERAL HOSPITAL ⊕

Year 19 94	Month June	Day	3	4	5	6	7	8
Medication Dosage and Interval			Initials* and Hours	Initials and Hours	Initials and Hours	Initials and Hours	Initials and Hours	Initials and Hours
Date started: 6/3/94 Dilantin 0.2 g po tid		I	AG	LA	LA			
		AM	10	10	10			
		I	AG AG	LA LA	LA LA			
Discontinued:		PM	2 – 6	2 – 6	2 – 6			
Date started: 6/3/94 amoxicillin 0.25 g po q6h		I	AG	LA LA	LA LA			
		AM	6	12 – 6	12 – 6			
Discontinued: 6/5/94 6:30 P.M.		I	AG AG	LR	LR			
		PM	12 – 6	12 – 6	12 – 6			
Date started: 6/3/94 carteolol HCl 0.01 g po daily		I	AG	LA	LA			
		AM	10	10	10			
		I						
Discontinued: 6/5/94		PM						

Allergies: (Specify)
none

Init*	Signature
AG	Anthony Giangrasso
LA	Leon Ablon
LR	Laura Reese

MEDICATION ADMINISTRATION RECORD

PATIENT IDENTIFICATION

705432 6/3/94
John Thompson 12/1/32
10-01 4th Ave. Muslim
Brooklyn, NY 11209 GHI-CBP
June Olsen, M.D.

Figure 7.11 *Medication administration record*

15. Your patient must receive grains V of allopurinol (Zyloprim), an anti-uric medication. Consult the label in Figure 7.12 and calculate how many tablets you will administer to your patient. ________

NDC 0555-0242-02
NSN 6505-01-004-3952
Lot No.:
Exp. Date:
N 3 0555-0242-02
BARR LABORATORIES, INC.
b
Allopurinol Tablets, USP
300 mg
Caution: Federal law prohibits dispensing without prescription.
100 Tablets
Usual Dosage: See package insert.
Dispense with child-resistant closure in a well-closed, light-resistant container as defined in the USP/NF.
Store at controlled room temperature 15°-30°C (59°-86°F).
BARR LABORATORIES, INC.
Pomona, NY 10970
R10-88

Figure 7.12 *Drug label for allopurinol*

Notes/Workspace

16. The prescriber ordered 500 milligrams po tid of penicillamine (Cuprimine), an anti-inflammatory drug used in the treatment of rheumatoid arthritis. The capsules are labeled 0.125 gram. How many capsules equal the prescribed dosage? ________

17. The order for Cuprimine in Problem 16 has been changed to 20 milligrams per kilogram per day. The patient weighs 50 kilograms. How many milligrams equal this dosage? ________

18. The order reads:

captopril 6.25 mg po tid

Each scored tablet contains 12.5 milligrams. How many tablets will you administer to the patient of this ACE (angiotensin converting enzyme) inhibitor drug? ________

19. A patient has been prescribed 0.01 gram po of loratine (Claratin). How many tablets of this antihistamine will you administer if each tablet is labeled 10 milligrams? ________

20. The order reads:

Bactocill 0.5 g po bid

Read the label in Figure 7.13 and calculate the number of tablets you would administer. ________

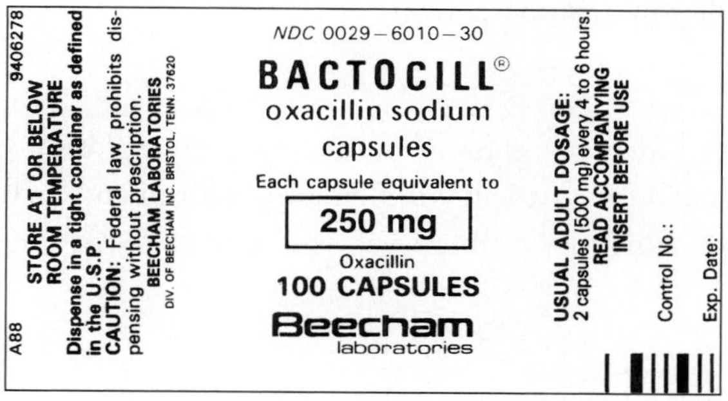

9406278
STORE AT OR BELOW ROOM TEMPERATURE
Dispense in a tight container as defined in the U.S.P.
CAUTION: Federal law prohibits dispensing without prescription.
BEECHAM LABORATORIES
DIV. OF BEECHAM INC. BRISTOL, TENN. 37620
A88
NDC 0029–6010–30
BACTOCILL®
oxacillin sodium
capsules
Each capsule equivalent to
250 mg
Oxacillin
100 CAPSULES
Beecham
laboratories
USUAL ADULT DOSAGE:
2 capsules (500 mg) every 4 to 6 hours.
READ ACCOMPANYING INSERT BEFORE USE
Control No.:
Exp. Date:

Figure 7.13 *Drug label for Bactocill*

Notes/Workspace

Cumulative Review Exercises

Review your mastery of earlier chapters.

1. The order for Margaret Jones is grain $\frac{1}{4}$ po of the sedative quazepam (Doral). What is the equivalent in milligrams if the label indicates that 1 tablet contains 15 milligrams? ________

2. The patient must receive 0.005 gram po of terbutaline sulfate (Brethine). How many tablets will you administer to this patient of this bronchodilating drug if each tablet contains 5 milligrams? ________

3. ℥ 10 = ʒ ________

4. 0.2 g = gr ________

5. The order is 250 milligrams of trimethobenzamide hydrochloride (Tigan). Give the equivalent in grains of this anti-emetic drug. ________

6. 40 mg = ________ g

7. 2500 mg = gr ________

8. 1 t = ♏ ________

9. 7500 mL = ________ L

10. gr $\overline{\text{VIISS}}$ = ________ mg

11. dr 3 = ________ t

12. The prescriber ordered 0.015 gram po of glipizide (Glucotrol), and the tablets contain 5 milligrams of the drug. How many tablets will you administer of this oral hypoglycemic drug? ________

13. The patient must receive 1000 milligrams po of the antibiotic sulfisoxazole (Gantrisin). The drug label reads 500 milligrams per 5 milliliters. How many milliliters will you give the patient? ________

14. If a prescriber orders 0.2 gram of the antihyperthyroid drug propylthiouracil (Propyl-Thyracil) for a patient with hyperthyroidism and each tablet contains 50 milligrams, how many tablets will you administer to the patient?

    ____

15. The patient has been prescribed 0.0625 milligram po of digoxin (Lanoxin), an anti-arrhythmic inotropic drug. The elixir is labeled 0.05 milligram per milliliter. How many milliliters will you administer to the patient?

    ____

chapter 8

Preparation of Solutions

Objectives

After completing this chapter, you will be able to

- *use the strength of a solution, given in ratio form or percent form, to calculate drug doses.*
- *do the calculations necessary to prepare solutions from pure drugs.*
- *do the calculations necessary to prepare solutions by diluting stock solutions.*
- *determine the amount of pure drug in a given amount of solution.*

In this chapter you will learn how to prepare solutions and how to determine the quantity of a pure drug in a solution. If the prescribed strength of a solution is not available, you must add a liquid (usually tap water or sterile water) to a pure drug or a stock solution to obtain the required strength of the solution. Although most solutions are prepared in the pharmacy by the pharmacist, nurses must be able to prepare solutions, especially in home-care situations.

Drugs are manufactured in both pure and diluted form. A pure drug contains only the drug and nothing else. A drug is frequently diluted by dissolving a quantity of pure drug in a liquid to form a solution. This solution is called a *stock solution.* The pure drug (either dry or

Notes/Workspace

liquid) is called the *solute.* The liquid added to the pure drug to form the solution is called the *solvent.* The solvents most commonly used are water and normal saline solution.

Strength of Solutions

The strength of a solution can be stated as a *ratio* or a *percentage.*

- The ratio 1:2 (read "1 to 2") means that there is 1 part of the drug in 2 parts of solution. This solution is also referred to as a $\frac{1}{2}$ strength solution.
- The ratio 1:40 (read "1 to 40") means that there is 1 part of the drug in 40 parts of solution.
- A 5% solution means that there are 5 parts of the drug in 100 parts of solution.
- A $2\frac{1}{2}$% solution means that there are $2\frac{1}{2}$ parts of the drug in 100 parts of solution.

Pure Drugs in Liquid Form

When a pure drug is in liquid form, the ratio 1:40 means there is 1 milliliter of pure drug in every 40 milliliters of solution. So 40 milliliters of a 1:40 acetic acid solution means that 1 milliliter of pure acetic acid is to be diluted with water to make a total of 40 milliliters of solution. You would prepare this solution by placing 1 milliliter of pure acetic acid in a graduated cylinder and adding water until the level in the graduated cylinder reaches 40 milliliters. See Figure 8.1.

A 1% solution means that there is 1 part of the drug in 100 parts of solution. So you would prepare 100 milliliters of a 1% creosol solution by placing 1 milliliter of pure creosol in a graduated cylinder and adding water until the level in the graduated cylinder reaches 100 milliliters. See Figure 8.2.

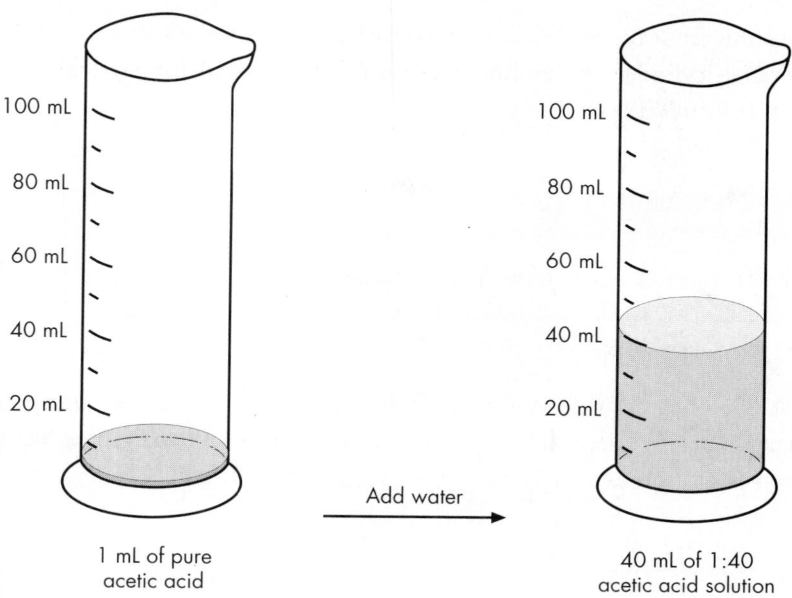

Figure 8.1 *Preparing a 1:40 solution of a pure liquid drug*

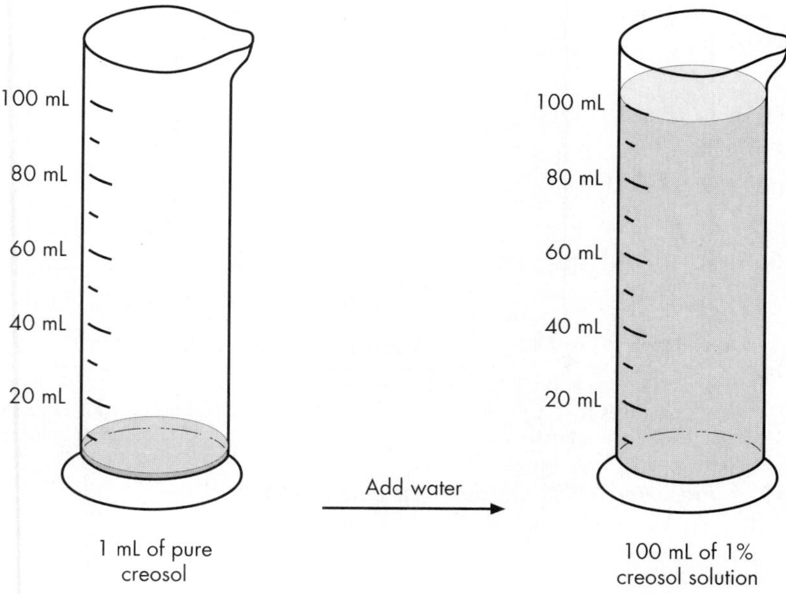

Figure 8.2 *Preparing a 1% solution of a pure liquid drug*

Notes/Workspace

Pure Drugs in Dry Form

The ratio 1:20 means 1 part of the pure drug in 20 parts of solution. When a pure drug is in *dry* form, the ratio 1:20 means 1 gram of pure drug in every 20 milliliters of solution. So 100 milliliters of a 1:20 potassium permanganate solution means 5 grams of pure potassium permanganate dissolved in water to make a total of 100 milliliters of the solution. If each tablet is 5 grams, then you would

Notes/Workspace

prepare this solution by placing 1 tablet of the pure potassium permanganate in a graduated cylinder and adding water until the level in the graduated cylinder reaches 100 milliliters.

By the way

A 1:20 solution is the same as a 5% solution.

A 5% potassium permanganate solution means 5 grams of pure potassium permanganate in 100 milliliters of solution. So a 5% potassium permanganate solution is written as $\frac{5\text{ g}}{100\text{ mL}}$ or $\frac{1\text{ g}}{20\text{ mL}}$. See Figure 8.3.

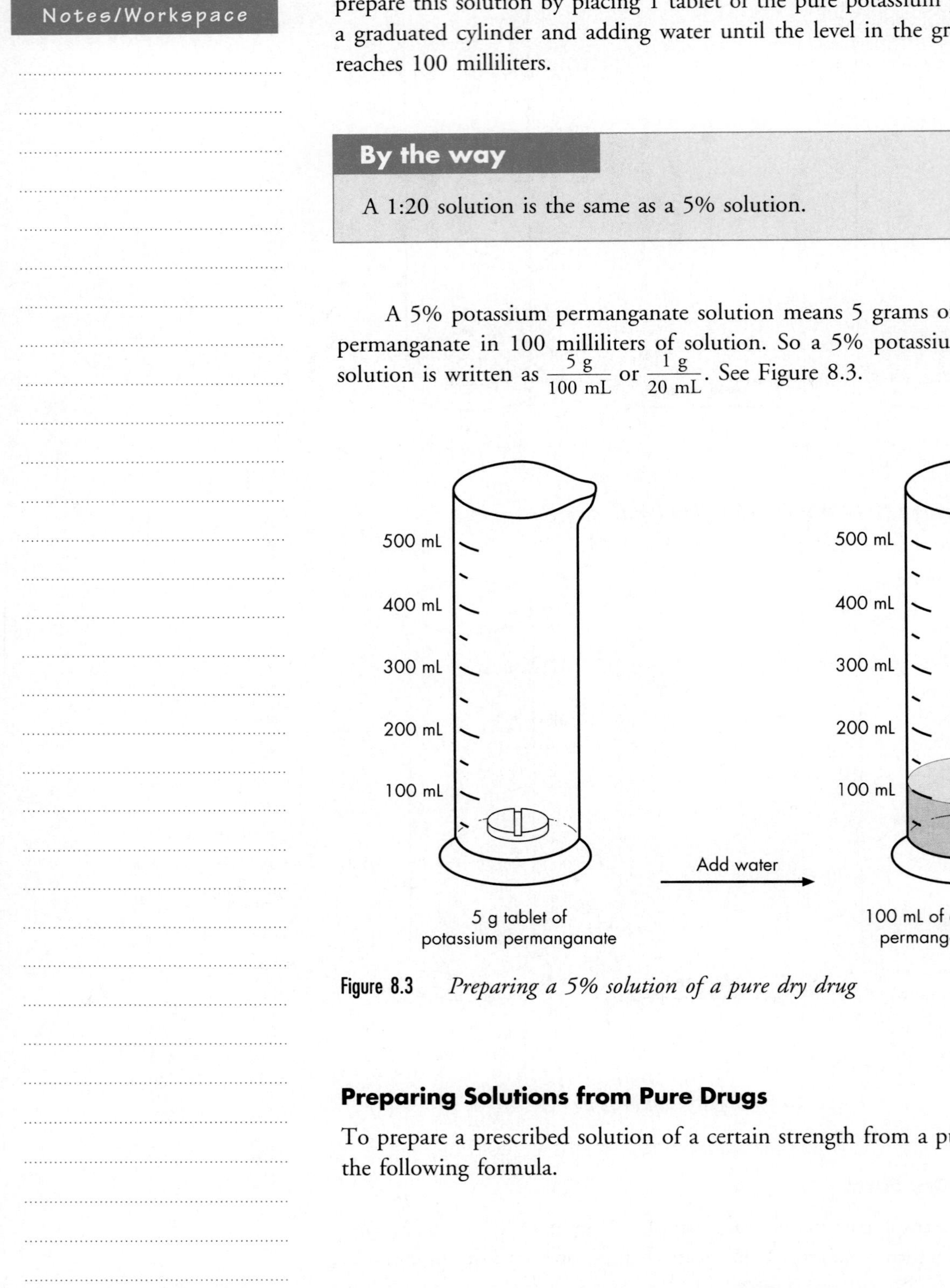

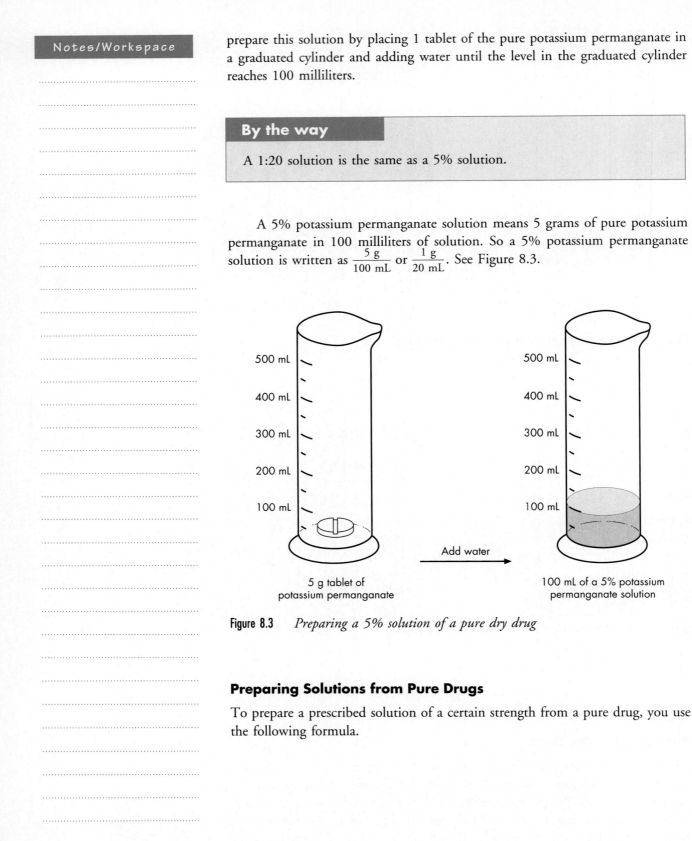

Figure 8.3 *Preparing a 5% solution of a pure dry drug*

Preparing Solutions from Pure Drugs

To prepare a prescribed solution of a certain strength from a pure drug, you use the following formula.

Note

Amount of solution × Strength = Amount of pure drug

Notes/Workspace

Amount of solution: Use **milliliters** (or **cubic centimeters**).
Strength: Always write as a fraction for calculations.

For liquids:

1:40 acetic acid solution is written as $\frac{1 \text{ mL}}{40 \text{ mL}}$.

5% acetic solution is written as $\frac{5 \text{ mL}}{100 \text{ mL}}$.

For tablets or powder:

1:20 potassium permanganate solution is written $\frac{1 \text{ g}}{20 \text{ mL}}$.

12% potassium permanganate solution is written as $\frac{12 \text{ g}}{100 \text{ mL}}$.

Amount of pure drug:

Use **milliliters** or **cubic centimeters** for liquids.
Use **grams** for tablets or powders.

Example 8.1

How many grams of magnesium sulfate (Epsom salts) would you need in order to prepare 100 milliliters of a 20% solution?

Since magnesium sulfate is in dry form, it is measured in grams. So a 20% solution means 20 grams of magnesium sulfate in 100 milliliters of solute.

Amount of solution is 100 milliliters.
Strength is 20% or $\frac{20}{100}$, so you use $\frac{20 \text{ g}}{100 \text{ mL}}$.

$$100 \text{ mL} \times \frac{20 \text{ g}}{100 \text{ mL}} = \text{Amount of pure drug}$$

$$\overset{1}{\cancel{100 \text{ mL}}} \times \frac{20 \text{ g}}{\underset{1}{\cancel{100 \text{ mL}}}} = 20 \text{ g}$$

So you need 20 grams of magnesium sulfate to prepare 100 milliliters of a 20% solution.

Notes/Workspace

Example 8.2

How many grams of dextrose would you need to prepare 1000 milliliters of a 5% solution?

Amount of solution is 1000 milliliters.
Strength is 5% or $\frac{5}{100}$, so you use $\frac{5\text{ g}}{100\text{ mL}}$.

$$1000\text{ mL} \times \frac{5\text{ g}}{100\text{ mL}} = \text{Amount of pure drug}$$

$$\overset{10}{\cancel{1000}\,\cancel{\text{mL}}} \times \frac{5\text{ g}}{\underset{1}{\cancel{100}\,\cancel{\text{mL}}}} = 50\text{ g}$$

So you need 50 grams of dextrose to prepare 1000 milliliters of a 5% solution.

Example 8.3

How would you prepare 2000 milliliters of a 1:10 Clorox solution?

Since Clorox is a liquid, it is measured in milliliters. So a 1:10 solution means 1 milliliter of Clorox in 10 milliliters of solution.

Amount of solution is 2000 milliliters.
Strength is 1:10 or $\frac{1}{10}$. You use $\frac{1\text{ mL}}{10\text{ mL}}$.

$$\overset{200}{\cancel{2000}\,\cancel{\text{mL}}} \times \frac{1\,\cancel{\text{mL}}}{\cancel{10}\,\cancel{\text{mL}}} = 200\text{ mL}$$

So you need 200 milliliters of Clorox to prepare 2000 milliliters of a 1:10 solution. This means that 200 milliliters of Clorox is diluted with water to 2000 milliliters of solution.

Example 8.4

How would you prepare 250 milliliters of a $\frac{1}{2}$% creosol solution? Creosol comes in liquid form, so a $\frac{1}{2}$% solution means 0.5 milliliter of creosol in 100 milliliters of solution. (*Remember:* $\frac{1}{2} = 0.5$.)

Amount of solution is 250 milliliters.
Strength is $\frac{1}{2}\%$ or $\frac{0.5}{100}$, so you use $\frac{0.5 \text{ mL}}{100 \text{ mL}}$.

$$\overset{5}{\cancel{250}} \text{ mL} \times \frac{0.5 \cancel{\text{mL}}}{\underset{2}{\cancel{100}} \cancel{\text{mL}}} = 1.25 \text{ mL}$$

So you need 1.25 milliliters of creosol to prepare 250 milliliters of a $\frac{1}{2}\%$ creosol solution. This means that 1.25 milliliters of creosol is diluted with water to 250 milliliters of solution.

Example 8.5

How would you prepare 3 liters of a 1% urinary antiseptic solution using 5 g tablets of Neosporin?

Since the pure Neosporin is in dry form, it is measured in grams. So a 1% solution means 1 gram of Neosporin in 100 milliliters of solution.

You must find the amount of pure drug necessary and convert to tablets.

Amount of solution is 3 liters.
Strength is 1% of $\frac{1}{100}$, so you use $\frac{1 \text{ g}}{100 \text{ mL}}$.

Since you are working in milliliters, change 3 liters to 3000 milliliters.
Since each tablet contains 5 grams, you use the fraction $\frac{1 \text{ tab}}{5 \text{ g}}$.

$$\overset{30}{\cancel{3000}} \cancel{\text{mL}} \times \frac{1 \cancel{\text{g}}}{\underset{1}{\cancel{100}} \cancel{\text{mL}}} \times \frac{1 \text{ tab}}{5 \cancel{\text{g}}} = 6 \text{ tab}$$

So you dissolve 6 tablets of Neosporin in water and dilute to 3000 milliliters.

Diluting Stock Solutions

A stock solution is one in which a pure drug is already dissolved in a liquid. The strength of each stock solution is written on the label. If the order is for a stronger solution, you will need to prepare a new solution. However, if the order is for a weaker solution, you can dilute the stock solution to the prescribed strength. To find out how much stock solution to mix, use the following formula.

Notes/Workspace

Notes/Workspace

Note

$$\frac{\text{Amount prescribed} \times \text{Strength prescribed}}{\text{Strength of stock}} = \text{Amount of stock}$$

Example 8.6

How would you prepare 1 liter of a 10% glucose solution from a 50% stock solution of glucose?

Amount prescribed is 1 liter, so you use 1000 milliliters.

Strength prescribed is 10%, so you use $\frac{10 \text{ mL}}{100 \text{ mL}}$.

Strength of stock is 50%, so you use $\frac{50 \text{ mL}}{100 \text{ mL}}$.

$$\frac{1000 \text{ mL} \times \frac{10 \cancel{\text{mL}}}{100 \cancel{\text{mL}}}}{\frac{50 \cancel{\text{mL}}}{100 \cancel{\text{mL}}}} = \text{Amount of stock}$$

$$1000 \text{ mL} \times \frac{10}{100} \div \frac{50}{100} =$$

$$1000 \text{ mL} \times \frac{\overset{1}{\cancel{10}}}{\underset{1}{\cancel{100}}} \times \frac{\overset{1}{\cancel{100}}}{\underset{5}{\cancel{50}}} = 200 \text{ mL}$$

So you would take 200 milliliters of the 50% stock solution of glucose and dilute it with water to 1000 milliliters.

Example 8.7

How would you prepare 2500 milliliters of a 1:10 boric acid solution from a 40% stock solution of this antiseptic?

Amount prescribed is 2500 milliliters.

Strength prescribed is 1:10, so you use $\frac{1 \text{ mL}}{10 \text{ mL}}$.

Strength of stock is 40%, so you use $\frac{40 \text{ mL}}{100 \text{ mL}}$.

$$\frac{2500 \text{ mL} \times \frac{1 \cancel{\text{mL}}}{10 \cancel{\text{mL}}}}{\frac{40 \cancel{\text{mL}}}{100 \cancel{\text{mL}}}} = \text{Amount of stock}$$

$$2500 \text{ mL} \times \frac{1}{10} \div \frac{40}{100} =$$

$$\overset{250}{\cancel{2500}} \text{ mL} \times \frac{1}{\underset{1}{\cancel{10}}} \times \frac{100}{40} = 625 \text{ mL}$$

So you would take 625 milliliters of the 40% stock solution of boric acid and dilute with water to 2500 milliliters.

Example 8.8

How would you prepare 500 milliliters of a 1:25 solution from a 1:4 stock solution of the antiseptic Argyrol?

Amount prescribed is 500 milliliters.

Strength prescribed is 1:25, so you use $\frac{1 \text{ mL}}{25 \text{ mL}}$.

Strength of stock is 1:4, so you use $\frac{1 \text{ mL}}{4 \text{ mL}}$.

$$\frac{500 \text{ mL} \times \frac{1 \cancel{\text{mL}}}{25 \cancel{\text{mL}}}}{\frac{1 \cancel{\text{mL}}}{4 \cancel{\text{mL}}}} = \text{Amount of stock}$$

$$500 \text{ mL} \times \frac{1}{25} \div \frac{1}{4} =$$

$$\overset{20}{\cancel{500}} \text{ mL} \times \frac{1}{\underset{1}{\cancel{25}}} \times \frac{4}{1} = 80 \text{ mL}$$

So you would take 80 milliliters of a 1:4 stock solution of Argyrol and dilute it with water to 500 milliliters.

Notes/Workspace

Notes/Workspace

Practice Sets

You will find the answers to the Try These for Practice, Exercises, and Cumulative Review Practice Sets in the Answer Section at the back of the book. Your instructor has the answers to the Additional Exercises.

Try These for Practice

Test your comprehension after reading the chapter.

1. How many grams of dextrose are needed to prepare 4000 milliliters of a 10% glucose solution? ________

2. Describe how you would prepare 500 milliliters of a 0.9% normal saline solution from the pure drug (sodium chloride). ________

3. How many grams of Epsom salts crystals are required to make 200 milliliters of a $2\frac{1}{2}\%$ solution? ________

4. How would you prepare 4000 milliliters of 5% potassium permanganate solution from 5 g tablets? ________

5. The prescriber has ordered 4 liters of a 1% neomycin solution for bladder irrigation. Calculate the amount needed from a 2% stock solution. ________

Exercises

Reinforce your understanding in class or at home.

1. Describe how you would prepare 1000 milliliters of a 2% solution of formaldehyde, a disinfectant, from a 100% solution.

____

____

____

Notes/Workspace

2. Explain how to prepare 500 milliliters of a 2% solution of Betadine from a 50% stock solution.

3. How would you prepare 2000 milliliters of a 10% Weskodyne solution, a disinfectant, from pure drug?

4. How would you prepare 1250 milliliters of a 0.45% solution from sodium chloride crystals?

5. Describe how you would prepare 5000 milliliters of a 1:1000 aluminum acetate (Burow's) solution, an antiseptic, from 0.5 g tablets.

6. You must prepare 100 milliliters of a 2% boric acid solution, a mild antiseptic. How would you prepare this from boric acid crystals?

7. Explain how to prepare a 1% ammonium chloride solution (1 liter) from 1 g tablets.

Notes/Workspace

8. Use the information found on the label in Figure 8.4 to determine the number of grams of calcium chloride contained in 5 milliliters of this solution.

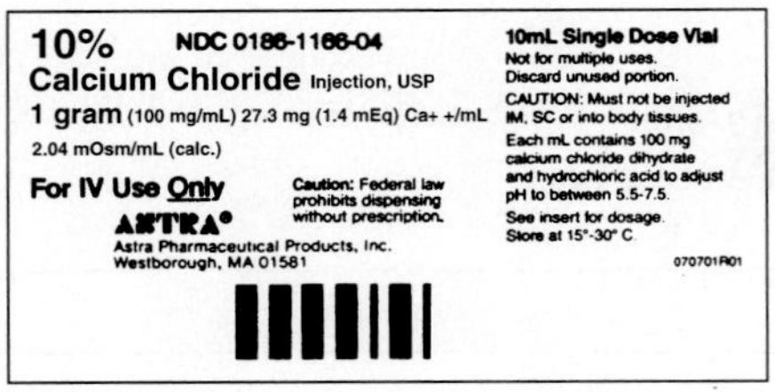

10% NDC 0186-1166-04
Calcium Chloride Injection, USP
1 gram (100 mg/mL) 27.3 mg (1.4 mEq) Ca+ +/mL
2.04 mOsm/mL (calc.)
For IV Use Only
Caution: Federal law prohibits dispensing without prescription.
ASTRA®
Astra Pharmaceutical Products, Inc.
Westborough, MA 01581
10mL Single Dose Vial
Not for multiple uses.
Discard unused portion.
CAUTION: Must not be injected IM, SC or into body tissues.
Each mL contains 100 mg calcium chloride dihydrate and hydrochloric acid to adjust pH to between 5.5-7.5.
See insert for dosage.
Store at 15°-30° C.
070701R01

Figure 8.4 *Drug label for 10% calcium chloride*

9. Describe how to prepare 1000 milliliters of a 2.5% solution from a 3% solution of the antiseptic hydrogen peroxide.

10. How would you prepare 100 milliliters of a 1% solution from a 20% solution?

11. Describe how to prepare 4000 milliliters of a 1:50 solution of the antiseptic potassium permanganate from 0.5 g tablets.

Notes/Workspace

12. How would you prepare 1000 milliliters of a 10% Lysol solution, a disinfectant, from a 25% stock solution?

______

______

______

13. How many grams of glucose are contained in 3 liters of a 10% glucose solution?

______

______

______

14. How would you prepare 4000 milliliters of a 1:40 solution from a 1:20 solution?

______

______

______

15. How would you prepare 1000 milliliters of a 1:750 solution of Zephiran Chloride (an antiseptic) from a 1:500 solution?

$\frac{1000\text{ m}}{1} \times \frac{1}{750} \times \frac{500}{1} = \frac{2000}{3}$ (handwritten; 750 and 500 crossed out, with 3 and 2 written beside them)

16. Describe how to prepare 500 milliliters of a 0.025% solution from a 1% solution.

______

______

______

17. If 1 gram of pure drug is added to a container of sterile water and the total amount is now 1000 milliliters, what would be the strength of this solution?

______

Notes/Workspace

18. How would you prepare 2000 milliliters of 10% aluminum acetate (Burow's) solution from 1 g tablets?

19. The information found in the second order on the physician's order sheet in Figure 8.5 is "cleanse abdominal wound with 1:750 Zephiran Chloride q shift" (q shift means "every shift"). Describe how you would prepare this solution from a 2% solution (500 milliliters).

GENERAL HOSPITAL

PRESS HARD WITH BALLPOINT PEN. WRITE DATE & TIME AND SIGN EACH ORDER

DATE	TIME	A.M. / P.M.
7/8/94	*3*	(P.M.)

1. Apply fluocinonide 0.05% to affected skin qid

2. Cleanse abdominal wound with 1:750 Zephiran Chloride q shift

3. Tube feeding: 1/3 strength Meritine 240 mL q4h via gastrostomy tube

SIGNATURE *L. Ablon* M.D.

IMPRINT
873667 7/8/94
Gene Martin 3/3/30
333 Ocean Pkwy Jewish
Huntington, NY Aetna
41001
Dr. Leon Ablon

ORDERS NOTED
DATE *7/8/94* TIME *3:10* A.M. (P.M.)
❑ MEDEX ❑ KARDEX
NURSE'S SIG. *A. Giangrasso*

FILLED BY DATE

PHYSICIAN'S ORDERS

Figure 8.5 *Physician's order sheet*

20. Read the information in the first order from the physician's order sheet in Figure 8.5. How would you prepare 250 milliliters of 0.05% fluocinonide (Lidex) solution from a 1% solution?

Additional Exercises

Now, on your own, test yourself! Ask your instructor to check your answers.

Notes/Workspace

1. Your patient is to have a tube feeding of $\frac{1}{2}$ strength Isocal, a nutritional supplement. Each can contains 240 milliliters. How many milliliters of water should be added to the Isocal for a $\frac{1}{2}$ strength solution? (*Hint:* $\frac{1}{2}$ strength means 50% solution.) ________

2. A 25% solution of serum albumin has been ordered for a patient. If the prescriber wants the patient to have 50 grams of serum albumin, how many milliliters will the patient receive? ________

3. If the serum albumin was a 25% solution and the order was 400 milliliters, how many grams of serum albumin would the patient receive? ________

4. The prescriber has requested that 500 milligrams of 2% lidocaine solution be added to 500 milliliters of 5% D/W. How many milliliters of lidocaine must be added to the 5% D/W? ________

5. A dentist is to inject a 1% solution of lidocaine as a nerve block for a patient. He will give the patient a total of 5 milliliters. How many grams of lidocaine will the patient receive? ________

6. The prescriber has ordered 10 ounces of 0.9% sodium chloride solution as a cleansing agent. How many grams of sodium chloride are necessary to make this solution? ________

7. How would you prepare 250 milliliters of a 10% magnesium sulfate solution from pure drug? ________

8. Describe how a 2.5% solution of hexachlorophene solution would be prepared from a 3% solution (200 milliliters). ________

9. The prescriber has ordered a norepinephrine (Levophed) lavage for a patient having a gastric bleed. Each ampule contains 4 milligrams per 4 milliliters of Levophed and the prescriber has ordered 1000 milliliters of normal saline

Notes/Workspace

with 0.04 gram of Levophed, how many milliliters of Levophed will be added to the normal saline? ________

10. Explain how to prepare 1000 milliliters of a 1:50,000 silver nitrate solution from a 1:1000 stock solution of silver nitrate. ________

11. You have a 100% Clorox solution available. How would you prepare 1 gallon of a 10% solution? ________

12. The order reads:

Meritine $\frac{1}{2}$ strength, 240 mL q4h via gastrostomy tube

How many grams of Meritine are contained in 240 milliliters of Meritine $\frac{1}{2}$ strength? ________

13. Read the physician's third order in Figure 8.5, page 154. How would you prepare the tube feeding from $\frac{1}{2}$ strength Meritine? ________

14. Read the information on the label in Figure 8.6 and calculate the amount of dextrose in 20 milliliters of the solution. ________

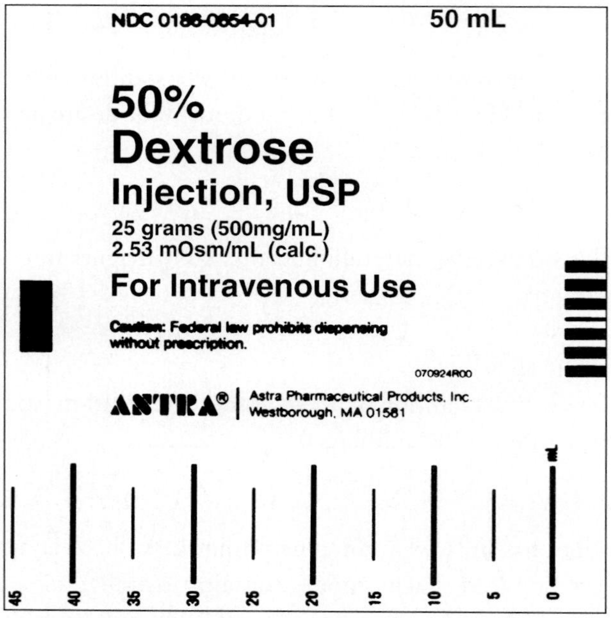

NDC 0186-0654-01 50 mL

50% Dextrose Injection, USP

25 grams (500mg/mL)
2.53 mOsm/mL (calc.)

For Intravenous Use

Caution: Federal law prohibits dispensing without prescription.

070924R00

ASTRA® | Astra Pharmaceutical Products, Inc. Westborough, MA 01581

45 40 35 30 25 20 15 10 5 0

Figure 8.6 *Drug label for 50% dextrose*

15. A physician has prescribed a 2% acetic acid solution to treat an external ear canal infection. How would you prepare 25 milliliters of this solution from a 100% acetic acid solution? _________

16. You have a 2.75% otic boric acid solution. How many grams of boric acid would be contained in 30 milliliters? _________

17. A patient has an accumulation of ear wax (cerumen) in the ear canal. A 6.5% solution of carbamide peroxide (Debrox), which is an otic solution, is prescribed. How many milligrams of Debrox will be contained in 50 milliliters? _________

18. The prescriber has ordered a 1.5 mL IV push of a 10% solution of magnesium sulfate. How many grams of magnesium sulfate will the patient receive? _________

19. How many grams of sodium chloride are in 500 milliliters of 0.45% normal saline? _________

20. An order requests that 100 milligrams of 2% lidocaine solution be added to an infusion of 5% D/W. How many milliliters of this solution contains 100 milligrams of lidocaine? _________

Notes/Workspace

Cumulative Review Exercises

Review your mastery of earlier chapters.

1. How do you prepare 250 milliliters of 2.5% boric acid solution (an antiseptic) from a 10% stock solution?

____

____

____

2. The pharmacist must prepare a $2\frac{1}{2}$% magnesium sulfate solution (an electrolyte). How many grams of pure magnesium sulfate are contained in 100 milliliters of this solution? _________

Notes/Workspace

3. Explain how to prepare 500 milliliters of a 5% solution from a pure liquid drug.

____

____

____

4. The order is 0.5 milligram of the anti-anxiety drug alprazolam (Xanax); the tablets on hand are grain $\frac{1}{120}$. How many tablets would you administer?

____

5. The physician orders 450 milligrams of clindamycin hydrochloride (Cleocin). The bottle label states that 1 tablet equals 0.15 gram. How many tablets are equal to 450 milligrams? ________

6. How many grain $\frac{1}{200}$ tablets of the anticholinergic drug atropine sulfate are needed when the tablets are 0.3 milligram each? ________

7. The order is dram 1 of theophylline (Elixophyllin). How many minims are contained in dram 1 of this drug, which has a bronchodilating action?

____

8. The order reads: Zithromax 0.5 g po qd. How many milligrams are contained in this dosage? ________

9. 750 mg = ________ g

10. 2500 mg = ________ g

11. 50 mg = gr ________

12. The order is for 4 milligrams po of benztropine mesylate (Cogentin). Each tablet contains 0.5 milligram. How many tablets of this antiparkinsonian drug would you administer? ________

13. The prescriber ordered 0.0006 gram sc of scopolamine hydrobromide, an anticholinergic drug. Convert this amount to milligrams. ________

14. gr V = ________ mg

15. $2\frac{1}{2}$ qt = ________ pt

chapter 9

Syringes

Objectives

After completing this chapter, you will be able to

- *identify the various types of syringes.*
- *identify the parts of a syringe.*
- *determine the amount of solution in a syringe.*
- *understand prepackaged cartridges.*
- *read and use USP units.*

A hypodermic syringe (inserted beneath the skin) is an instrument used in parenteral therapy for the administration of sterile liquid medications by injection. The medication is introduced into a body space such as a vein (IV), a muscle (IM), subcutaneous tissue (sc), cardiac muscle, subarachnoid space, or bone tissue. Figure 9.1 illustrates the parts of a syringe: the plunger, barrel, and hollow needle, which must all be connected separately. The plunger and needle must always be kept sterile.

Notes/Workspace

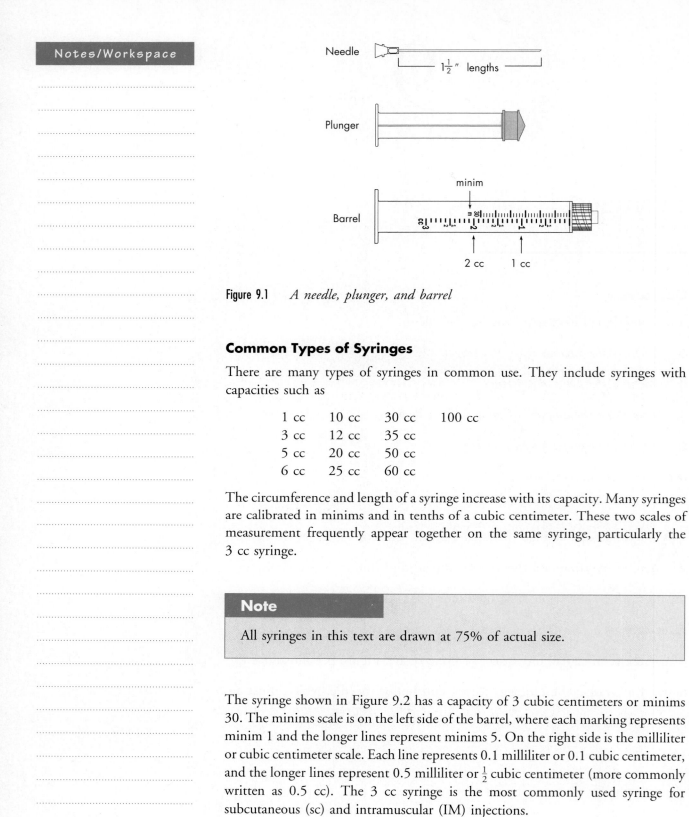

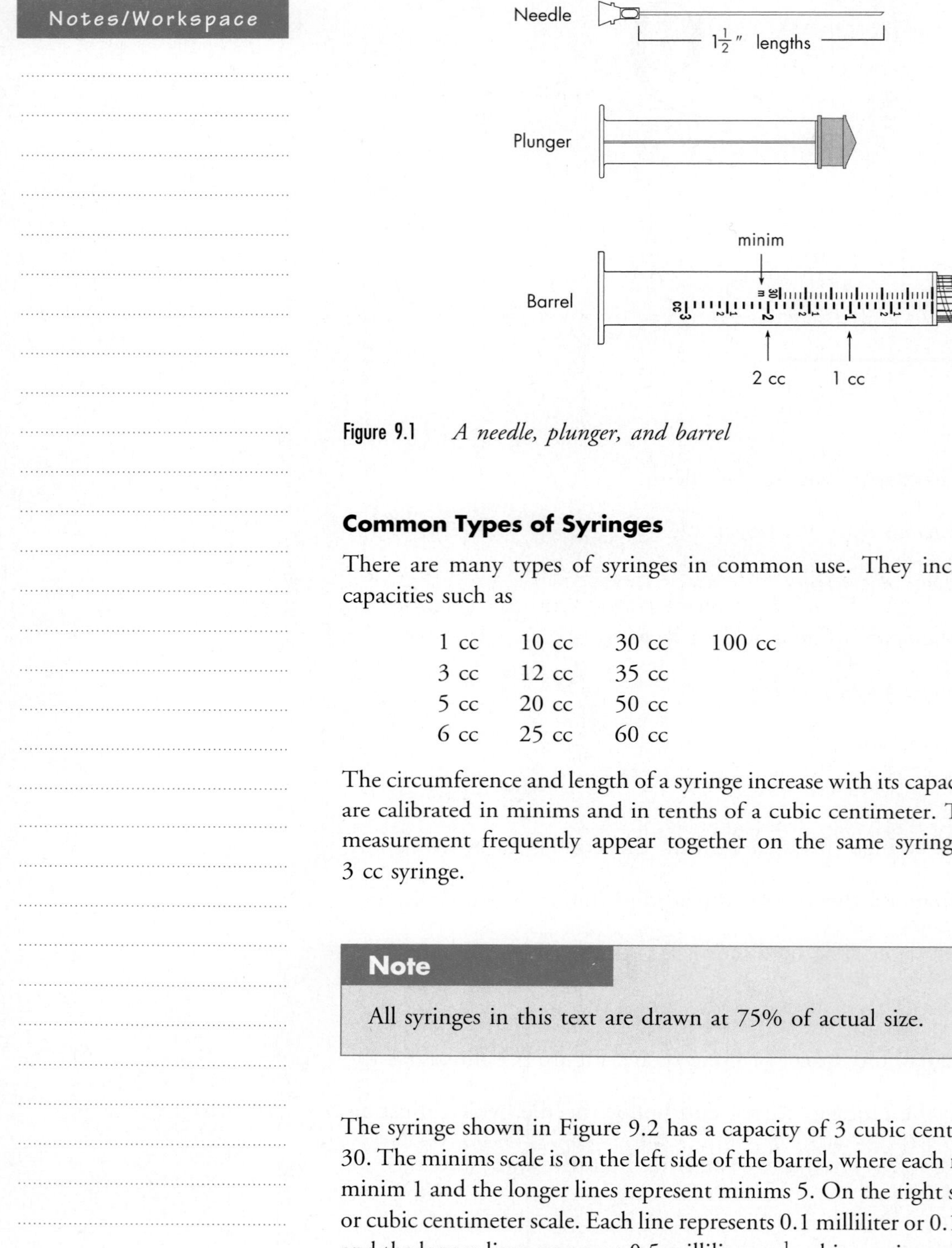

Figure 9.1 *A needle, plunger, and barrel*

Common Types of Syringes

There are many types of syringes in common use. They include syringes with capacities such as

1 cc	10 cc	30 cc	100 cc
3 cc	12 cc	35 cc	
5 cc	20 cc	50 cc	
6 cc	25 cc	60 cc	

The circumference and length of a syringe increase with its capacity. Many syringes are calibrated in minims and in tenths of a cubic centimeter. These two scales of measurement frequently appear together on the same syringe, particularly the 3 cc syringe.

Note

All syringes in this text are drawn at 75% of actual size.

The syringe shown in Figure 9.2 has a capacity of 3 cubic centimeters or minims 30. The minims scale is on the left side of the barrel, where each marking represents minim 1 and the longer lines represent minims 5. On the right side is the milliliter or cubic centimeter scale. Each line represents 0.1 milliliter or 0.1 cubic centimeter, and the longer lines represent 0.5 milliliter or $\frac{1}{2}$ cubic centimeter (more commonly written as 0.5 cc). The 3 cc syringe is the most commonly used syringe for subcutaneous (sc) and intramuscular (IM) injections.

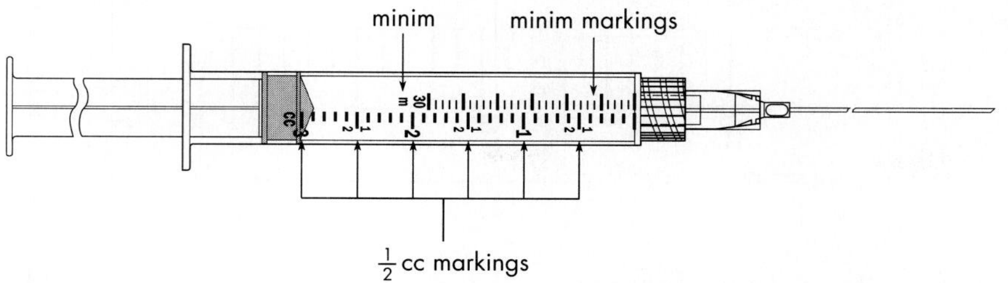

Figure 9.2 *A 3 cc syringe*

Remember

A cubic centimeter is the same as a milliliter:

1 cc = 1 mL

Figure 9.3 shows a 10 cc syringe. Notice that this syringe has neither incremental markings of 0.5 cubic centimeter nor a minims scale. Each line represents 0.2 cubic centimeter, and the longer lines represent 1 cubic centimeter. This syringe can be used to draw venous or arterial blood as well as to add sterile diluent to a vial or ampule of powdered medication.

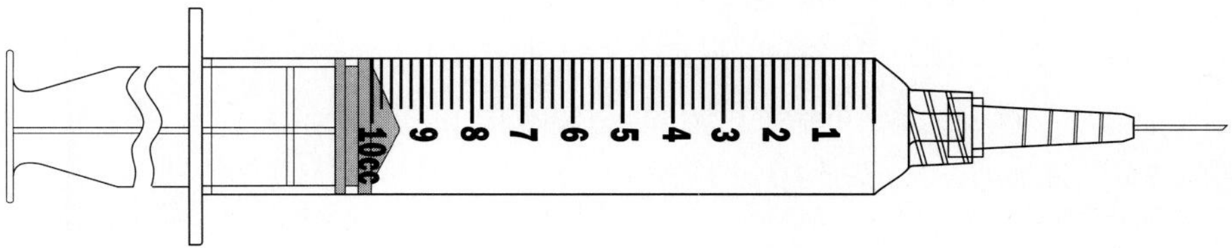

Figure 9.3 *A 10 cc syringe*

A 20 cc syringe is shown in Figure 9.4. Each line on the scale represents 1 cubic centimeter, and the longer line indicates 5 cubic centimeters. The 20 cc syringe can be used to inject large volumes of sterile liquids. Figure 9.5 shows a 20 cc syringe filled with liquid up to the 12 cc mark.

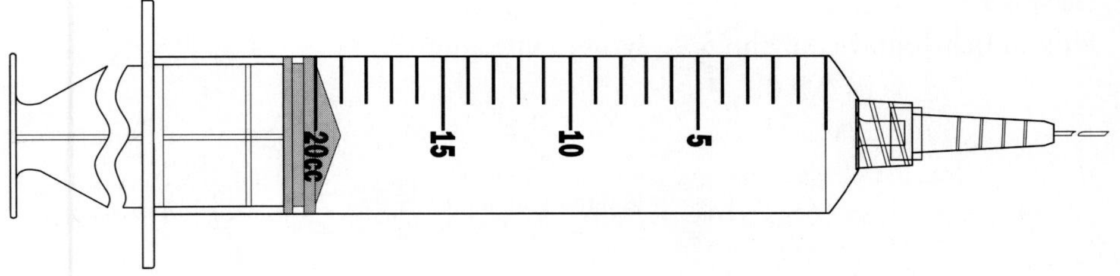

Figure 9.4 *A 20 cc syringe*

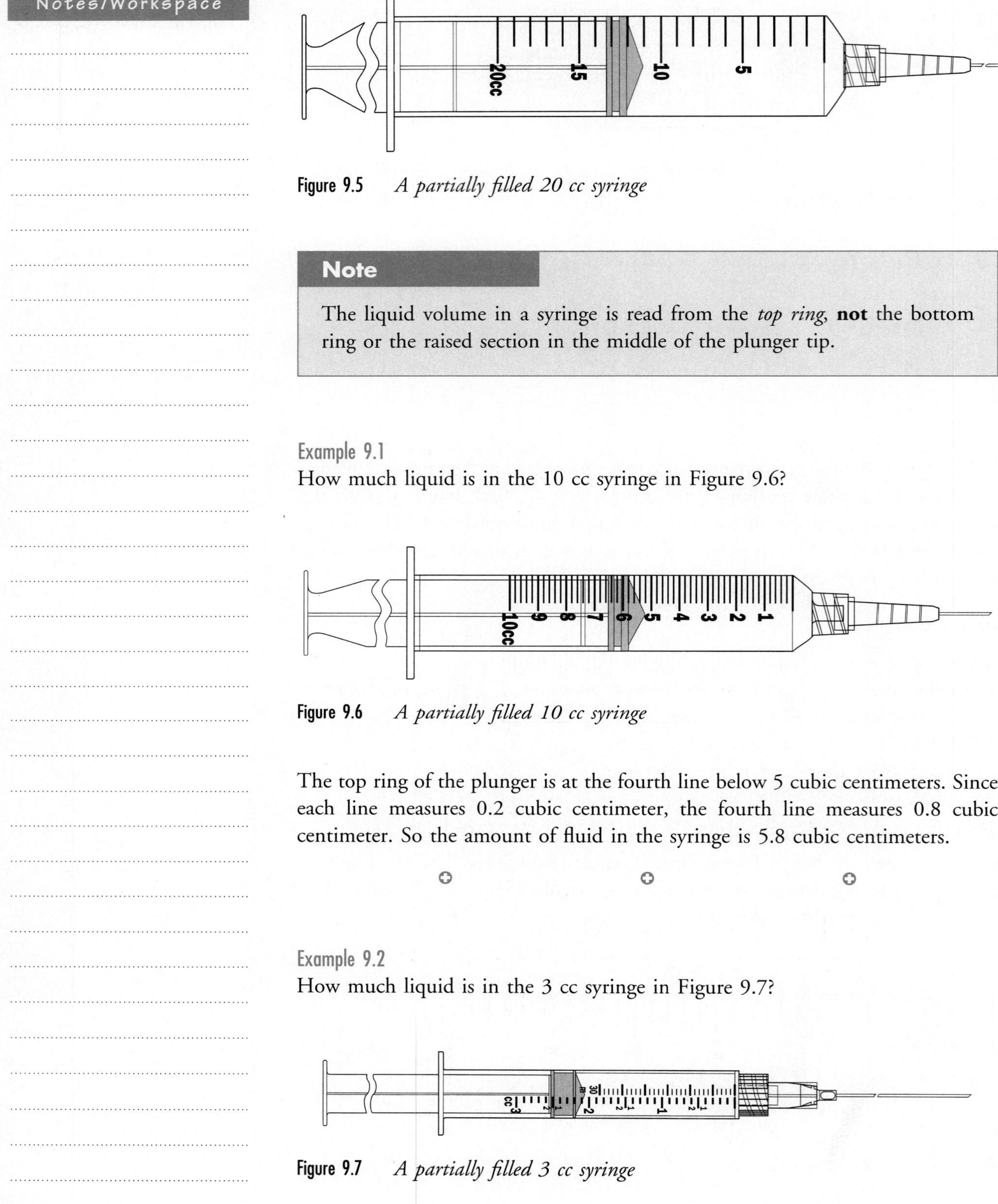

Figure 9.5 *A partially filled 20 cc syringe*

Note

The liquid volume in a syringe is read from the *top ring*, **not** the bottom ring or the raised section in the middle of the plunger tip.

Example 9.1

How much liquid is in the 10 cc syringe in Figure 9.6?

Figure 9.6 *A partially filled 10 cc syringe*

The top ring of the plunger is at the fourth line below 5 cubic centimeters. Since each line measures 0.2 cubic centimeter, the fourth line measures 0.8 cubic centimeter. So the amount of fluid in the syringe is 5.8 cubic centimeters.

Example 9.2

How much liquid is in the 3 cc syringe in Figure 9.7?

Figure 9.7 *A partially filled 3 cc syringe*

Notes/Workspace

The top ring of the plunger is at the second line below 2 cubic centimeters. Since each line measures 0.1 cubic centimeter, the two lines measure 0.2 cubic centimeter. So the amount of liquid in the syringe is 2.2 cubic centimeters.

Example 9.3

How much liquid is in the 3 cc syringe in Figure 9.8?

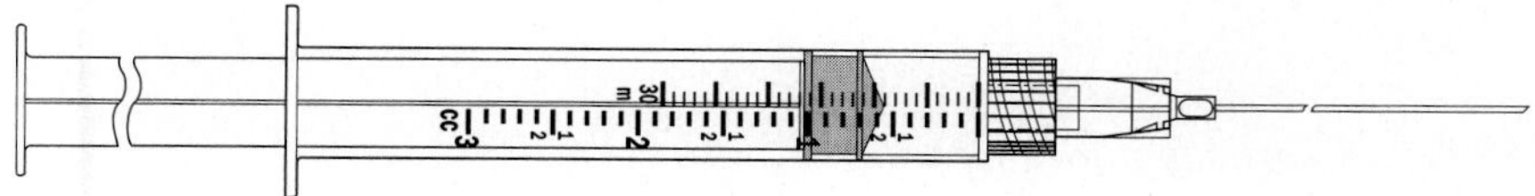

Figure 9.8 *A partially filled 3 cc syringe*

The top ring of the plunger is at the second line below $\frac{1}{2}$ cubic centimeter. Since each short line measures 0.1 cubic centimeter, the two lines measure 0.2 cubic centimeter. So the amount of liquid in the syringe is 0.7 cubic centimeter.

Other Types of Syringes

Other types of syringes that are available for the administration of medications include the prepackaged cartridge, the tuberculin syringe, and the insulin syringe.

A *prepackaged cartridge* is a syringe that is prefilled with medication. If the medication order is for the exact amount of drug in the prepackaged cartridge, the possibility of measurement error by the medication administrator is eliminated. The prepackaged cartridge syringe shown in Figure 9.9 is calibrated so that each line measures 0.1 milliliter and the thicker lines measure 0.5 milliliter.

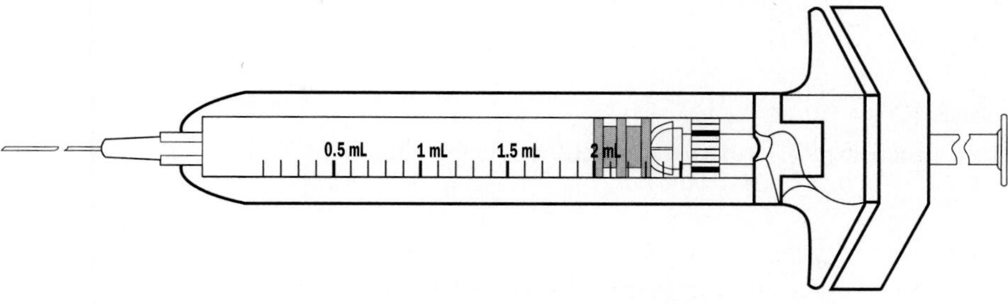

Figure 9.9 *A prepackaged cartridge*

Notes/Workspace

Example 9.4

How much liquid is in the prepackaged cartridge shown in Figure 9.10?

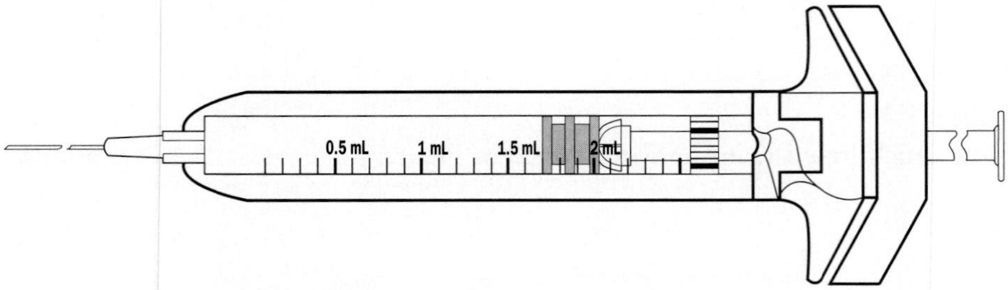

Figure 9.10 *A partially filled prepackaged 2 mL syringe*

The top of the plunger is at two lines above 1.5 milliliters. Since each line measures 0.1 milliliter, the two lines measure 0.2 milliliter. So the prepackaged cartridge contains 1.7 milliliters.

The *tuberculin syringe* shown in Figure 9.11 is a small, slender syringe used to inject small quantities of liquids. It has a capacity of 1 cubic centimeter. Each line on the syringe represents 0.01 cubic centimeter, and the longer lines represent 0.05 cubic centimeter. This syringe is used for intradermal injection (directly beneath the skin) as well as for injection of small quantities of medication that might be prescribed for pediatric or adult patients.

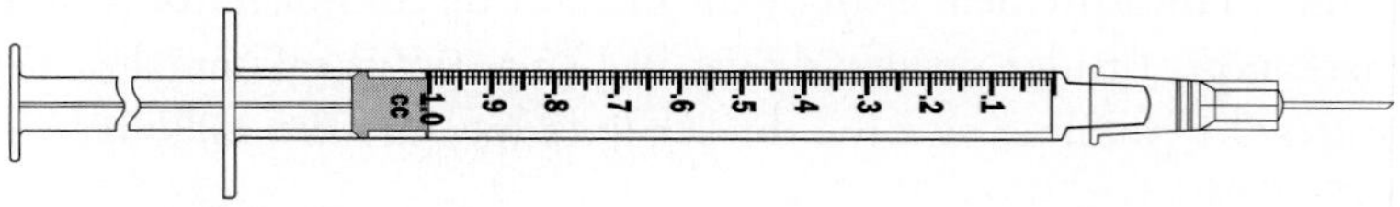

Figure 9.11 *A tuberculin syringe*

Example 9.5

How much liquid is in the tuberculin syringe shown in Figure 9.12?

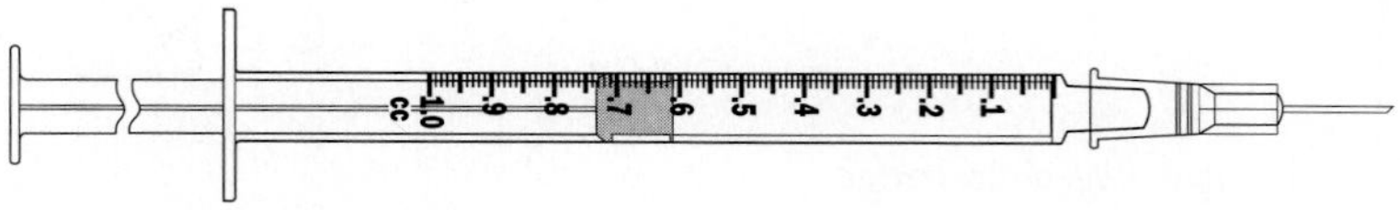

Figure 9.12 *A partially filled tuberculin syringe*

The top ring of the plunger is at one line above 0.60 milliliter. Since each line represents 0.01 milliliter, the amount of liquid in the syringe is 0.61 milliliter.

The *insulin syringe* is used to measure insulin. Insulin is a hormone used to treat patients with insulin-dependent diabetes mellitus (IDDM). It is available in both short-acting and long-acting preparations. Insulin can also be prescribed for patients who are hyperglycemic as a result of certain medical therapies. Insulin is supplied in standardized units of potency rather than by weight or volume. These standardized units are called *USP units*, which is often shortened to *units* and abbreviated u.

The insulin syringe is calibrated in units. Figure 9.13 shows an insulin syringe with a capacity of 50 units ($\frac{1}{2}$ cubic centimeter), where each line on the scale measures 1 unit (0.01 cubic centimeter). A 100 u insulin syringe is shown in Figure 9.14. Each line on its scale measures 2 units (0.02 cubic centimeter).

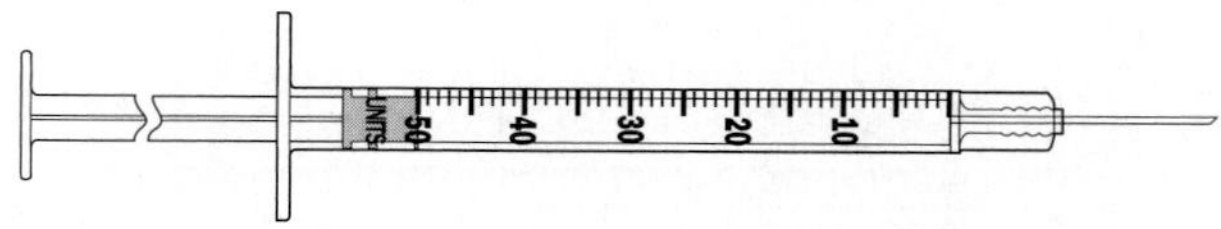

Figure 9.13 *A 50 u insulin syringe*

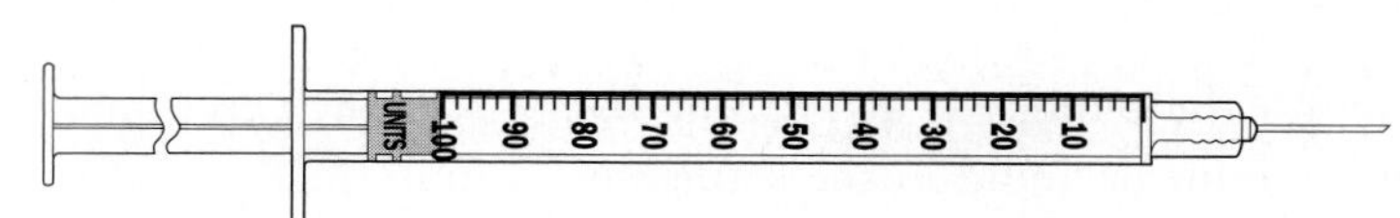

Figure 9.14 *A 100 u insulin syringe*

Note

The top ring of an insulin syringe plunger is flat. As mentioned earlier, other types of syringes have a peak in the center of the top ring. With both types of syringes, the liquid volume is measured from the *top ring*.

Notes/Workspace

Notes/Workspace

Example 9.6

How much liquid is in the 50 u insulin syringe shown in Figure 9.15?

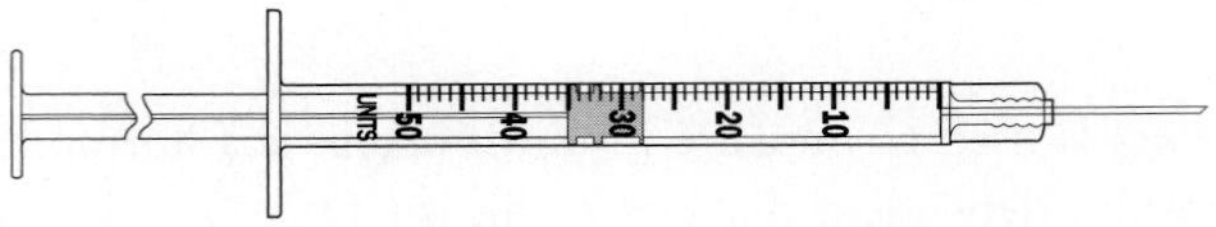

Figure 9.15 *A partially filled 50 u insulin syringe*

The top ring of the plunger is at three lines above 25. Since each line represents 1 unit, the amount of liquid in the syringe is 28 units.

Example 9.7

How much liquid is in the 100 u insulin syringe shown in Figure 9.16?

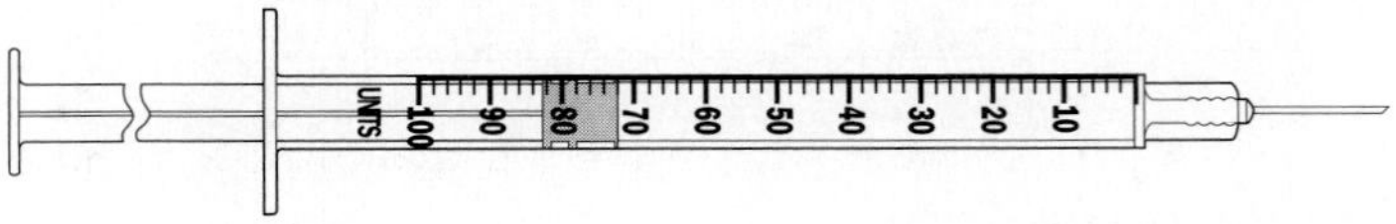

Figure 9.16 *A partially filled 100 u insulin syringe*

The top ring of the plunger is at one line above 70. Since each line represents 2 units, the amount of liquid in the syringe is 72 units.

Example 9.8

Explain what you would do to fill a medication order for 55 units of NPH insulin.

There are no calculations necessary. You would simply draw 55 units into an insulin syringe as shown in Figure 9.17.

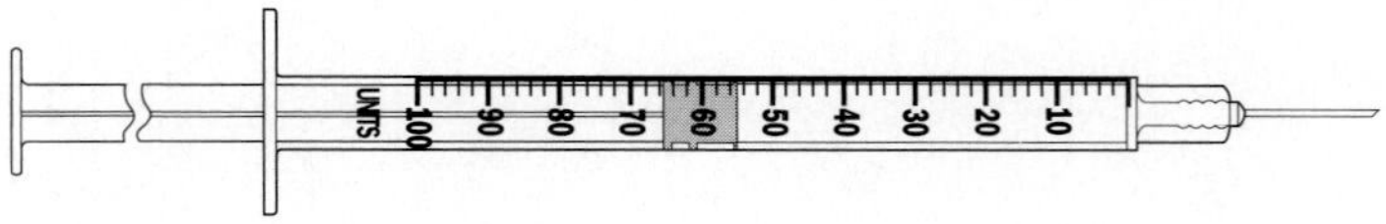

Figure 9.17 *The correctly filled insulin syringe*

Example 9.9

Explain what you would do to fill a medication order for 26 units of Humulin R insulin.

There are no calculations necessary. You would draw 26 units into an insulin syringe as shown in Figure 9.18.

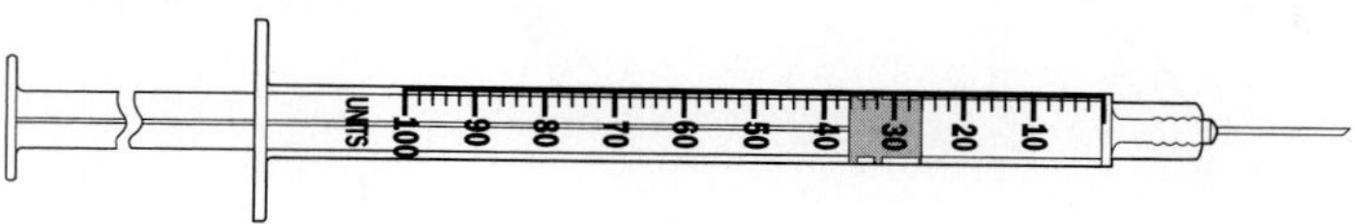

Figure 9.18 *The correctly filled insulin syringe*

Example 9.10

The prescriber ordered 15 units of Humulin R insulin and 45 units of NPH insulin in the same syringe for a total of 60 units sc. Explain how you would fill this order.

You would first draw 15 units of Humulin R insulin into a 100 u insulin syringe and then draw 45 units of NPH insulin into the same syringe as shown in the four steps of Figure 9.19a and 9.19b.

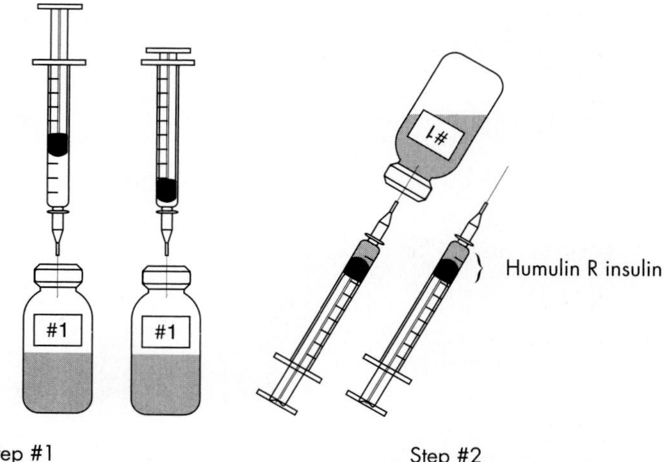

Figure 9.19a *Filling the insulin syringe: Humulin R insulin from vial #1. (See Figure 9.19b on next page.)*

Notes/Workspace

Notes/Workspace

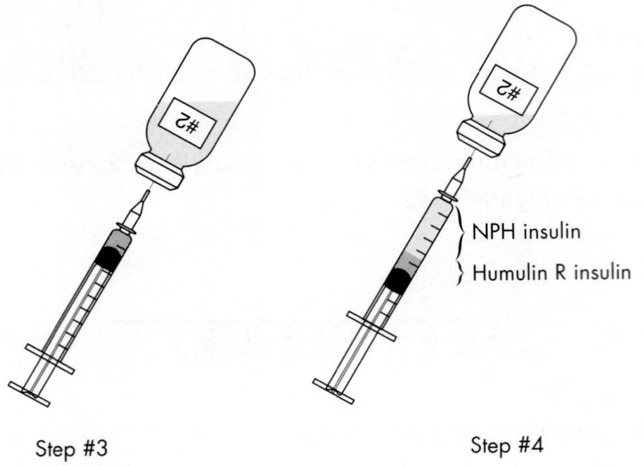

Step #3

Step #4

NPH insulin

Humulin R insulin

Figure 9.19b *The correctly filled insulin syringe: Adding NPH insulin from vial #2.*

By the way

It is recommended that Humulin R insulin be drawn into the syringe first.

Practice Sets

You will find the answers to the Try These for Practice, Exercises, and Cumulative Review Practice Sets in the Answer Section at the back of the book. Your instructor has the answers to the Additional Exercises.

Try These for Practice

Test your comprehension after reading the chapter.

In each of the following problems, identify the type of syringe shown in the figure. Then for each quantity place an arrow at the appropriate level of measurement on the syringe.

1. 3 cc syringe; ♏ 15

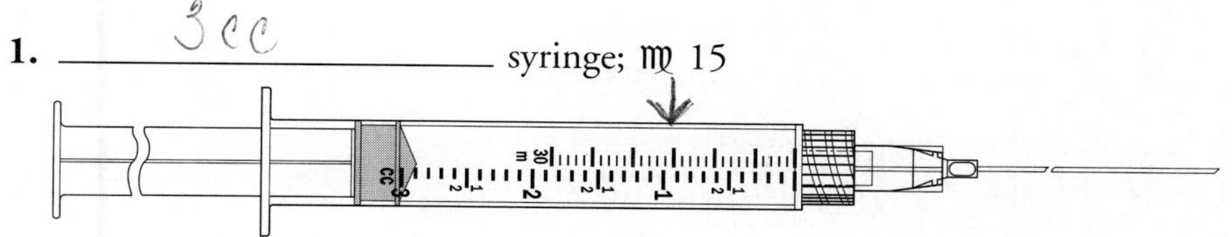

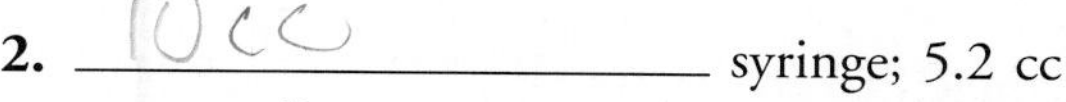

2. 10 cc syringe; 5.2 cc

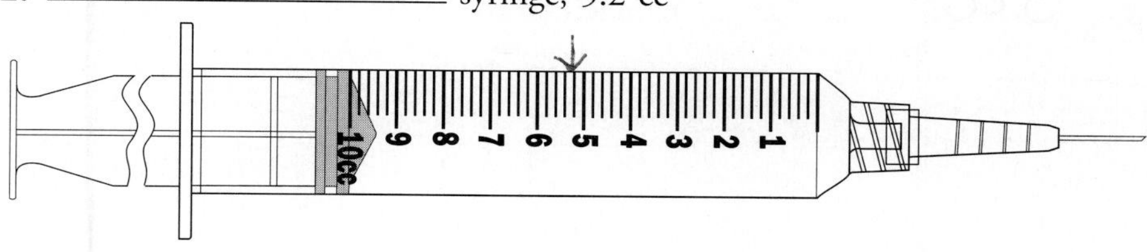

3. Insulin syringe; 12 u

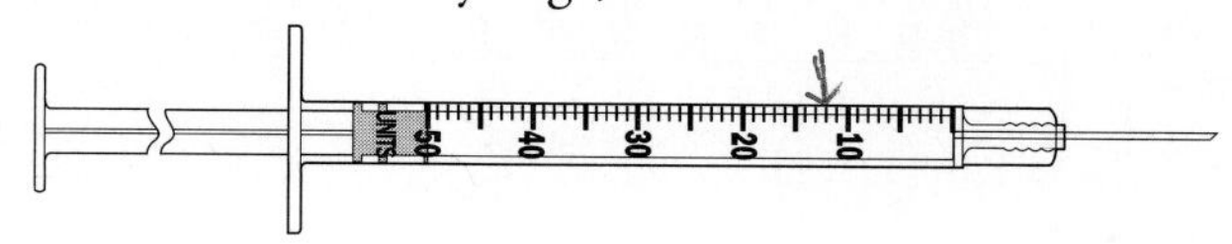

4. Insulin syringe; 22 u

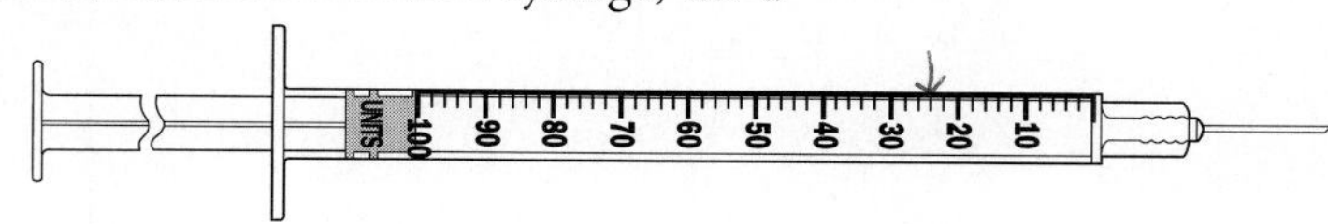

5. TB or Subcutaneous syringe; 0.3 cc

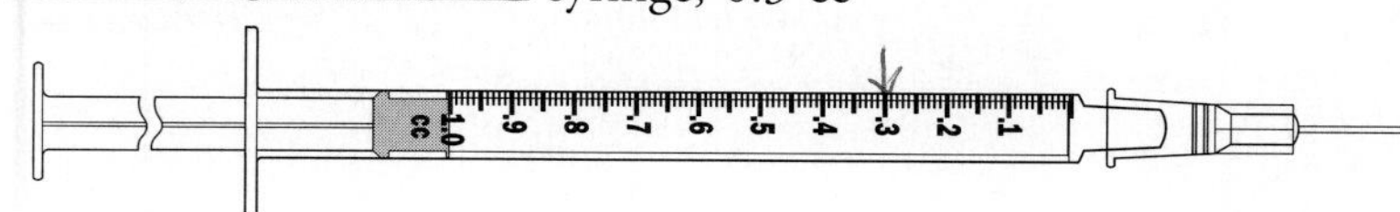

Notes/Workspace

Notes/Workspace

Exercises

Reinforce your understanding in class or at home.

In each of the following problems, identify the type of syringe shown in the figure. Then for each quantity place an arrow at the appropriate level of measurement on the syringe.

1. ______________ syringe; 9.8 cc

2. ______________ syringe; 1.2 cc

3. ______________ syringe; 0.8 mL

4. ______________ syringe; 40 u

5. ______________ syringe; 35 u

6. ______________ syringe; ♏ 8

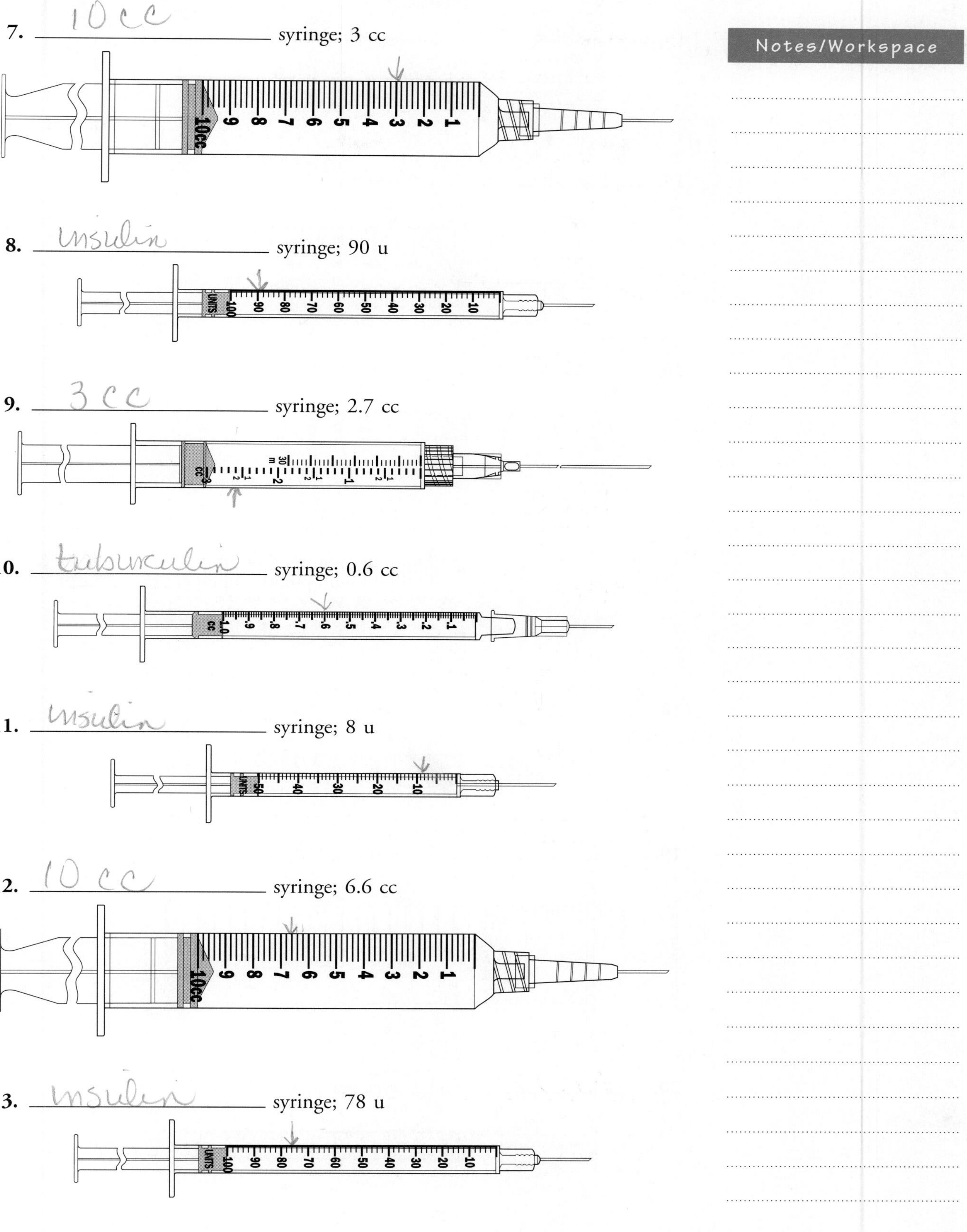

7. 10 cc syringe; 3 cc

8. insulin syringe; 90 u

9. 3 cc syringe; 2.7 cc

10. tuberculin syringe; 0.6 cc

11. insulin syringe; 8 u

12. 10 cc syringe; 6.6 cc

13. insulin syringe; 78 u

Notes/Workspace

Notes/Workspace

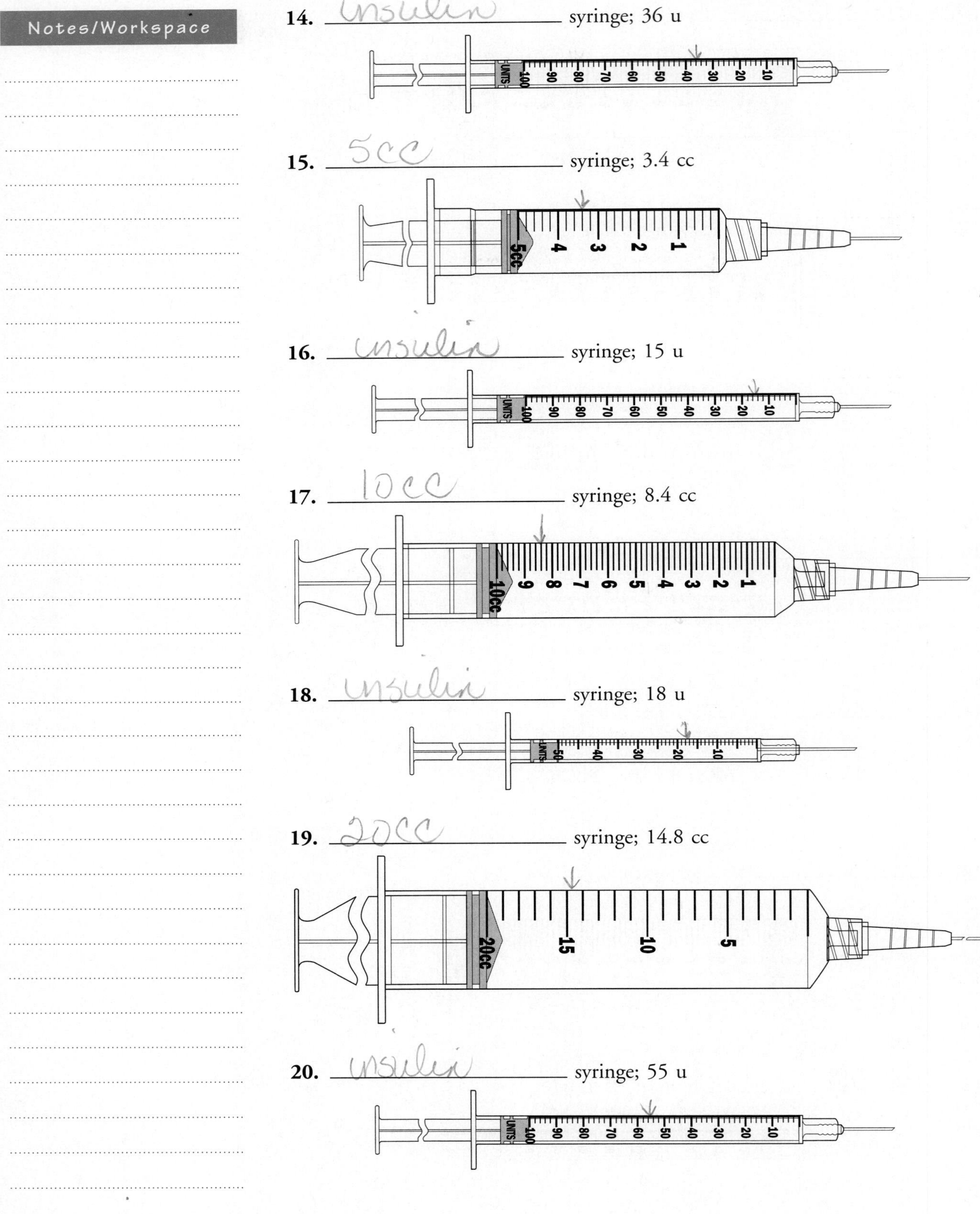

14. [insulin] syringe; 36 u

15. [5cc] syringe; 3.4 cc

16. [insulin] syringe; 15 u

17. [10cc] syringe; 8.4 cc

18. [insulin] syringe; 18 u

19. [20cc] syringe; 14.8 cc

20. [insulin] syringe; 55 u

Additional Exercises

Now, on your own, test yourself! Ask your instructor to check your answers.

In each of the following problems, identify the type of syringe shown in the figure. Then for each quantity place an arrow at the appropriate level of measurement on the syringe.

1. insulin syringe; 42 u

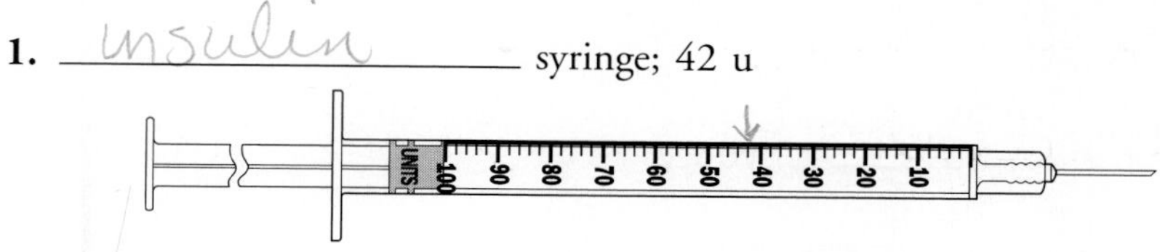

2. insulin syringe; 30 u

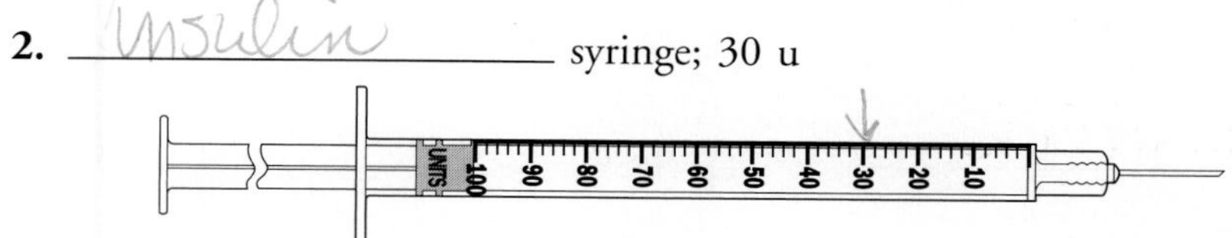

3. 5cc syringe; 3.4 cc

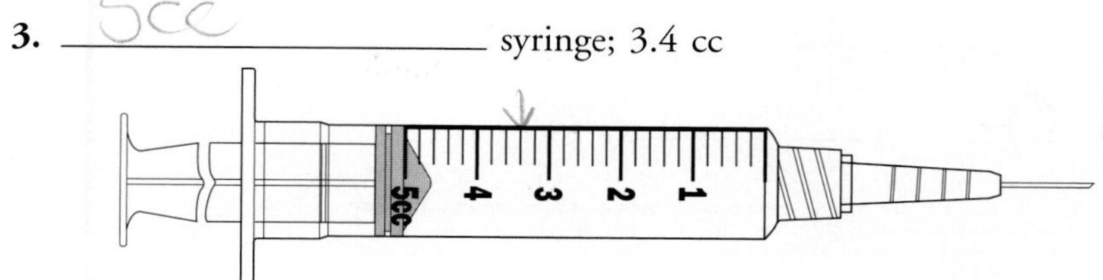

4. 3 cc syringe; 1.6 cc

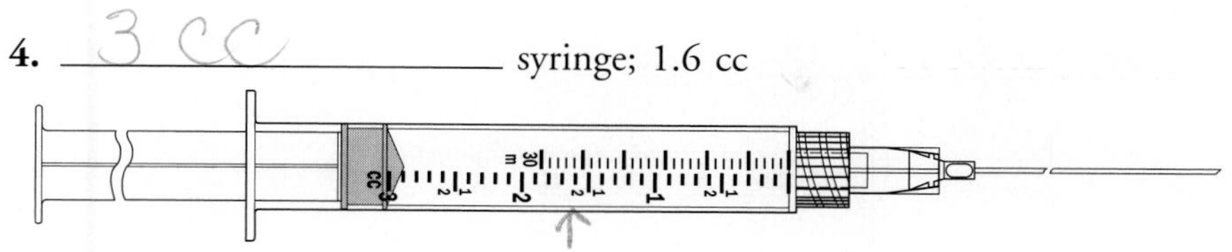

5. 20cc syringe; 11 cc

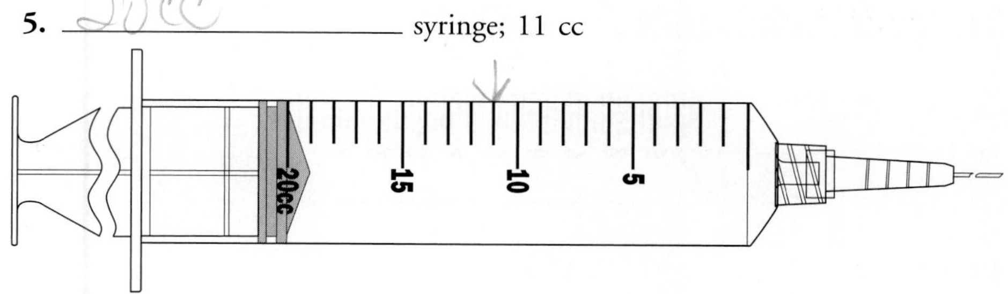

Notes/Workspace

Notes/Workspace

6. 20cc ______________ syringe; 18 cc

7. insulin ______________ syringe; 22 u

8. insulin ______________ syringe; 48 u

9. 1 cc ______________ syringe; 0.4 cc

10. insulin ______________ syringe; 12 u

11. 10cc ______________ syringe; 6.8 cc

Notes/Workspace

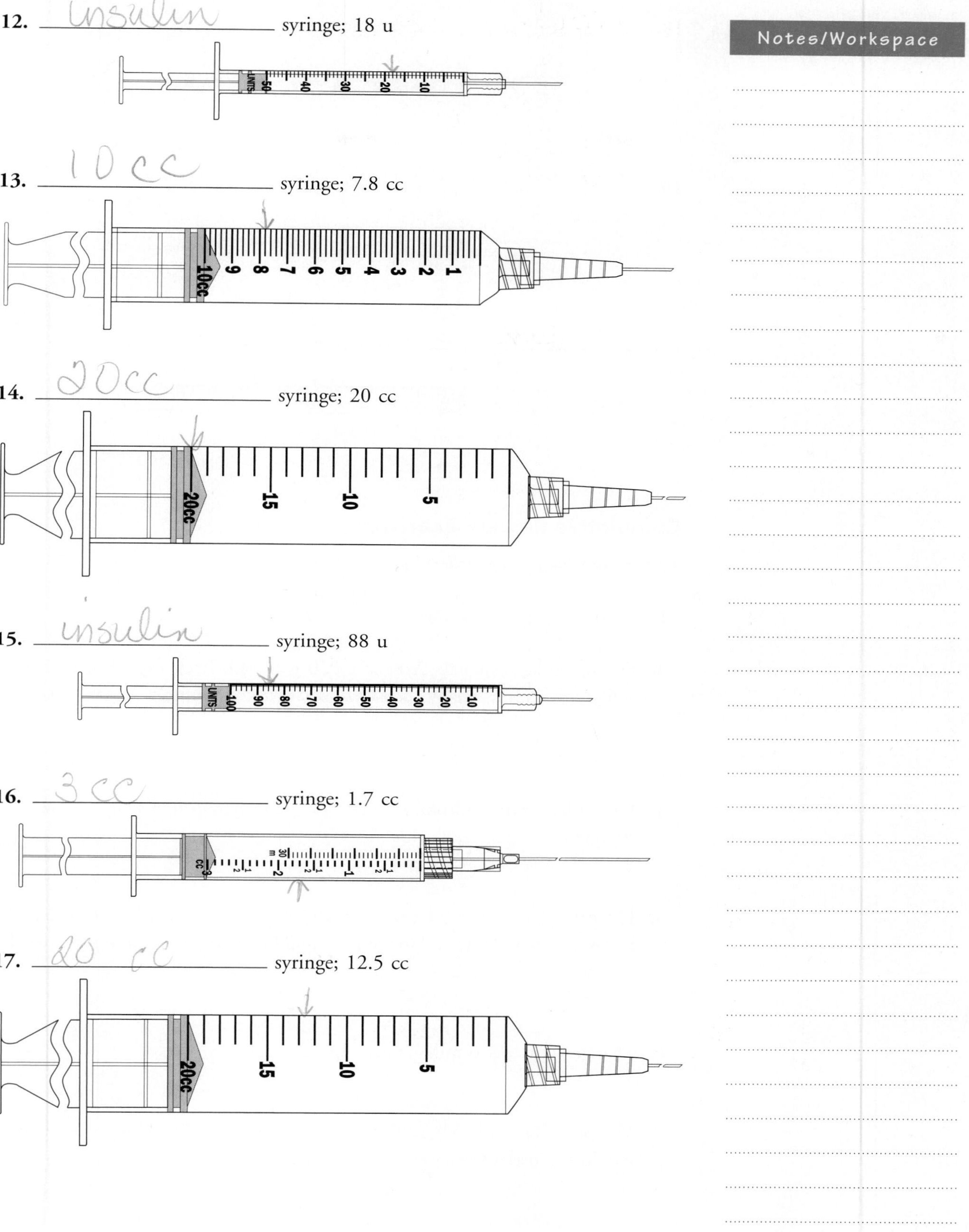

12. insulin syringe; 18 u

13. 10 cc syringe; 7.8 cc

14. 20cc syringe; 20 cc

15. insulin syringe; 88 u

16. 3 cc syringe; 1.7 cc

17. 20 cc syringe; 12.5 cc

Notes/Workspace

18. ______________ syringe; 6 u

19. ______________ syringe; 0.25 cc

20. ______________ syringe; 30 u

Cumulative Review Exercises

Review your mastery of earlier chapters.

1. gr 10 = ________ mg

2. 1200 mL = ________ L

3. The prescriber ordered: Prilosec 0.020 g po qd. Each capsule contains 20 milligrams. How many capsules will you administer to the patient? ________

4. The order reads: morphine sulfate gr $\frac{1}{6}$ IM q4h prn. Change grain $\frac{1}{6}$ to milligrams. ________

5. The prescriber ordered: Ceclor 250 mg po q12h. The label reads 375 milligrams per 5 milliliters. How many milliliters will you administer to the patient? ________

6. Change grain $\frac{1}{240}$ to milligrams. ________

7. The prescriber ordered: 120 mL H_2O po q2h for 12h. How many ounces should the patient receive? ________

8. ʒ 16 = ℥ ________ **9.** 0.6 mg = gr ________

10. 0.004 g = gr ________

11. The prescriber ordered: Feldene 20 mg po qd. Each capsule contains 0.02 gram. How many capsules will you administer to the patient? ________

12. The prescriber ordered 0.3 milligram of clonidine hydrochloride. If each tablet contains 0.1 milligram, how many tablets will you administer to the patient? ________

13. Read the information on the label in Figure 9.20 and calculate the number of tablets equal to 0.6 gram. ________

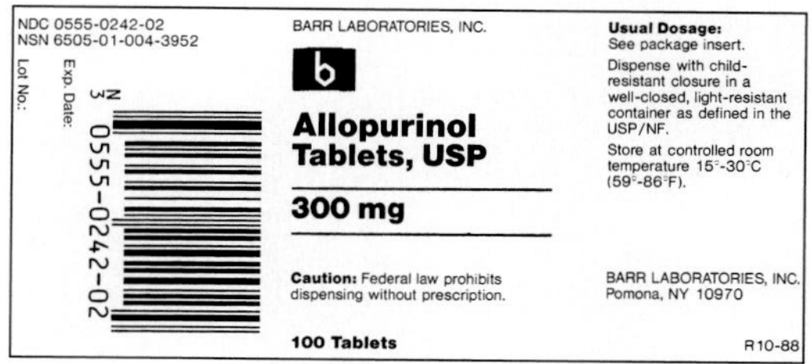

NDC 0555-0242-02
NSN 6505-01-004-3952
BARR LABORATORIES, INC.
b
Allopurinol Tablets, USP
300 mg
Caution: Federal law prohibits dispensing without prescription.
100 Tablets
Usual Dosage: See package insert.
Dispense with child-resistant closure in a well-closed, light-resistant container as defined in the USP/NF.
Store at controlled room temperature 15°-30°C (59°-86°F).
BARR LABORATORIES, INC. Pomona, NY 10970
R10-88
Lot No.:
Exp. Date:
N 3 0555-0242-02

Figure 9.20 *Drug label for allopurinol*

14. Each tablet of haloperidol in Figure 9.21 contains 0.5 milligram. Calculate the number of tablets required to make 2 milligrams. ________

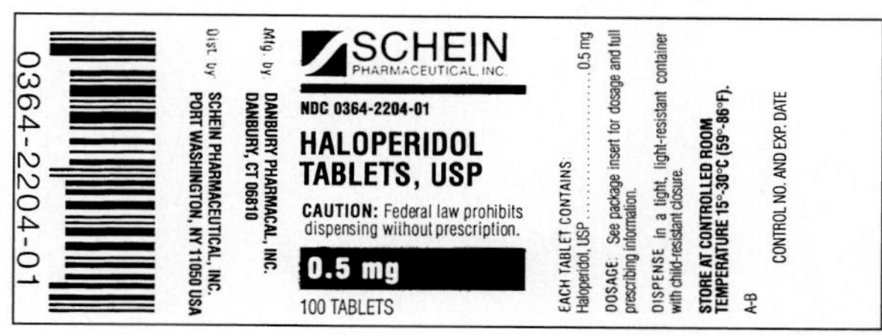

0364-2204-01
Dist. by SCHEIN PHARMACEUTICAL, INC. PORT WASHINGTON, NY 11050 USA
Mfg. by DANBURY PHARMACAL, INC. DANBURY, CT 06810
SCHEIN PHARMACEUTICAL, INC.
NDC 0364-2204-01
HALOPERIDOL TABLETS, USP
CAUTION: Federal law prohibits dispensing without prescription.
0.5 mg
100 TABLETS
EACH TABLET CONTAINS Haloperidol, USP .... 0.5 mg
DOSAGE: See package insert for dosage and full prescribing information.
DISPENSE in a tight, light-resistant container with child-resistant closure.
STORE AT CONTROLLED ROOM TEMPERATURE 15°-30°C (59°-86°F).
A-B
CONTROL NO. AND EXP. DATE

Figure 9.21 *Drug label for haloperidol*

Notes/Workspace

Notes/Workspace

15. The prescriber ordered:

Moderil 500 μg po qd

Read the label in Figure 9.22. How many tablets equal 500 micrograms? ________

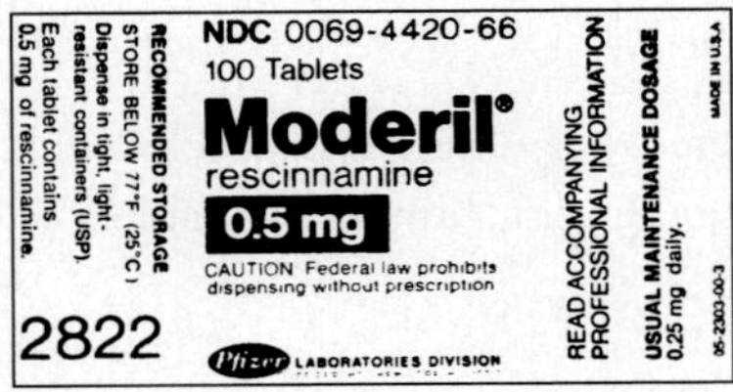
RECOMMENDED STORAGE
STORE BELOW 77°F (25°C)
Dispense in tight, light-resistant containers (USP).
Each tablet contains 0.5 mg of rescinnamine.
2822
NDC 0069-4420-66
100 Tablets
Moderil®
rescinnamine
0.5 mg
CAUTION Federal law prohibits dispensing without prescription
Pfizer LABORATORIES DIVISION
READ ACCOMPANYING PROFESSIONAL INFORMATION
USUAL MAINTENANCE DOSAGE
0.25 mg daily.
MADE IN U.S.A.
05-2303-00-3

Figure 9.22 *Drug label for Moderil*

chapter 10

Parenteral Medications

Objectives

After completing this chapter, you will be able to

- *do the calculations necessary to prepare medications for injection from drugs supplied in liquid form in vials and ampules.*
- *do the calculations necessary to prepare medications for injection from drugs supplied in powdered form in vials.*
- *do calculations involving units.*

Parenteral medications are supplied in sterile liquid form in vials and ampules (Figure 10.1). They can also be supplied in powdered form in a sealed vial or ampule. Powdered drugs must be dissolved in sterile water or 0.9% sodium chloride (normal saline) prior to injection. This chapter introduces you to the calculations you will use to administer parenteral medications safely.

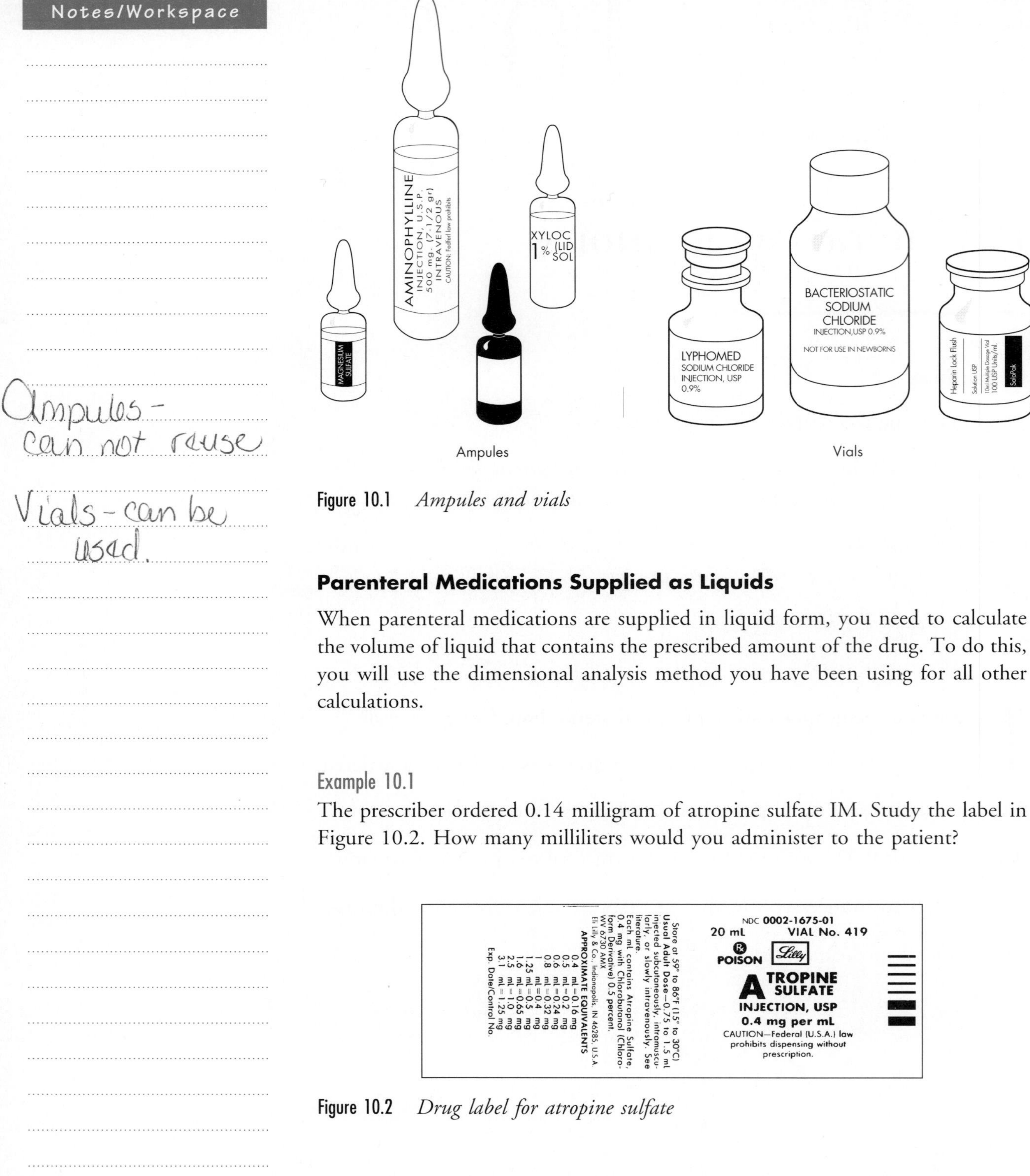

Ampules - can not reuse

Vials - can be used.

Figure 10.1 *Ampules and vials*

Parenteral Medications Supplied as Liquids

When parenteral medications are supplied in liquid form, you need to calculate the volume of liquid that contains the prescribed amount of the drug. To do this, you will use the dimensional analysis method you have been using for all other calculations.

Example 10.1

The prescriber ordered 0.14 milligram of atropine sulfate IM. Study the label in Figure 10.2. How many milliliters would you administer to the patient?

Figure 10.2 *Drug label for atropine sulfate*

Notes/Workspace

Begin by finding out how many milliliters of the liquid in the ampule contains the prescribed quantity of the drug (0.14 milligram of atropine sulfate). That is, you want to convert 0.14 milligram to an equivalent in milliliters.

$$0.14 \text{ mg} = ? \text{ mL}$$

You cancel the milligrams and obtain the equivalent quantity in milliliters.

$$0.14 \text{ mg} \times \frac{? \text{ mL}}{? \text{ mg}} = ? \text{ mL}$$

The label reads 0.4 milligram per milliliter, which means 0.4 mg = 1 mL. So the equivalent fraction is $\frac{1 \text{ mL}}{0.4 \text{ mg}}$.

$$0.14 \cancel{\text{mg}} \times \frac{1 \text{ mL}}{0.4 \cancel{\text{mg}}} = \frac{0.14}{0.4} \text{ mL} = 0.35 \text{ mL}$$

So 0.35 milliliter contains 0.14 milligram of atropine sulfate, and you would administer 0.35 milliliter of the drug to your patient.

Example 10.2

A drug vial reads 2500 milligrams per minims 150. How many minims would you administer if the medication order reads 500 milligrams IM of the drug?

You want to convert the order (500 milligrams) to its equivalent in minims.

$$500 \text{ mg} = \text{♏} \ ?$$

You cancel the milligrams and obtain the equivalent amount in minims.

$$500 \text{ mg} \times \frac{\text{♏} \ ?}{? \text{ mg}} = \text{♏} \ ?$$

The label reads 2500 milligrams per minims 150. So the equivalent fraction is $\frac{\text{♏ } 150}{2500 \text{ mg}}$.

$$\overset{1}{\cancel{500 \text{ mg}}} \times \frac{\text{♏ } 150}{\underset{5}{\cancel{2500 \text{ mg}}}} = \text{♏} \frac{150}{5} = \text{♏ } 30$$

So minims 30 contains 500 milligrams, and you would administer minims 30 IM of the drug to your patient.

Example 10.3

The prescriber ordered 0.004 gram of hydromorphone HCl (Dilaudid) IM. Read the label in Figure 10.3 and calculate how many milliliters of this narcotic you would administer.

Notes/Workspace

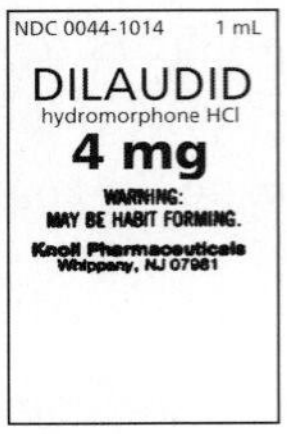

NDC 0044-1014 1 mL
DILAUDID
hydromorphone HCl
4 mg
WARNING:
MAY BE HABIT FORMING.
Knoll Pharmaceuticals
Whippany, NJ 07981

Figure 10.3 *Drug label for Dilaudid*

The label shows Dilaudid in milligrams per milliliter, so you want to convert 0.004 gram to its equivalent in milligrams and then change milligrams to milliliters.

$$0.004 \text{ g} \rightarrow \text{? mg} \rightarrow \text{? mL}$$

Do this on one line as follows:

$$0.004 \text{ g} \times \frac{\text{? mg}}{\text{? g}} \times \frac{\text{? mL}}{\text{? mg}} = \text{? mL}$$

The first equivalent fraction is $\frac{1000 \text{ mg}}{1 \text{ g}}$.

The label reads 4 milligrams per milliliter, which means 4 mg = 1 mL. So the second fraction is $\frac{1 \text{ mL}}{4 \text{ mg}}$.

$$0.004 \cancel{\text{g}} \times \frac{1000 \cancel{\text{mg}}}{1 \cancel{\text{g}}} \times \frac{1 \text{ mL}}{4 \cancel{\text{mg}}} = 1 \text{ mL}$$

You would administer 1 milliliter of hydromorphone HCl IM, which would contain 0.004 gram of hydromorphone HCl.

Example 10.4

The medication order reads 0.9 milligram of naloxone HCl (Narcan) IV. Read the label in Figure 10.4 and calculate how much of this narcotic antagonist you would administer.

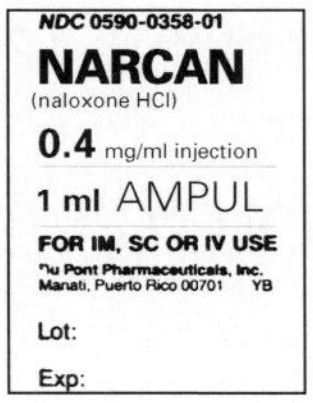

NDC 0590-0358-01
NARCAN
(naloxone HCl)
0.4 mg/ml injection
1 ml AMPUL
FOR IM, SC OR IV USE
Du Pont Pharmaceuticals, Inc.
Manati, Puerto Rico 00701 YB
Lot:
Exp:

Figure 10.4 *Drug label for Narcan*

Notes/Workspace

Because this drug is available in milligrams per milliliter, you want to convert the order (0.9 milligram) to its equivalent in milliliters.

$$0.9 \text{ mg} = ? \text{ mL}$$

You cancel the milligrams and obtain the equivalent amount in milliliters.

$$0.9 \text{ mg} \times \frac{? \text{ mL}}{? \text{ mg}} = ? \text{ mL}$$

Since the label reads 0.4 milligram per milliliter, you use the equivalent fraction $\frac{1 \text{ mL}}{0.4 \text{ mg}}$.

$$0.9 \cancel{\text{mg}} \times \frac{1 \text{ mL}}{0.4 \cancel{\text{mg}}} = \frac{0.9}{0.4} \text{ mL} = 2.25 \text{ mL}$$

So 2.25 milliliters contain 0.9 milligram of Narcan, and you would administer 2.25 milliliters IV to your patient.

Example 10.5

Mr. Jones is to receive grain $\frac{1}{600}$ of atropine sulfate sc. The ampule of liquid is labeled grain $\frac{1}{150}$ per minims 15. How many minims of this anticholinergic drug should be administered to the patient?

You want to convert the order of grain $\frac{1}{600}$ to its equivalent in minims.

$$\text{gr } \frac{1}{600} = ♏ \ ?$$

You cancel the grains and obtain the equivalent amount in minims.

$$\text{gr } \frac{1}{600} \times \frac{♏ \ ?}{\text{gr } ?} = ♏ \ ?$$

Because the label on the ampule reads grain $\frac{1}{150}$ per minims 15, the equivalent fraction is $\frac{♏ \ 15}{\text{gr } \frac{1}{150}}$.

$$\cancel{\text{gr}} \frac{1}{600} \times \frac{♏ \ 15}{\cancel{\text{gr}} \frac{1}{150}} = ♏ \ \frac{1 \times 15}{\frac{600}{150}} = ♏ \ \frac{15}{4} = ♏ \ 3\frac{3}{4}$$ = 4 minums

Do round to minums.

So minims $3\frac{3}{4}$ of this solution contains grain $\frac{1}{600}$ of atropine sulfate. Normally, you would give the patient minims 4, since three-fourths of a minim is too small to measure into the syringe (Figure 10.5).

Notes/Workspace

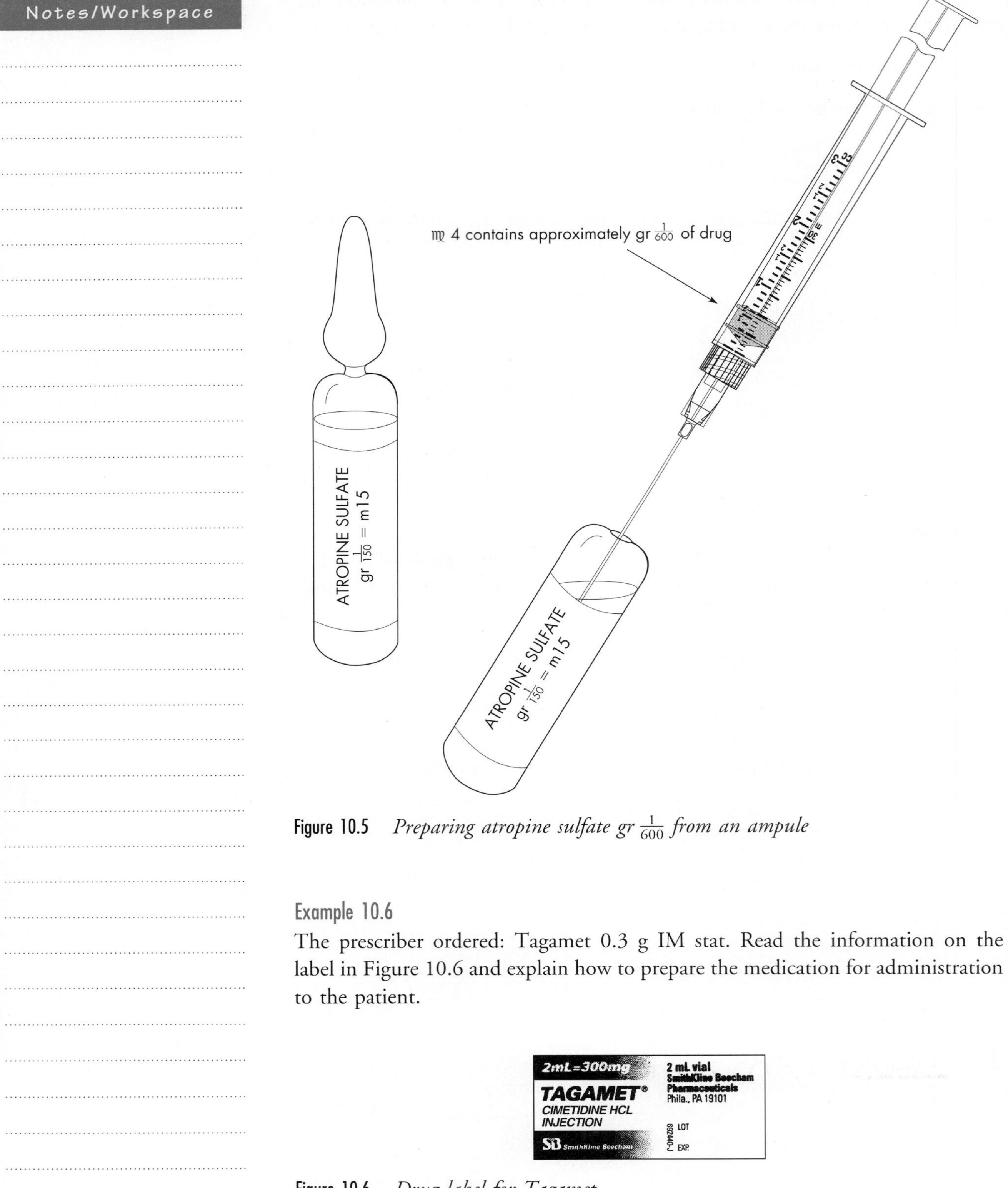

♏ 4 contains approximately gr $\frac{1}{600}$ of drug
ATROPINE SULFATE
gr $\frac{1}{150}$ = m15
ATROPINE SULFATE
gr $\frac{1}{150}$ = m15
2mL=300mg
TAGAMET®
CIMETIDINE HCL
INJECTION
SB SmithKline Beecham
2 mL vial
SmithKline Beecham
Pharmaceuticals
Phila., PA 19101
LOT
EXP.

Figure 10.5 *Preparing atropine sulfate gr $\frac{1}{600}$ from an ampule*

Example 10.6

The prescriber ordered: Tagamet 0.3 g IM stat. Read the information on the label in Figure 10.6 and explain how to prepare the medication for administration to the patient.

Figure 10.6 *Drug label for Tagamet*

Notes/Workspace

Because the vial contains medication measured in milligrams per milliliter, you want to convert 0.3 gram to milligrams and then find the amount in milliliters.

$$0.3 \text{ g} \rightarrow ? \text{ mg} \rightarrow ? \text{ mL}$$

$$0.3 \text{ g} \times \frac{? \text{ mg}}{? \text{ g}} \times \frac{? \text{ mL}}{? \text{ mg}} = ? \text{ mL}$$

The first equivalent fraction is $\frac{1000 \text{ mg}}{1 \text{ g}}$.

The label reads 300 milligrams per 2 milliliters, so the second equivalent fraction is $\frac{2 \text{ mL}}{300 \text{ mg}}$.

$$0.3 \cancel{\text{g}} \times \frac{\overset{10}{\cancel{1000 \text{ mg}}}}{1 \cancel{\text{g}}} \times \frac{2 \text{ mL}}{\underset{3}{\cancel{300 \text{ mg}}}} = 2 \text{ mL}$$

So 2 milliliters contains 0.3 gram of Tagamet, and you would administer 2 milliliters IM to your patient.

Example 10.7

Examine the label in Figure 10.7 and determine the quantity of solution to be withdrawn from the vial if the medication order reads 250 milligrams of 10% calcium chloride.

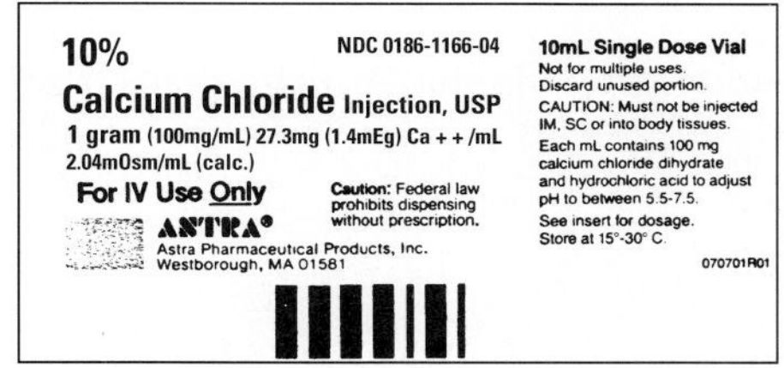
10%
NDC 0186-1166-04
Calcium Chloride Injection, USP
1 gram (100mg/mL) 27.3mg (1.4mEg) Ca + + /mL
2.04mOsm/mL (calc.)
For IV Use Only
Caution: Federal law prohibits dispensing without prescription.
ASTRA®
Astra Pharmaceutical Products, Inc.
Westborough, MA 01581
10mL Single Dose Vial
Not for multiple uses.
Discard unused portion.
CAUTION: Must not be injected IM, SC or into body tissues.
Each mL contains 100 mg calcium chloride dihydrate and hydrochloric acid to adjust pH to between 5.5-7.5.
See insert for dosage.
Store at 15°-30° C.
070701R01

Figure 10.7 *Drug label for calcium chloride*

You want to convert milligrams to milliliters.

$$250 \text{ mg} \rightarrow ? \text{ mL}$$

$$250 \text{ mg} \times \frac{? \text{ mL}}{? \text{ mg}} = ? \text{ mL}$$

The label 10% calcium chloride means that 10 grams of calcium chloride are in 100 milliliters, or 100 milligrams of calcium chloride are in 1 milliliter. So the equivalent fraction is $\frac{1 \text{ mL}}{100 \text{ mg}}$.

$$\overset{5}{\cancel{250 \text{ mg}}} \times \frac{1 \text{ mL}}{\underset{2}{\cancel{100 \text{ mg}}}} = 2.5 \text{ mL}$$

Notes/Workspace

So you would withdraw 2.5 milliliters from the vial.

Example 10.8

The prescriber ordered 40 units of NPH insulin (Humulin N) sc for a patient, and you must use a standard syringe since no insulin syringe is available. What would the dose be in milliliters? The label on the vial is shown in Figure 10.8.

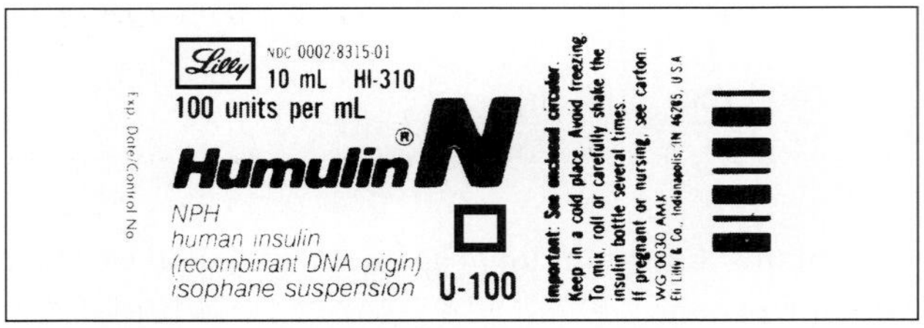

Figure 10.8 *Drug label for Humulin N*

You want to convert 40 units to milliliters.

$$40 \text{ u} = ?\text{ mL}$$

You cancel the units and obtain the equivalent amount in milliliters.

$$40 \text{ u} \times \frac{?\text{ mL}}{?\text{ u}} = ?\text{ mL}$$

The label reads 100 units per milliliter, which means 100 u = 1 mL. So the equivalent fraction is $\frac{1\text{ mL}}{100\text{ u}}$.

$$\overset{4}{\cancel{40}}\ \cancel{\text{u}} \times \frac{1\text{ mL}}{\underset{10}{\cancel{100}}\ \cancel{\text{u}}} = 0.4\text{ mL}$$

So 40 units would be contained in 0.4 milliliter, and you would draw 0.4 milliliter into the standard syringe.

Heparin

Heparin is an anticoagulant (clot-preventing) medication that can be administered to a patient by subcutaneous injection, intermittent intravenous injection, and by continuous intravenous infusion. Like insulin, penicillin, and some other medications, heparin is supplied in *USP units*, which are often shortened (as noted in Chapter 9) to *units* and abbreviated u. Vials of heparin are prepared by the manufacturer in a variety of strengths. Some examples of heparin preparations are shown in Table 10.1.

Notes/Workspace

Table 10.1 *USP Unit Potencies of Heparin*

Supplied Form	Potency per mL
Vials	1000 units
	5000 units
	20,000 units
	40,000 units
Ampules	1000 units
	5000 units
	10,000 units

Heparin is also available in premixed intravenous solutions—for example, 12,500 units in 250 milliliters of 5% D/W; 25,000 units in 500 milliliters of 0.45% saline solution. With a premixed parenteral solution, the nurse has to convert the physician's order to the volume of solution that contains the amount of heparin ordered.

Example 10.9

The prescriber ordered:

heparin 5000 u sc q12h

The label on the vial (Figure 10.9) reads 10,000 units per milliliter. How many milliliters will you administer to the patient?

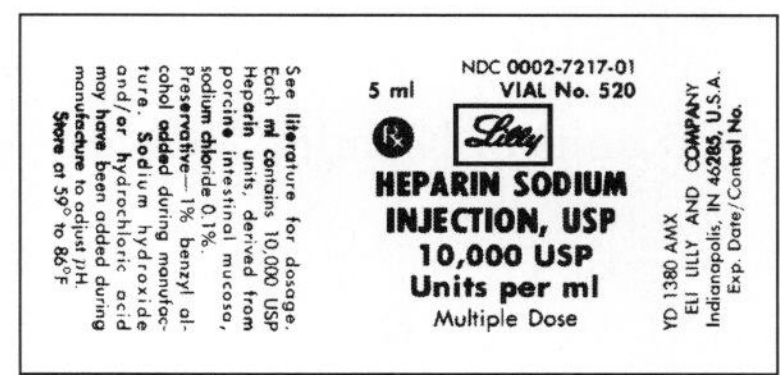

Figure 10.9 *Drug label for heparin*

You want to convert units to milliliters.

$$5000 \text{ u} = ? \text{ mL}$$

You cancel the units and obtain the equivalent amount in milliliters.

$$5000 \text{ u} \times \frac{? \text{ mL}}{? \text{ u}} = ? \text{ mL}$$

Notes/Workspace

The label on the vial reads 10,000 units per milliliter, so the equivalent fraction is $\frac{1\text{ mL}}{10{,}000\text{ u}}$.

$$\overset{1}{\cancel{5000\text{ u}}} \times \frac{1\text{ mL}}{\underset{2}{\cancel{10{,}000\text{ u}}}} = 0.5\text{ mL}$$

So 0.5 milliliter contains 10,000 units of heparin, and you would administer 0.5 milliliter to the patient sc.

Example 10.10

The prescriber ordered:

heparin 8000 u sc q8h

If the label on the drug vial reads 10,000 units per minims 15, how many minims equal 8000 units?

You want to convert 8000 units to minims.

$$8000\text{ u} = \text{♏ } ?$$

You cancel the units and obtain the equivalent amount in minims.

$$8000\text{ u} \times \frac{\text{♏ } ?}{?\text{ u}} = \text{♏ } ?$$

The label on the vial reads 10,000 units per minims 15, so the fraction is $\frac{\text{♏ } 15}{10{,}000\text{ u}}$.

$$\overset{8}{\cancel{8000\text{ u}}} \times \frac{\text{♏ } 15}{\underset{10}{\cancel{10{,}000\text{ u}}}} = \frac{\text{♏ } 120}{10} = \text{♏ } 12$$

So minims 12 contains 8000 units of heparin, and you would administer minims 12 sc to your patient.

Parenteral Medications Supplied in Powdered Form

Some parenteral medications are supplied in powdered form in sealed vials (Figure 10.10). The powder cannot be removed from these vials. You must add sterile water or saline to the vial and dissolve the powder to form a solution. You then inject the liquid volume of prepared solution that contains the proper amount of the drug.

Notes/Workspace

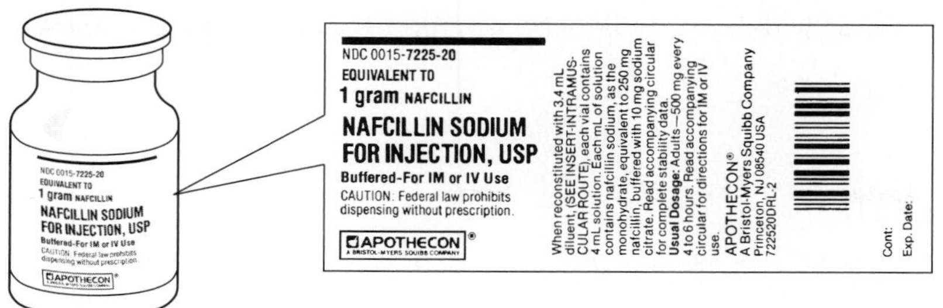

Figure 10.10 *A sealed vial of nafcillin sodium in powdered form with label detail*

The pharmaceutical manufacturer provides instructions that specify the amount of sterile liquid that must be injected into the vial of powder to make a solution of a given strength. After preparing the solution, you need to calculate the volume that contains the prescribed amount of the drug.

Example 10.11

The prescriber ordered 100 milligrams of cyclophosphamide (Cytoxan) IV. Read the label shown in Figure 10.11. How would you prepare this dose?

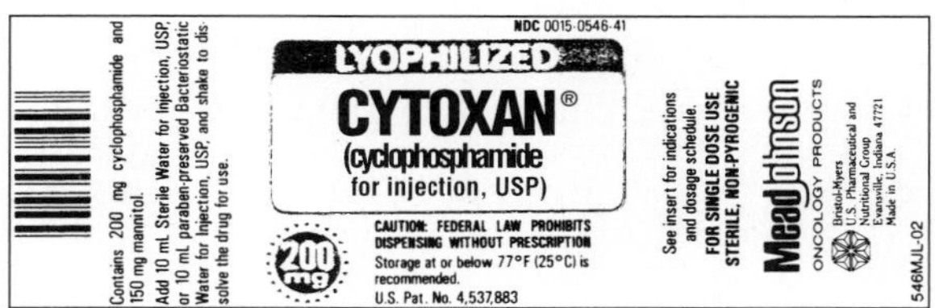

Figure 10.11 *Drug label for Cytoxan*

First, follow the instructions on the label to prepare the solution. Inject 10 milliliters of sterile water into the vial. Now the vial contains a solution in which

$$10 \text{ mL} = 200 \text{ mg}$$

To calculate the amount of this solution, you need to convert milligrams to milliliters.

$$100 \text{ mg} \times \frac{? \text{ mL}}{? \text{ mg}} = ? \text{ mL}$$

The vial now contains 200 milligrams per 10 milliliters, so the equivalent fraction is $\frac{10 \text{ mL}}{200 \text{ mg}}$.

$$\overset{1}{\cancel{100 \text{ mg}}} \times \frac{10 \text{ mL}}{\underset{2}{\cancel{200 \text{ mg}}}} = 5 \text{ mL}$$

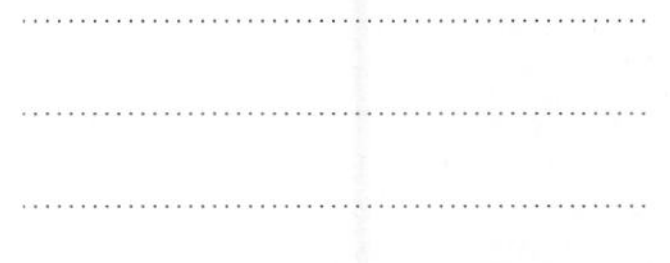

Notes/Workspace

So you would withdraw 5 milliliters from the vial and administer it to the patient.

Example 10.12

The prescriber has ordered 0.25 gram of the antibiotic ampicillin sodium (Polycillin-N). The label on the vial reads 250 milligrams per milliliter. How many milliliters of the solution would contain the prescribed dose?

You want to convert 0.25 gram to milliliters. This is a two-step problem.

$$0.25 \text{ g} \rightarrow ? \text{ mg} \rightarrow ? \text{ mL}$$

$$0.25 \text{ g} \times \frac{? \text{ mg}}{? \text{ g}} \times \frac{? \text{ mL}}{? \text{ mg}} = ? \text{ mL}$$

The first equivalent fraction is $\frac{1000 \text{ mg}}{1 \text{ g}}$.

Since the prepared solution is 1 mL = 250 mg, the second equivalent fraction is $\frac{1 \text{ mL}}{250 \text{ mg}}$.

$$0.25 \cancel{\text{g}} \times \frac{\overset{4}{\cancel{1000 \text{ mg}}}}{1 \cancel{\text{g}}} \times \frac{1 \text{ mL}}{\underset{1}{\cancel{250 \text{ mg}}}} = 1 \text{ mL}$$

So 1 milliliter of the solution contains 0.25 gram of ampicillin sodium.

Example 10.13

The prescriber ordered: cefoxitin sodium 0.75 g IM q12h. The vial of cefoxitin sodium, an antibiotic, contains 5 grams of powder. The instructions are as follows: Add 13.2 mL of sterile water to the vial, 3 mL = 1 g. How many milliliters of the solution would contain the prescribed dose?

You want to change 0.75 gram to milliliters.

$$0.75 \text{ g} \times \frac{? \text{ mL}}{? \text{ g}} = ? \text{ mL}$$

Since the prepared solution is 3 mL = 1 g, the equivalent fraction is $\frac{3 \text{ mL}}{1 \text{ g}}$.

$$0.75 \cancel{\text{g}} \times \frac{3 \text{ mL}}{1 \cancel{\text{g}}} = 2.25 \text{ mL}$$

So 2.25 milliliters of the prepared solution contains 0.75 gram of cefoxitin sodium.

Practice Sets

You will find the answers to the Try These for Practice, Exercises, and Cumulative Review Practice Sets in the Answer Section at the back of the book. Your instructor has the answers to the Additional Exercises.

Try These for Practice

Test your comprehension after reading the chapter.

1. The prescriber ordered: cefazolin sodium 0.44 g IM q8h. The directions state: Add 2.5 mL of sterile water to a vial labeled 1 g, 1 mL = 330 mg. How many milliliters equal 0.44 gram? ________

2. The prescriber ordered: low-dose insulin 0.54 u/kg sc qd. The label on the vial reads 100 units per milliliter. How many milliliters will you give your patient whose weight is 50 kilograms? ________

3. Your patient is to receive grain $\frac{1}{400}$ of atropine sulfate. The label on the vial reads 0.1 milligram per milliliter. How many milliliters equal grain $\frac{1}{400}$? ________

4. An ampule of digoxin is labeled 0.125 milligram per milliliter. How many milliliters equal 0.25 milligram? ________

5. If your patient's medication order is for 5000 units of heparin and the vial is labeled 10,000 units per milliliter, how many minims equal 5000 units? ________

Exercises

Reinforce your understanding in class or at home.

1. A patient is to receive 25 units of the hormonal drug vasopressin (Pitressin) IM. If the label reads 50 units per 2 milliliters, how many milliliters will you administer to the patient? ________

Notes/Workspace

Notes/Workspace

2. The order reads: calcitonin 2 u/kg sc daily. The label reads 100 units per milliliter. How many milliliters will you administer to the patient if the weight of the patient is 64 kilograms? ________

3. The order reads: amitriptyline HCl 0.03 g IM tid. If the drug vial is labeled 10 milligrams per milliliter, how many milliliters will you prepare for the patient? ________

4. The prescriber ordered: cefoxitin sodium 500 mg IM q6h. The instructions state: Add 5 mL of sterile water to 1 g vial, 1 mL = 400 mg. How many milliliters will equal 500 milligrams? ________

5. Read the first medication order in Figure 10.12. The vial of furosemide is labeled 10 milligrams per milliliter. How many milliliters would you prepare for a patient who weighs 45 kilograms? ________

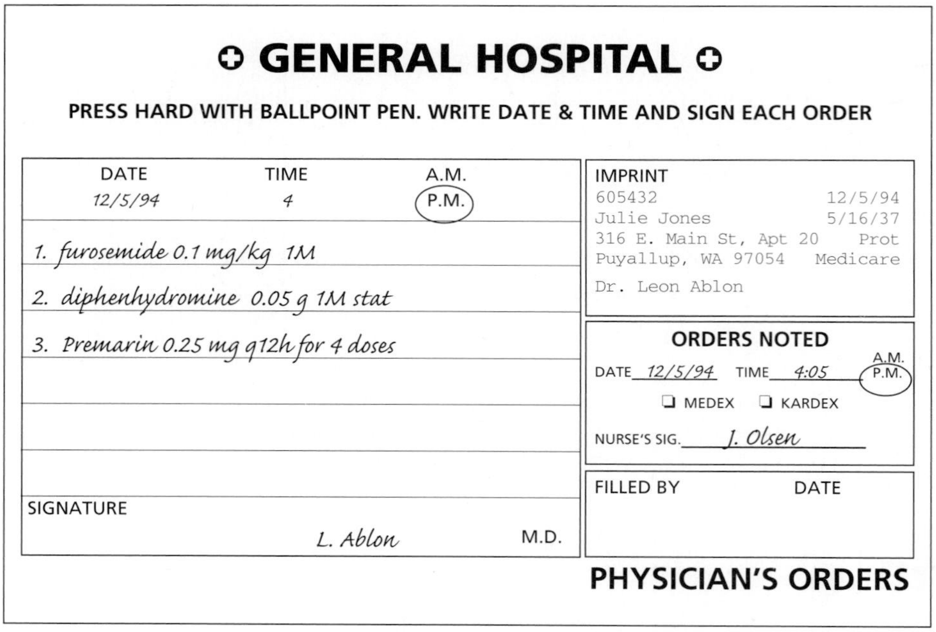

GENERAL HOSPITAL

PRESS HARD WITH BALLPOINT PEN. WRITE DATE & TIME AND SIGN EACH ORDER

DATE	TIME	A.M. / P.M.
12/5/94	4	P.M. (circled)
1. *furosemide 0.1 mg/kg 1M*		
2. *diphenhydromine 0.05 g 1M stat*		
3. *Premarin 0.25 mg q12h for 4 doses*		
SIGNATURE	*L. Ablon*	M.D.

IMPRINT
605432 12/5/94
Julie Jones 5/16/37
316 E. Main St, Apt 20 Prot
Puyallup, WA 97054 Medicare
Dr. Leon Ablon

ORDERS NOTED
DATE *12/5/94* TIME *4:05* A.M. P.M. (circled)
❑ MEDEX ❑ KARDEX
NURSE'S SIG. *J. Olsen*

FILLED BY DATE

PHYSICIAN'S ORDERS

Figure 10.12 *Physician's order sheet*

6. In the second medication order in Figure 10.12, the patient must receive 0.05 gram of the antihistamine diphenhydramine (Benadryl) IM stat. The vial is labeled 50 milligrams per milliliter. How many milliliters will you administer to this patient? ________

Notes/Workspace

7. Read the information in the third medication order in Figure 10.12. If the vial of Premarin is labeled 0.025 gram per 5 milliliters, how many milliliters equal the prescribed single dose? _________

8. The dose of dobutamine (Dobutrex) ordered by the prescriber is 100 micrograms per kilogram. If the patient weighs 75 kilograms and the vial is labeled 12.5 milligrams per milliliter, how many milliliters would you prepare? _________

9. The order reads: cosyntropin 0.5 mg IM once only. The vial is labeled 0.25 milligram per milliliter. Calculate the amount in milliliters required for this dose. _________

10. The label on the vial of verapamil HCl reads 10 milligrams per 4 milliliters. If the medication order is 7.5 milligrams, calculate the amount in milliliters you would prepare for this patient. _________

11. The label on a vial reads: penicillin G 1,000,000 u. The instructions are as follows: Add 19.6 mL of sterile diluent to vial, 1 mL = 50,000 u. How many milliliters contain 100,000 units? _________

12. The prescriber ordered: Dolophine HCl 0.015 g IM q4h prn. Read the label in Figure 10.13. How many milliliters will you prepare for this patient? _________

1 mL POISON No. 456 CII
DOLOPHINE®
HCl
METHADONE
HCl 10 mg
Sub. Q. or I.M.
YU 6001 AMU
LILLY, INDPLS.

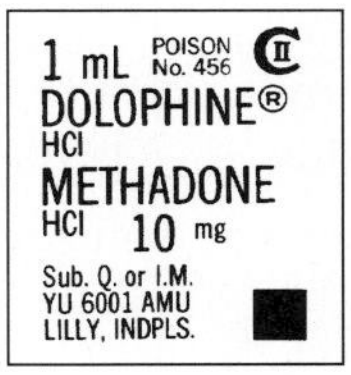

Figure 10.13 *Drug label for Dolophine HCl*

Notes/Workspace

13. Read the label in Figure 10.14. Calculate how many milliliters of insulin you will prepare if the order reads: NPH insulin 40 u sc at breakfast. _________

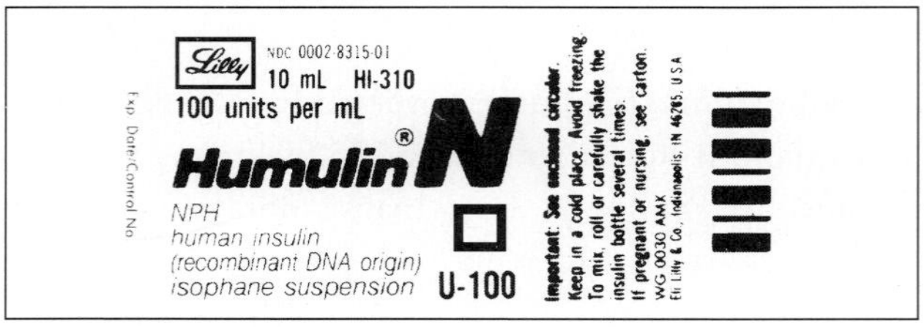

Figure 10.14 *Drug label for Humulin N*

14. The order reads: Terramycin 10 mg/kg IM q12h. Read the label in Figure 10.15. How many milliliters will you prepare for a patient who weighs 25 kilograms? _________

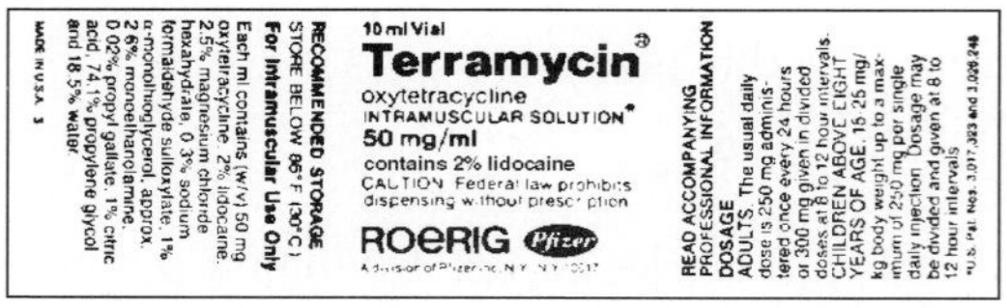

Figure 10.15 *Drug label for Terramycin*

15. The patient must receive 250 milligrams of cephaloridine (Loridine) IM. The 1 g vial has the following directions: Add 4.2 mL of sterile water, 1 mL = 200 mg. How many minims of this antibiotic will you administer to the patient? _________

16. Your patient is to receive 75 milligrams of hydrocortisone acetate (Biosone), injected into a joint by the physician. If the vial is labeled 25 milligrams per milliliter, how many milliliters will you prepare? _________

17. The order reads: phenytoin 0.2 g IM stat. The drug label reads 200 milligrams per 2 milliliters. How many milliliters of this anticonvulsant will you administer to your patient? _________

18. Your patient has been prescribed 1.3 milliliters of the antineoplastic methotrexate sodium (Folex) IM per day. The recommended dose is 3.3 milligrams per square meter per day. The label on the vial reads 25 milligrams per milliliter. If this patient's body surface area (BSA) is 1.66 square meters, is this an appropriate dose? ________

Notes/Workspace

19. Prepare 1550 milligrams of ticarcillin (Ticar) from a vial that has the following directions: Add 13 mL of sterile water to vial, 200 mg = 1 mL. How many milliliters contain this dose? ________

20. The order reads: methylergonovine maleate 0.0002 g IM q4h for five doses. The drug label reads 0.2 milligram per milliliter. How many milliliters will you administer in one dose? What is the total number of milligrams this patient will receive in five doses? ________ ; ________

Additional Exercises

Now, on your own, test yourself! Ask your instructor to check your answers.

1. Describe how to prepare 6500 units sc of heparin from a vial labeled 2500 units per milliliter.

   ____

   ____

2. The prescriber ordered: epinephrine HCl 0.5 mg IM stat. The label on the vial reads 1:1000. How many milliliters will you administer to the patient? ________

3. The medication order reads: atropine sulfate gr $\frac{1}{150}$ sc @ 7 A.M. The drug ampule reads 0.5 milligram per milliliter. How many milliliters will you administer to the patient? ________

4. The prescriber ordered: furosemide 60 mg IV push, stat. The label on the vial reads 50 milligrams per milliliter. How many milliliters will you prepare of this drug? ________

Notes/Workspace

5. Read the first medication order in Figure 10.16. The ampule for this medication reads 1 mL = 25 mg meperidine HCl and 25 mg promethazine. How many milliliters will you administer to your patient? ________

⊕ GENERAL HOSPITAL ⊕

PRESS HARD WITH BALLPOINT PEN. WRITE DATE & TIME AND SIGN EACH ORDER

DATE	TIME
9/9/94	*12 noon*
1. meperidine HCL 50 mg } *IM stat*	
promethazine 50 mg }	
2. Irrigate PICC (peripherally inserted central	
catheter) q12h with 5000 u of urokinase	
3. estrone 0.001 g IM qd x 5	
SIGNATURE *J. Olsen* M.D.	

IMPRINT
407553 9/9/94
Joshua Kelley 3/21/48
1505 M Street Jewish
Los Angeles, CA 93120 BC
Dr. J. Olsen

ORDERS NOTED
DATE *9/9/94* TIME *12:10* A.M. (P.M.)
❑ MEDEX ❑ KARDEX
NURSE'S SIG. *A. Giangrasso*

FILLED BY DATE

PHYSICIAN'S ORDERS

Figure 10.16 *Physician's order sheet*

6. The second medication order in Figure 10.16 is for 5000 units of urokinase. If the label on the drug vial reads 5000 units per milliliter, how many milliliters of this thrombolytic drug will you use in 24 hours? ________

7. The third medication order in Figure 10.16 is prepackaged in a vial labeled 5 milligrams per milliliter. How many milliliters of this hormone will you administer to your patient? ________

8. The patient must receive 600 milligrams of clindamycin phosphate. The label reads: Add 4.8 mL of sterile water to vial, 0.4 g = 1 mL. How many milliliters equal the prescribed dose? ________

9. The order reads: Premarin 0.25 mg IM qd. The label reads 2.5 milligrams per 5 milliliters. How many milliliters of this hormone will you administer to the patient? ________

Notes/Workspace

10. The medication order reads 20 units of regular (Humulin R) insulin sc. How many milliliters would equal this dose if the label on the vial reads 100 units per milliliter? ________

11. The order reads: vitamin B_{12} 400 mcg IM stat. The drug vial is labeled 1 milligram per milliliter. How many milliliters will you administer to your patient? ________

12. The order reads: Cleocin Phosphate 175 mg IM stat. Read the information on the drug label in Figure 10.17 and calculate the amount of medication in milliliters you will administer to your patient. ________

NDC 0009-0728-05
6505-01-246-8718
60 ml Pharmacy Bulk Package
Not for direct infusion
Cleocin Phosphate®
Sterile Solution
clindamycin phosphate injection, USP
Equivalent to clindamycin
150 mg per ml
For intramuscular or intravenous use
Caution: Federal law prohibits dispensing without prescription.
Upjohn The Upjohn Company Kalamazoo, MI 49001, USA

See package insert for complete product information.
Warning—If given intravenously, dilute before use.
Swab vial closure with an antiseptic solution. Dispense aliquots from the vial via a suitable dispensing device into infusion fluids under a laminar flow hood using aseptic technique. DISCARD VIAL WITHIN 24 HOURS AFTER INITIAL ENTRY.
Store at controlled room temperature 15°-30° C (59°-86° F)
Each ml contains: clindamycin phosphate equivalent to clindamycin 150 mg; also disodium edetate, 0.5 mg; benzyl alcohol 9.45 mg added as preservative. When necessary, pH was adjusted with sodium hydroxide and/or hydrochloric acid.
813 718 201 DATE/TIME ENTERED ....

Figure 10.17 *Drug label for Cleocin Phosphate*

13. The prescriber ordered: Humulin L insulin 65 u sc 2 A.M. Read the label in Figure 10.18 and calculate the amount in minims you would prepare for this order. ________

Important: See enclosed circular. Keep in a cold place. Avoid freezing. To mix, roll or carefully shake the insulin bottle several times. If pregnant or nursing, see carton.
VV 4210 AMX
Eli Lilly & Co., Indianapolis, IN 46285, U.S.A.
Exp. Date/Control No.

Lilly 10 mL HI-410
NDC 0002-8415-01
100 units per mL
U-100
Humulin® L
LENTE®
human insulin
(recombinant DNA origin)
zinc suspension

Figure 10.18 *Drug label for Humulin L*

Notes/Workspace

14. Your patient has an order for 0.5 unit per kilogram of Semilente Iletin I. The patient weighs 70 kilograms. According to the label in Figure 10.19, how many units will you administer to your patient? _________

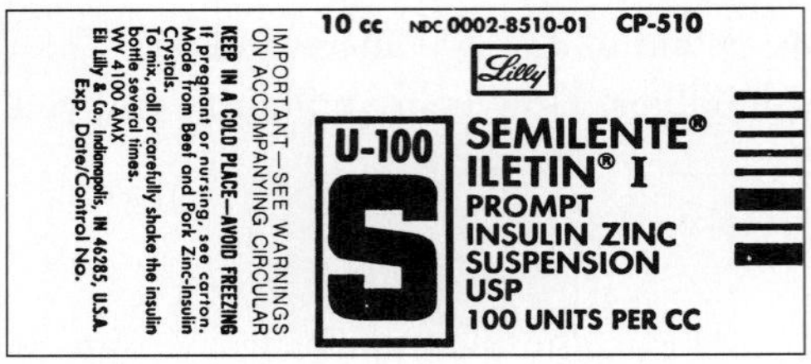

Figure 10.19 *Drug label for Semilente Iletin I*

15. The patient is to receive 15 milligrams of furosemide IM. Read the information on the label in Figure 10.20 and determine the amount in milliliters you will give your patient. _________

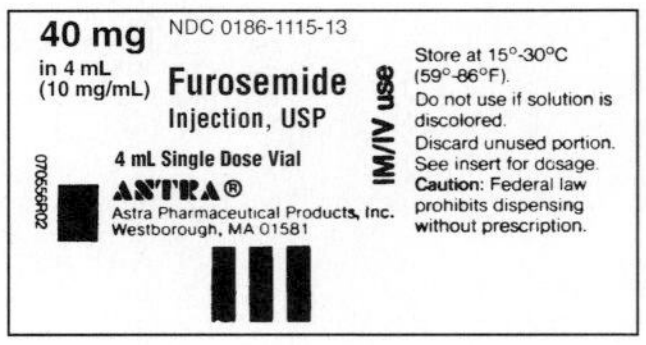

Figure 10.20 *Drug label for furosemide*

16. Your client must receive grain $\frac{1}{600}$ of atropine sulfate sc. The ampule reads 1 milligram per 10 milliliters. How many milliliters contain grain $\frac{1}{600}$?

____

17. If the order for magnesium sulfate is 1200 milligrams IM, how many milliliters would you administer from a vial labeled 50% magnesium sulfate?

____

18. The prescriber has ordered 100 units per kilogram of erythropoietin sc tiw for a patient in endstage renal disease. The patient weighs 88 kilograms, and the label on the vial reads 6000 units per milliliter. How many minims will you administer? _________

Notes/Workspace

19. If you were to prepare grain $\frac{1}{400}$ atropine sulfate from a vial labeled 0.4 milligram per milliliter, how many minims would equal this dose?

____

20. The order reads: quinidine 0.6 g IM stat. The label on the vial reads 200 milligrams per milliliter. How many milliliters contain this dose?

____

Cumulative Review Exercises

Review your mastery of earlier chapters.

1. The medication order is for 180 milligrams per 35 kilograms of zidovudine (Retrovir). How many milligrams are contained in this dose if the patient weighs 54 kilograms? __________

2. The medication order is for grain $\frac{1}{3}$ po of dicyclomine HCl (Bentyl), an antispasmodic drug. The tablets on hand are 10 milligrams. How many tablets would you administer? __________

3. The medication order reads 0.09 gram qd of nifedipine (Procardia XL), an anti-anginal drug. Each tablet contains 30 milligrams. How many tablets would you administer? __________

4. The medication order for a mucolytic agent, saturated solution of potassium iodine, is dram 1 po. How many teaspoons would you administer?

____

5. A vial is labeled meperidine HCl (Demerol), 50 milligrams per milliliter. The prescriber orders 12.5 milligrams IM. How many minims of this analgesic narcotic would you administer? __________

6. The medication order is for 0.15 milligram IM of digoxin. The label reads 0.5 milligram in 2 milliliters. How many minims of this cardiac glycoside would you administer to the patient? __________

Notes/Workspace

7. The prescriber ordered: norfloxacin 0.4 g po. The drug label reads 1 tab = 400 mg. How many tablets of this oral antibiotic would you administer?

____

8. The medication order is for 60 milligrams IM of furosemide (Lasix), a potent diuretic. The drug label reads 40 milligrams per milliliter. How many milliliters would you administer to the patient? ________

9. The medication order is for 0.4 gram po of acebutolol HCl (Sectral), an antihypertensive drug. Each capsule contains 200 milligrams. How many capsules would you administer to the patient? ________

10. The drug vial contains 1,000,000 units of penicillin G. The label directions state: Add 2.3 mL of sterile water to the vial, 1.2 mL = 500,000 u. How many milliliters equal 200,000 units? ________

11. gr $\frac{1}{400}$ = ________ g

12. 0.003 g = ________ mg

13. 180 mg = gr ________

14. $2\frac{1}{2}$ t = ________ gtt

15. 0.04 mg = gr ________

Unit Four

Specialized Medication Preparations

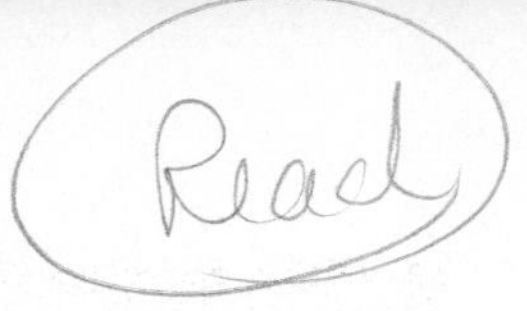

chapter 11

Calculating Flow Rates for Intravenous Infusions and Enteral Solutions

Objectives

After completing this chapter, you will be able to

- *understand intravenous (IV) flow rates and drop factors.*
- *calculate the flow rate of an IV solution.*
- *calculate the flow rate of intravenous piggyback medications.*
- *calculate the flow rate of enteral solutions.*
- *calculate the infusion time of an IV solution.*
- *calculate IV flow rates based on body weight.*
- *calculate IV flow rates based on body surface area.*

This chapter introduces the use of dimensional analysis for calculating flow rates and duration of flow for intravenous infusions and enteral solutions.

Notes/Workspace

A prescriber orders a specific amount of drug in solution or an enteral solution to be given over a specific period of time. An IV infusion is a solution given slowly to a patient through a vein over a period of time (see Figure 11.1). An enteral solution is given slowly through a tube inserted into the alimentary tract. For example, an IV medication order might read:

Add 10,000 u heparin to 250 mL 5% D/W, infuse at rate of 50 u/hr

or

1000 mL of 5% D/W per 8 h IV

An enteral solution order might read:

Isocal 50 mL/hr via nasogastric tube

Each of these medication orders must be converted to a *flow rate* expressed in drops per minute. The flow rate is then adjusted by counting the number of drops in 1 minute.

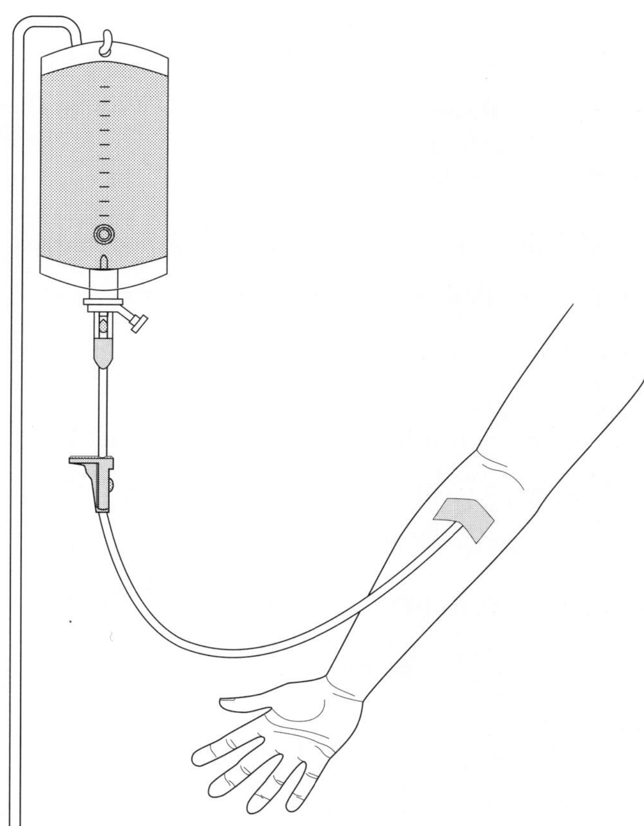

Figure 11.1 *Primary IV infusion*

Notes/Workspace

The size of the drop that IV tubing delivers is not standard; it depends on the way the tubing is designed. Manufacturers specify the number of drops that equal 1 milliliter for their particular tubing. This equivalent is called the tubing's *drop factor*; see Table 11.1. You must know the tubing's drop factor when calculating the flow rate of solutions in drops per minute (gtt/min) or microdrops per minute (μgtt/min).

Table 11.1 *Common Drop Factors*

10 gtt	=	1 mL
15 gtt	=	1 mL
20 gtt	=	1 mL
60 μgtt	=	1 mL

Calculating the Flow Rate of Infusions

Example 11.1

The prescriber ordered 240 cubic centimeters of 5% D/W to be given IV over a 12-hour period. The drop factor is 15 drops per cubic centimeter. How many drops per minute would you administer?

The notation "240 cubic centimeters in a 12 hour period" means $\frac{240\text{ cc}}{12\text{ hr}}$. You want to convert cubic centimeters per hour to drops per minute.

$$\frac{240\text{ cc}}{12\text{ hr}} \rightarrow \frac{?\text{ gtt}}{?\text{ min}}$$

This is a two-step problem, which you do in one line as follows:

$$\frac{240\text{ cc}}{12\text{ hr}} \times \frac{?\text{ gtt}}{?\text{ cc}} \times \frac{?\text{ hr}}{?\text{ min}} = ?\ \frac{\text{gtt}}{\text{min}}$$

Since 15 gtt = 1 cc, the first equivalent fraction is $\frac{15\text{ gtt}}{1\text{ cc}}$. Since 60 min = 1 hr, the second equivalent fraction is $\frac{1\text{ hr}}{60\text{ min}}$.

$$\frac{\overset{20}{\cancel{240}}\ \cancel{\text{cc}}}{\underset{1}{\cancel{12}}\ \cancel{\text{hr}}} \times \frac{\overset{1}{\cancel{15}}\text{ gtt}}{1\ \cancel{\text{cc}}} \times \frac{1\ \cancel{\text{hr}}}{\underset{4}{\cancel{60}}\text{ min}} = \frac{20\text{ gtt}}{4\text{ min}} = 5\ \frac{\text{gtt}}{\text{min}}$$

So 240 cubic centimeters given over a 12 hour period would be administered at the rate of 5 drops per minute.

Notes/Workspace

Example 11.2

The medication order reads:

250 mL 0.9% NS in 16h IV

The drop factor is 60 microdrops per milliliter. How many microdrops per minute would you administer?

The notation "250 milliliters in a 16 hour period" means $\frac{250 \text{ mL}}{16 \text{ hr}}$. You want to convert milliliters per hour to microdrops per minute:

$$\frac{250 \text{ mL}}{16 \text{ hr}} \rightarrow \frac{? \ \mu\text{gtt}}{? \text{ min}}$$

This is a two-step problem, which you do on one line, as follows:

$$\frac{250 \text{ mL}}{16 \text{ hr}} \times \frac{? \ \mu\text{gtt}}{? \text{ mL}} \times \frac{? \text{ hr}}{? \text{ min}} = ? \ \frac{\text{gtt}}{\text{min}}$$

Since 60 μgtt = 1 mL, the first equivalent fraction is $\frac{60 \ \mu\text{gtt}}{1 \text{ mL}}$. Since 60 min = 1 hr, the second equivalent fraction is $\frac{1 \text{ hr}}{60 \text{ min}}$.

$$\frac{250 \cancel{\text{mL}}}{16 \cancel{\text{hr}}} \times \frac{\overset{1}{\cancel{60}} \ \mu\text{gtt}}{1 \cancel{\text{mL}}} \times \frac{1 \cancel{\text{hr}}}{\underset{1}{\cancel{60}} \text{ min}} = \frac{250 \ \mu\text{gtt}}{16 \text{ min}} = 15.6 \ \frac{\mu\text{gtt}}{\text{min}}$$

So 16 microdrops per minute would be administered.

Sometimes, the infusion flow rate, due to a variety of reasons, can change. This will affect the prescribed duration of time in which the solution will be administered. Therefore, the nurse must assess the flow rate periodically and make any necessary adjustments.

Example 11.3

The medication order is for 500 milliliters of 5% D/W to infuse in 5 hours. The flow rate was calculated to be 25 drops per minute. When the nurse checked the infusion, 400 milliliters remained to be absorbed in 3 hours. Calculate the new flow rate if the drop factor is 15 drops per milliliter.

In this example, the problem is to determine the flow rate for the remaining 400 milliliters.

You want to convert milliliters per hour to drops per minute.

Notes/Workspace

$$\frac{400 \text{ mL}}{3 \text{ hr}} \rightarrow ? \frac{\text{gtt}}{\text{min}}$$

Do this on one line as follows:

$$\frac{400 \text{ mL}}{3 \text{ hr}} \times \frac{? \text{ gtt}}{? \text{ mL}} \times \frac{? \text{ hr}}{? \text{ min}}$$

Since 15 gtt = 1 mL, the first equivalent fraction is $\frac{15 \text{ gtt}}{1 \text{ mL}}$. Since 60 min = 1 hr, the second equivalent fraction is $\frac{1 \text{ hr}}{60 \text{ min}}$.

$$\frac{400 \cancel{\text{mL}}}{3 \cancel{\text{hr}}} \times \frac{\overset{1}{\cancel{15}} \text{ gtt}}{1 \cancel{\text{mL}}} \times \frac{1 \cancel{\text{hr}}}{\underset{4}{\cancel{60}} \text{ min}} = \frac{400 \text{ gtt}}{12 \text{ min}} = 33.3 \frac{\text{gtt}}{\text{min}}$$

So the new flow rate would be 33 drops per minute.

Example 11.4

The prescriber ordered 500 milliliters of 5% D/W with 20,000 units of heparin at 21 drops per minute. If the drop factor is 10 drops per milliliter, how many milliliters per hour will the patient receive?

In this example you need to change the flow rate, which is given in drops per minute, to milliliters per hour. Notice that the information in the order, 20,000 units in 500 milliliters, does not enter into our calculations because the flow rate indicates the amount of solution (in drops) rather than the amount of drug (in units) administered over a period of time.

You want to convert drops per minute to milliliters per hour.

$$\frac{21 \text{ gtt}}{1 \text{ min}} \rightarrow ? \frac{\text{mL}}{\text{hr}}$$

Do this on one line as follows:

$$\frac{21 \text{ gtt}}{1 \text{ min}} \times \frac{? \text{ mL}}{? \text{ gtt}} \times \frac{? \text{ min}}{? \text{ hr}} = ? \frac{\text{mL}}{\text{hr}}$$

Since 10 gtt = 1 mL and 60 min = 1 hr, the two equivalent fractions are $\frac{1 \text{ mL}}{10 \text{ gtt}}$ and $\frac{60 \text{ min}}{1 \text{ hr}}$.

$$\frac{21 \cancel{\text{gtt}}}{1 \cancel{\text{min}}} \times \frac{1 \text{ mL}}{\underset{1}{\cancel{10}} \cancel{\text{gtt}}} \times \frac{\overset{6}{\cancel{60}} \cancel{\text{min}}}{1 \text{ hr}} = 126 \frac{\text{mL}}{\text{hr}}$$

So the patient would receive 126 milliliters per hour.

Notes/Workspace

Example 11.5

The medication order reads:

1000 mL 5% D/W with 500 mg lidocaine at 1 mg/min

Calculate the flow rate if the drop factor is 15 drops per milliliter. In this example the prescriber has specified the solution (1000 milliliters of 5% D/W containing 500 milligrams of the drug lidocaine) and also the amount of lidocaine per minute (1 milligram per minute) that the patient is to receive.

You want to change the flow rate from milligrams per minute to drops per minute.

$$1 \frac{\text{mg}}{\text{min}} \rightarrow ? \frac{\text{gtt}}{\text{min}}$$

Do this on one line as follows:

$$\frac{1 \text{ mg}}{1 \text{ min}} \times \frac{? \text{ mL}}{? \text{ mg}} \times \frac{? \text{ gtt}}{? \text{ mL}} = ? \frac{\text{gtt}}{\text{min}}$$

Since 1000 milliliters contain 500 milligrams and since 15 gtt = 1 mL, the equivalent fractions are

$$\frac{1 \cancel{\text{mg}}}{1 \text{ min}} \times \frac{\overset{2}{\cancel{1000}} \cancel{\text{mL}}}{\underset{1}{\cancel{500}} \cancel{\text{mg}}} \times \frac{15 \text{ gtt}}{1 \cancel{\text{mL}}} = 30 \frac{\text{gtt}}{\text{min}}$$

So you would administer 30 drops per minute.

Example 11.6

The prescriber writes an order for 1000 milliliters of 5% D/W with 10 units of synthetic oxytocin (Pitocin). Your patient must receive 10 milliunits of this drug. The drop factor is 60 microdrops per milliliter. Calculate the flow rate in microdrops per minute.

You want to change the flow rate from milliunits per minute to microdrops per minute.

$$10 \frac{\text{mU}}{\text{min}} \rightarrow ? \frac{\mu\text{gtt}}{\text{min}}$$

Do this on one line as follows:

$$\frac{10 \text{ mU}}{1 \text{ min}} \times \frac{? \text{ u}}{? \text{ mU}} \times \frac{? \text{ mL}}{? \text{ u}} \times \frac{? \ \mu\text{gtt}}{? \text{ mL}} = ? \frac{\mu\text{gtt}}{\text{min}}$$

Notes/Workspace

Since 1000 mU = 1 u, 1000 mL = 10 u, and 60 μgtt = 1 mL, the equivalent fractions are

$$\frac{\overset{1}{\cancel{10}}\ \cancel{\text{mU}}}{1\ \text{min}} \times \frac{1\ \cancel{\text{u}}}{\underset{1}{\cancel{1000}}\ \cancel{\text{mU}}} \times \frac{\overset{1}{\cancel{1000}}\ \cancel{\text{mL}}}{\underset{1}{\cancel{10}}\ \cancel{\text{u}}} \times \frac{60\ \mu\text{gtt}}{1\ \cancel{\text{mL}}} = 60\ \frac{\mu\text{gtt}}{\text{min}}$$

So you will administer 60 microdrops per minute.

Note

1000 milliunits (mU) = 1 unit (u)

Example 11.7

Calculate the flow rate in milliliters per hour if the medication order reads: Add 10,000 u of heparin to 1000 mL 5% D/W. Your patient is to receive 250 units of this anticoagulant per hour via an infusion pump (see Figure 11.2).

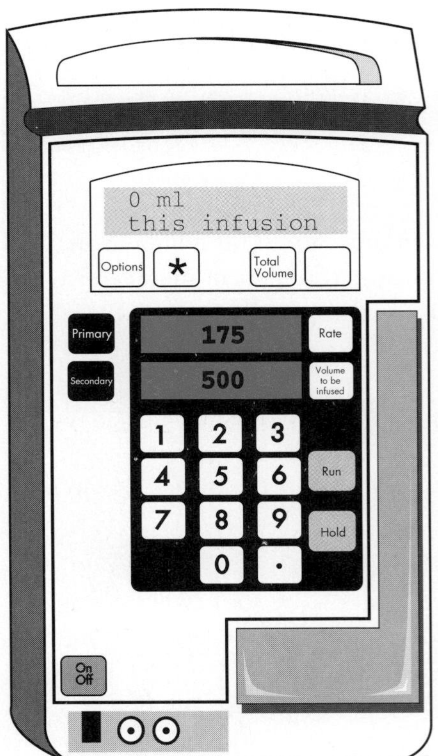

Figure 11.2 *Typical infusion pump*

You want to change the flow rate from units per hour to milliliters per hour.

$$\frac{250\text{ u}}{1\text{ hr}} \rightarrow ?\ \frac{\text{mL}}{\text{hr}}$$

Do this on one line as follows:

$$\frac{250\ \cancel{\text{u}}}{1\text{ hr}} \times \frac{\overset{1}{\cancel{1000}}\text{ mL}}{\underset{10}{\cancel{10{,}000}}\ \cancel{\text{u}}} = \frac{250\text{ mL}}{10\text{ hr}} = 25\ \frac{\text{mL}}{\text{hr}}$$

So your patient will receive 25 milliliters per hour.

⊕ ⊕ ⊕

Example 11.8

The medication order reads:

> 500 mL 5% D/W with 24,000 u of heparin, infuse at rate of 10 milliliters per hour

How many units is your patient receiving per hour?

You want to convert the flow rate from milliliters per hour to units per hour.

$$\frac{10\text{ mL}}{1\text{ hr}} \rightarrow ?\ \frac{\text{u}}{\text{hr}}$$

Do this on one line as follows:

$$\frac{10\ \cancel{\text{mL}}}{1\text{ hr}} \times \frac{24{,}000\text{ u}}{500\ \cancel{\text{mL}}} = 480\ \frac{\text{u}}{\text{hr}}$$

So your patient is receiving 480 units of heparin per hour.

⊕ ⊕ ⊕

Example 11.9

Your patient is receiving an IV of 1000 milliliters of 0.9% NS with 1000 milligrams of the bronchodilator aminophylline (Somophyllin). The flow rate is 35 milliliters per hour. How many milligrams per hour is your patient receiving?

You want to convert the flow rate from milliliters per hour to milligrams per hour.

$$\frac{35\text{ mL}}{1\text{ hr}} \rightarrow ?\ \frac{\text{mg}}{\text{hr}}$$

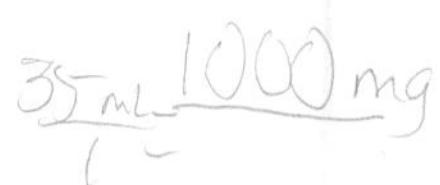

Notes/Workspace

Notes/Workspace

Do this on one line as follows:

$$\frac{35\ \cancel{\text{mL}}}{1\ \text{hr}} \times \frac{\overset{1}{\cancel{1000}}\ \text{mg}}{\underset{1}{\cancel{1000}}\ \cancel{\text{mL}}} = 35\ \frac{\text{mg}}{\text{hr}}$$

So your patient is receiving 35 milligrams of aminophylline per hour.

⭘ ⭘ ⭘

Example 11.10

The prescriber ordered:

750 mL of 0.9 NS IV in 8 h

The label on the box containing the intravenous set to be used for this infusion is shown in Figure 11.3. Calculate the flow rate in drops per minute.

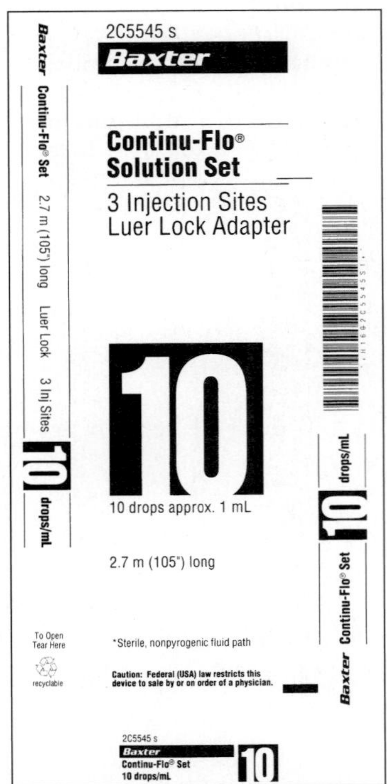

Figure 11.3 *Continu-Flo solution set box label*

You want to convert the flow rate from milliliters per hour to drops per minute.

$$\frac{750\text{ mL}}{8\text{ hr}} \rightarrow ?\ \frac{\text{gtt}}{\text{min}}$$

Do this on one line as follows:

$$\frac{750\ \cancel{\text{mL}}}{8\ \cancel{\text{hr}}} \times \frac{1\ \cancel{\text{hr}}}{\overset{}{\underset{6}{\cancel{60}}}\text{ min}} \times \frac{\overset{1}{\cancel{10}}\text{ gtt}}{1\ \cancel{\text{mL}}} = \frac{750\text{ gtt}}{48\text{ min}} = 15.6\ \frac{\text{gtt}}{\text{min}}$$

So the flow rate will be 16 drops per minute.

Intravenous Piggyback Medications

Patients can receive a drug through a port in an existing IV line. This is called an *intravenous piggyback (IVPB)*; see Figure 11.4.

For example, a patient who is already receiving 5% D/W via an IV line is to receive 1 gram of cefazolin (Ancef) every 4 hours. The prescriber's order reads:

Ancef 1 g IVPB q4h

This indicates that your patient will receive 1 gram of Ancef in solution via a secondary IV line that is attached to a port (piggyback) on the primary line.

Example 11.11

The prescriber ordered:

Ancef 1 g IVPB q4h

The package insert information is as follows: Add 50 mL sterile water to the bag of Ancef 1 g and infuse in 30 min. The tubing is labeled 20 drops per milliliter. Calculate the flow rate for this antibiotic.

You want to change the flow rate from milliliters per minute to drops per minute.

$$\frac{50\text{ mL}}{30\text{ min}} \rightarrow ?\ \frac{\text{gtt}}{\text{min}}$$

Do this on one line as follows:

$$\frac{\overset{5}{\cancel{50}}\ \cancel{\text{mL}}}{\underset{3}{\cancel{30}}\text{ min}} \times \frac{20\text{ gtt}}{1\ \cancel{\text{mL}}} = \frac{100\text{ gtt}}{3\text{ min}} = 33.3\ \frac{\text{gtt}}{\text{min}}$$

So the flow rate is 33 drops per minute.

Notes/Workspace

Notes/Workspace

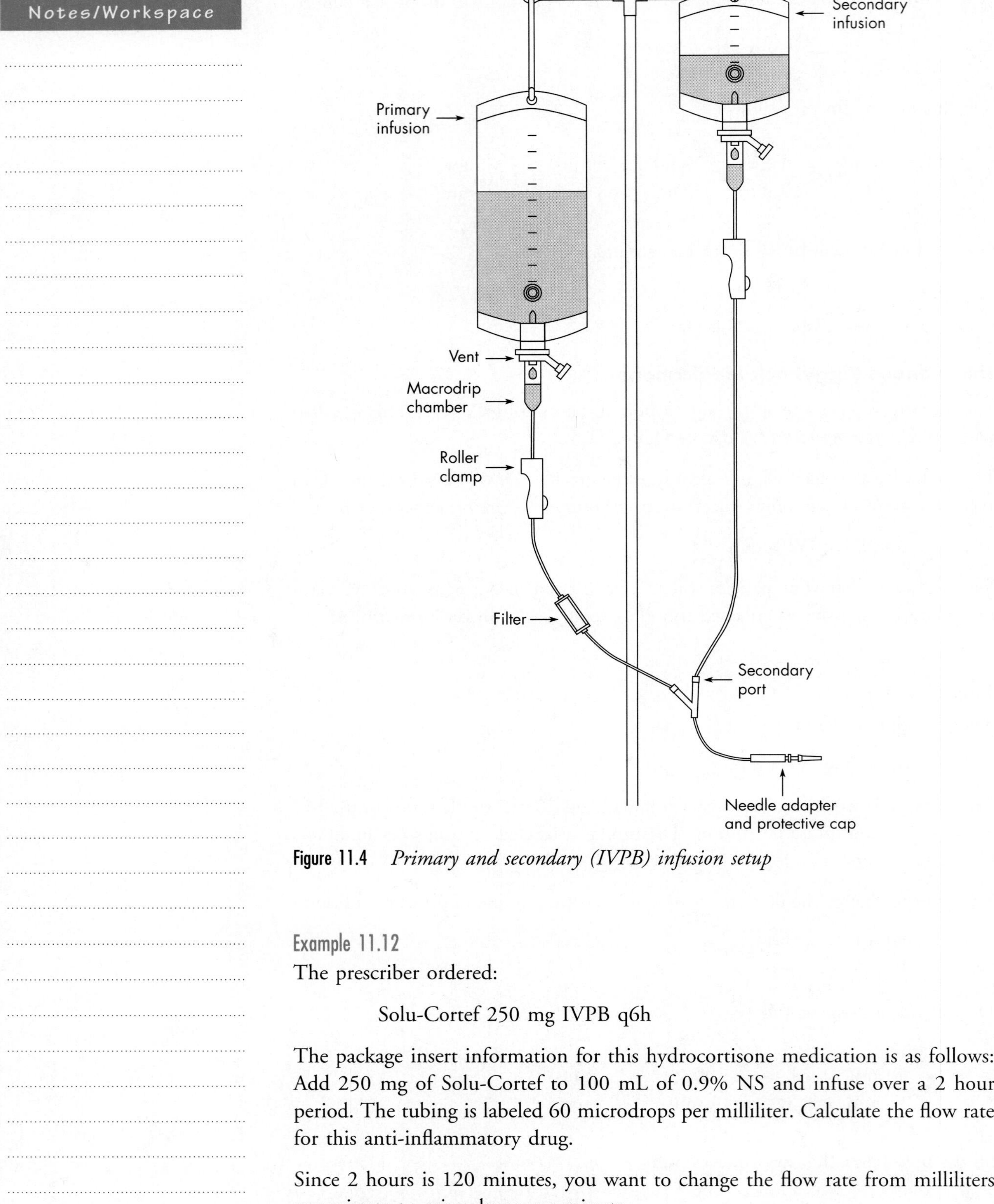

Figure 11.4 *Primary and secondary (IVPB) infusion setup*

Example 11.12

The prescriber ordered:

Solu-Cortef 250 mg IVPB q6h

The package insert information for this hydrocortisone medication is as follows: Add 250 mg of Solu-Cortef to 100 mL of 0.9% NS and infuse over a 2 hour period. The tubing is labeled 60 microdrops per milliliter. Calculate the flow rate for this anti-inflammatory drug.

Since 2 hours is 120 minutes, you want to change the flow rate from milliliters per minute to microdrops per minute.

$$\frac{100\text{ mL}}{120\text{ min}} \rightarrow ?\ \frac{\mu\text{gtt}}{\text{min}}$$

Do this on one line as follows:

$$\frac{100\ \cancel{\text{mL}}}{\underset{2}{\cancel{120}}\ \text{min}} \times \frac{\overset{1}{\cancel{60}}\ \mu\text{gtt}}{1\ \cancel{\text{mL}}} = 50\ \frac{\mu\text{gtt}}{\text{min}}$$

So the flow rate is 50 microdrops per minute.

Calculating the Flow Rate of Enteral Solutions

A patient can be fed nutrients enterally—that is, by way of a tube in the alimentary canal. The flow rate of the nutrient (enteral solution) is calculated in drops per minute or milliliters per hour.

Example 11.13

A patient must receive a tube-feeding of Ensure, 240 milliliters in 60 minutes. The calibration of the tubing is 20 drops per milliliter. Calculate the flow rate in drops per minute.

You want to convert milliliters per minute to drops per minute.

$$\frac{240\text{ mL}}{60\text{ min}} \rightarrow ?\ \frac{\text{gtt}}{\text{min}}$$

Do this on one line as follows:

$$\frac{\overset{4}{\cancel{240}}\ \cancel{\text{mL}}}{\underset{1}{\cancel{60}}\ \text{min}} \times \frac{20\text{ gtt}}{1\ \cancel{\text{mL}}} = 80\ \frac{\text{gtt}}{\text{min}}$$

So the flow rate is 80 drops per minute.

Calculating the Duration of Flow for IV and Enteral Solutions

In the following examples, you will determine the length of time it will take to complete an infusion.

Example 11.14

An infusion of 0.9% NS has solution remaining in the bag (see Figure 11.5). It is infusing at a rate of 20 drops per minute. If the drop factor is 12 drops per milliliter, how many hours will it take for the remaining solution in the bag to infuse?

Notes/Workspace

Notes/Workspace

You can see that 500 milliliters of solution were originally in the bag and that the patient has received 200 milliliters. Therefore, 300 milliliters remain to be infused.

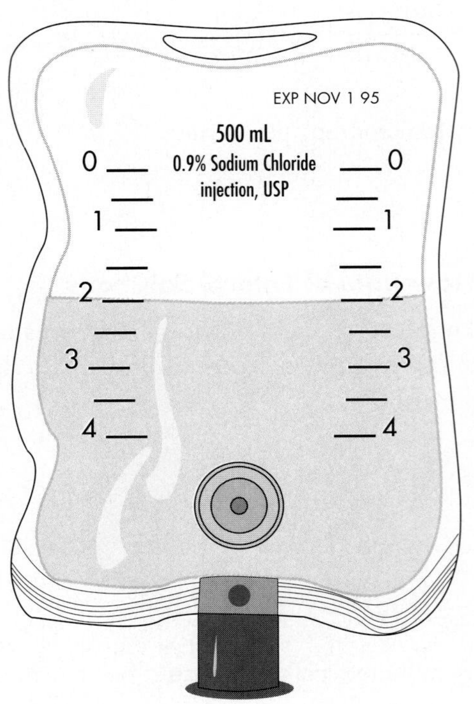

Figure 11.5 *0.9% sodium chloride intravenous solution*

You want to convert milliliters to hours.

$$300 \text{ mL} \rightarrow ? \text{ gtt} \rightarrow ? \text{ min} \rightarrow ? \text{ hr}$$

Do this on one line as follows:

$$300 \text{ mL} \times \frac{? \text{ gtt}}{? \text{ mL}} \times \frac{? \text{ min}}{? \text{ gtt}} \times \frac{? \text{ hr}}{? \text{ min}} = ? \text{ hr}$$

Since 12 gtt = 1 mL, 20 gtt = 1 min, and 60 min = 1 hr, these become the equivalent fractions.

$$\overset{15}{\cancel{300} \, \cancel{\text{mL}}} \times \frac{\overset{1}{\cancel{12} \, \cancel{\text{gtt}}}}{1 \, \cancel{\text{mL}}} \times \frac{1 \, \cancel{\text{min}}}{\underset{1}{\cancel{20} \, \cancel{\text{gtt}}}} \times \frac{1 \text{ hr}}{\underset{5}{\cancel{60} \, \cancel{\text{min}}}} = 3 \text{ hr}$$

So it will take 3 hours to infuse this solution.

Notes/Workspace

Example 11.15

A patient is receiving an IV of 1000 milliliters of 5% D/W. The flow rate is 32 drops per minute. If the drop factor is 10 drops per milliliter, how many hours will it take for this infusion to finish?

You want to convert milliliters to hours.

$$1000 \text{ mL} \rightarrow ? \text{ gtt} \rightarrow ? \text{ min} \rightarrow ? \text{ hr}$$

Do this on one line as follows:

$$1000 \text{ mL} \times \frac{? \text{ gtt}}{? \text{ mL}} \times \frac{? \text{ min}}{? \text{ gtt}} \times \frac{? \text{ hr}}{? \text{ min}} = ? \text{ hr}$$

Since 10 gtt = 1 mL, 32 gtt = 1 min, and 60 min = 1 hr, these become the equivalent fractions.

$$1000 \cancel{\text{mL}} \times \frac{\overset{1}{\cancel{10}} \cancel{\text{gtt}}}{1 \cancel{\text{mL}}} \times \frac{1 \cancel{\text{min}}}{32 \cancel{\text{gtt}}} \times \frac{1 \text{ hr}}{\underset{6}{\cancel{60}} \cancel{\text{min}}} = 5.2 \text{ hr}$$

Convert the portion of an hour to minutes—that is, convert 0.2 hour to minutes.

$$0.2 \cancel{\text{hr}} \times \frac{60 \text{ min}}{1 \cancel{\text{hr}}} = 12 \text{ min}$$

So the infusion will take 5 hours and 12 minutes.

Example 11.16

An IV of 1000 milliliters of 5% D/W 0.9% NS is started at 1 P.M. The flow rate is 17 drops per minute, and the drop factor is 10 drops per milliliter. At what time will this infusion finish?

You want to convert milliliters to hours.

$$1000 \text{ mL} \rightarrow ? \text{ gtt} \rightarrow ? \text{ min} \rightarrow ? \text{ hr}$$

Do this on one line as follows:

$$1000 \text{ mL} \times \frac{? \text{ gtt}}{? \text{ mL}} \times \frac{? \text{ min}}{? \text{ gtt}} \times \frac{? \text{ hr}}{? \text{ min}} = ? \text{ hr}$$

Since 10 gtt = 1 mL, 17 gtt = 1 min, and 60 min = 1 hr, these become the equivalent fractions.

$$1000 \cancel{\text{mL}} \times \frac{\overset{1}{\cancel{10}} \cancel{\text{gtt}}}{1 \cancel{\text{mL}}} \times \frac{1 \cancel{\text{min}}}{17 \cancel{\text{gtt}}} \times \frac{1 \text{ hr}}{\underset{6}{\cancel{60}} \cancel{\text{min}}} = 9.8 \text{ hr}$$

Notes/Workspace

You then convert 0.8 hour to minutes.

$$0.8\ \cancel{\text{hr}} \times \frac{60\ \text{min}}{1\ \cancel{\text{hr}}} = 48\ \text{min}$$

So the IV will infuse for 9 hours and 48 minutes. Since the infusion started at 1 P.M., it will finish at 10:48 P.M.

Example 11.17

An IV of 1500 milliliters of 10% D/W is to infuse at a rate of 40 drops per minute. The drop factor is 15 drops per milliliter. If this IV solution begins to infuse at 10:15 A.M., at what time will it finish?

You want to convert milliliters to hours.

$$1500\ \text{mL} \rightarrow ?\ \text{gtt} \rightarrow ?\ \text{min} \rightarrow ?\ \text{hr}$$

Do this on one line as follows:

$$1500\ \text{mL} \times \frac{?\ \text{gtt}}{?\ \text{mL}} \times \frac{?\ \text{min}}{?\ \text{gtt}} \times \frac{?\ \text{hr}}{?\ \text{min}} = ?\ \text{hr}$$

Since 15 gtt = 1 mL, 40 gtt = 1 min, and 60 min = 1 hr, these become the equivalent fractions.

$$1500\ \cancel{\text{mL}} \times \frac{\overset{1}{\cancel{15}}\ \cancel{\text{gtt}}}{1\ \cancel{\text{mL}}} \times \frac{1\ \cancel{\text{min}}}{40\ \cancel{\text{gtt}}} \times \frac{1\ \text{hr}}{\underset{4}{\cancel{60}}\ \cancel{\text{min}}} = 9.4\ \text{hr}$$

You then convert 0.4 hour to minutes.

$$0.4\ \cancel{\text{hr}} \times \frac{60\ \text{min}}{1\ \cancel{\text{hr}}} = 24\ \text{min}$$

So the IV will infuse for 9 hours and 24 minutes. Since the infusion started at 10:15 A.M., it will finish at 7:39 P.M.

Calculating Flow Rates Based on Body Weight

Some IV and enteral medications are prescribed based on your patient's weight. For example, the medication order might read:

0.02 mg/kg/min

This means that each minute, your patient is to receive 0.02 milligram of the drug for every kilogram of body weight. This can also be written as $\frac{0.02\ \text{mg}}{\text{kg} \times \text{min}}$.

Notes/Workspace

Example 11.18

The prescriber ordered:

1000 mL 5% D/W with 500 mg lidocaine, 0.02 mg/kg/min

The patient weighs 70 kilograms, and the drop factor is 20 drops per milliliter. Calculate the flow rate.

Since the amount of drug ordered is based on the weight of the patient (kilograms), the weight will determine the flow rate (drops per minute). You want to convert kilograms to drops per minute. You have the following information:

- The patient weighs 70 kg
- The order is 0.02 mg/kg/min
- 500 mg = 1000 mL
- 20 gtt = 1 mL

Do this problem on one line as follows:

$$70\ \cancel{\text{kg}} \times \frac{0.02\ \cancel{\text{mg}}}{\cancel{\text{kg}} \times \text{min}} \times \frac{\overset{2}{\cancel{1000\ \text{mL}}}}{\underset{1}{\cancel{500\ \text{mg}}}} \times \frac{20\ \text{gtt}}{1\ \cancel{\text{mL}}} = 56\ \frac{\text{gtt}}{\text{min}}$$

So the flow rate is 56 drops per minute.

Example 11.19

The medication order reads:

Yutopar 0.0018 mg/kg/min

The package insert directions for this tocolytic drug are as follows: Add 150 mg (10 mL) of Yutopar to 500 mL 5% D/W. The patient weighs 60 kilograms. How many milligrams per hour will your patient receive?

The concentration of the drug is 150 milligrams in the 10 milliliters of solution. So the total volume of the infusion is 510 milliliters. You have the following information:

- The patient weighs 60 kg
- The order is 0.0018 mg/kg/min
- 510 mL = 150 mg

Notes/Workspace

Do this problem on one line as follows:

$$60\,\cancel{\text{kg}} \times \frac{0.0018\,\cancel{\text{mg}}}{\cancel{\text{kg}} \times \cancel{\text{min}}} \times \frac{510\text{ mL}}{\underset{5}{\cancel{150}}\,\cancel{\text{mg}}} \times \frac{\overset{2}{\cancel{60}}\,\cancel{\text{min}}}{1\text{ hr}} = 22.03\,\frac{\text{mL}}{\text{hr}}$$

So your patient will receive 22.03 milliliters per hour.

Calculating Flow Rates Based on Body Surface Area

As you know, certain medications are ordered based on body surface area (BSA). Chapter 12 discusses how to determine a child's BSA, and you will find a pediatric nomogram, the chart that enables you to do this, in Appendix F.

The following examples show how to calculate flow rates for this type of medication order.

Example 11.20

The prescriber ordered 500 milligrams of cyclophosphamide (Cytoxan), an antineoplastic drug, in 250 milliliters 0.9% NS, to be infused at a rate of 50 milligrams per square meter per hour (see the label in Figure 11.6 for drug information). Your patient's BSA is 1.5 square meters. How many milliliters per hour should your patient receive?

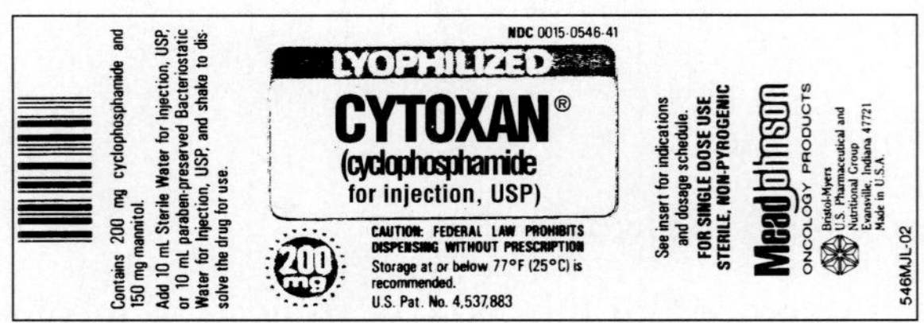

Figure 11.6 *Drug label for Cytoxan*

Since the medication order is based on the BSA of the patient, it will determine the flow rate (milliliters per hour). You have the following information:

- The BSA of the patient is 1.5 m^2
- The order is 50 mg/m^2/hr
- 275 mL = 500 mg (250 mL + 25 mL of Cytoxan = 275 mL)

Do this problem on one line as follows:

$$1.5\,\cancel{m^2} \times \frac{\overset{1}{\cancel{50\text{ mg}}}}{\cancel{m^2} \times \text{hr}} \times \frac{275\text{ mL}}{\underset{10}{\cancel{500\text{ mg}}}} = 41.3\text{ mL/hr}$$

So your patient should receive 41.3 milliliters per hour.

Example 11.21

The prescriber ordered:

vinblastine sulfate 0.03 mg/m^2/min

The package insert directions are as follows: Add 10 mg (10 mL) to 250 mL 5% D/W. Calculate the flow rate in milliliters per hour if the patient's BSA is 1.6 square meters.

You have the following information:

- The BSA of the patient is 1.6 m^2
- The order is 0.03 mg/m^2/min
- 10 mg = 260 mL (250 mL + 10 mL)

Do this problem on one line as follows:

$$1.6\,\cancel{m^2} \times \frac{0.03\,\cancel{\text{mg}}}{\cancel{m^2} \times \cancel{\text{min}}} \times \frac{260\text{ mL}}{\underset{1}{\cancel{10\text{ mg}}}} \times \frac{\overset{6}{\cancel{60\text{ min}}}}{1\text{ hr}} = 74.9\,\frac{\text{mL}}{\text{hr}}$$

So the flow rate is 74.9 milliliters per hour.

Notes/Workspace

Notes/Workspace

Practice Sets

You will find the answers to the Try These for Practice, Exercises, and Cumulative Review Practice Sets in the Answer Section at the back of the book. Your instructor has the answers to the Additional Exercises.

Try These for Practice

Test your comprehension after reading the chapter.

1. The prescriber ordered:

500 mL 5% D/W in 4 h IV

Calculate the flow rate when the drop factor is 10 drops per milliliter. ________

2. The prescriber ordered:

1000 mL 0.9% NS in 8 h IV

The flow rate is 21 drops per minute. When the nurse assessed the infusion, 400 milliliters had infused in 4 hours. Calculate the new flow rate if the drop factor is 15 drops per milliliter. ________

3. The patient is to receive 1200 units of heparin q1h IV. If the order is 250 milliliters of 5% D/W with 10,000 units of heparin, how many milliliters per hour will your patient receive of this drug (see Figure 11.7)? ________

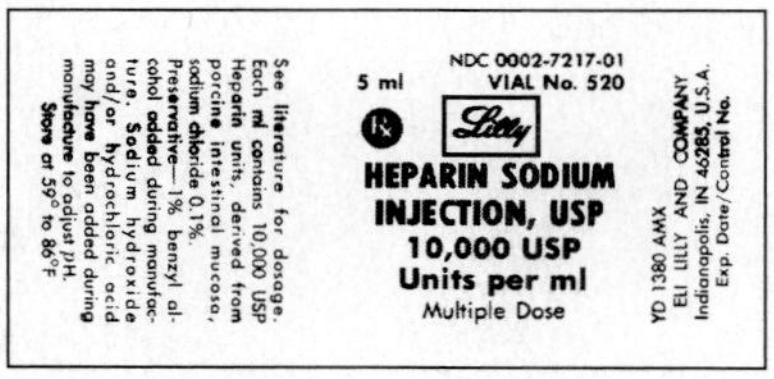

NDC 0002-7217-01
5 ml VIAL No. 520
Lilly
HEPARIN SODIUM INJECTION, USP
10,000 USP Units per ml
Multiple Dose

Figure 11.7 *Drug label for heparin*

4. A patient has an IV of 500 milliliters of 5% D/W. The flow rate is 19 microdrops per minute. If the drop factor is 60 microdrops per milliliter, how many hours will it take for this infusion to finish? ________

5. Read the first medication order in Figure 11.8. The label for this drug reads:

clindamycin phosphate 900 mg/2 mL

a. How many milliliters of clindamycin phosphate would you add to a 50 mL bag of 5% D/W? ________

b. Calculate the infusion rate in microdrops per minute when the total time of this infusion is 1 hour. ________

⊕ GENERAL HOSPITAL ⊕

PRESS HARD WITH BALLPOINT PEN. WRITE DATE & TIME AND SIGN EACH ORDER

DATE	TIME	A.M. (circled) / P.M.
9/30/94	*10*	

1. *clindamycin phosphate 600 mg IVPB q8h x 5 days*
2. *Solu-Medrol 1 g in 250 mL 5% D/W, infuse 20 mg/hr*
3. *aminophylline 1 g in 250 mL 5% D/W, infuse 0.15 g/hr*

SIGNATURE *A. Giangrasso* M.D.

IMPRINT
506713 9/30/94
Jason O'Mooter 6/22/40
26 Marin Dr. RC
Thousand Oaks, Ore. Aetna
80413
Dr. A. Giangrasso

ORDERS NOTED
DATE *9/30/94* TIME *10* A.M. (circled) P.M.
❑ MEDEX ❑ KARDEX
NURSE'S SIG. *L. Ablon*

FILLED BY DATE

PHYSICIAN'S ORDERS

Figure 11.8 *Physician's order sheet*

Notes/Workspace

Exercises

Reinforce your understanding in class or at home.

1. The medication order states that 12,000 units of heparin are to be added to 250 milliliters of 5% D/W. The patient is to receive 1200 units per hour IV. How many milliliters per hour will your patient receive? ________

2. The prescriber has ordered 3.1 grams of ticarcillin disodium (Timentin), an antibiotic, IVPB in 100 milliliters of 5% D/W. The directions are as follows: Add 13 mL to vial, 15 mL = 3.1 g. (Total amount of fluid IV: 115 milliliters.) This IV is to be infused in 60 minutes; the drop factor is 15 drops per milliliter. Calculate the flow rate. ________

Notes/Workspace

3. A patient is to receive 500 milliliters of 5% D/W with 20 units of synthetic oxytocin (Pitocin) IV at a rate of 0.002 unit per minute. How many milliliters per hour will your patient receive? ________

4. The patient has an IV of 1000 milliliters of 5% D/0.45% NS infusing at a rate of 28 drops per minute; the drop factor is 10 drops per milliliter. How many milliliters per hour is your patient receiving? ________

5. The prescriber has ordered 500 milliliters of 5% D/W in 2 hours IV. The drop factor is 15 drops per milliliter. Calculate the flow rate. ________

6. An IV of 500 milliliters of 5% D/W is infusing at a rate of 27 drops per minute; the drop factor is 15 drops per milliliter. If this infusion was started at 6 P.M., at what time will it finish? ________

7. Calculate the flow rate in milliliters per hour for a patient receiving an IV of 250 milliliters of 5% D/W with 250 milligrams of aminophylline. The medication order is 0.06 milligram per kilogram per minute and the patient weighs 66 kilograms. ________

8. The prescriber has ordered 250 milliliters of 5% D/W with 2500 units of heparin; the patient is to receive 50 milliliters per hour IV. How many units per hour will your patient receive? ________

9. The order states that 200 milligrams of morphine are to be added to 250 milliliters of 5% D/W, and this solution is to be infused at a rate of 10 milligrams per hour. How many milliliters per hour will your patient receive? ________

10. The medication order is for 180 milligrams of morphine sulfate to be added to 250 milliliters of 5% D/W. If your patient is to receive 0.005 milligram per kilogram per minute IV, how many milligrams per hour should a patient who weighs 100 pounds receive? ________

11. The anti-arrhythmic drug bretylium tosylate has been prescribed for a 70 kg patient at 30 micrograms per kilogram per minute IV. Read the label in Figure 11.9. The mixing instructions are as follows: Add bretylium tosylate

solution to 250 mL of 5% D/W. Calculate the flow rate in milliliters per hour. ________

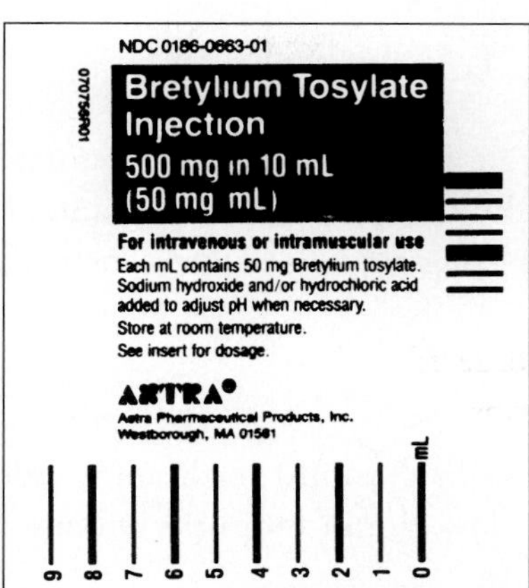

Figure 11.9 *Drug label for bretylium tosylate*

12. The prescriber ordered dopamine hydrochloride (Intropin) at a rate of 0.003 milligram per kilogram per minute; the patient weighs 122 pounds. The directions are as follows: Add 160 mg (1 mL) to 250 mL of 5% D/W. Calculate the flow rate in milliliters per hour for this infusion. ________

13. A medication order states that 50 milliliters of asparaginase (Elspar) are to be added to 100 milliliters of 5% D/W (total 150 milliliters). Calculate the flow rate in microdrops so that your patient, who weighs 60 kilograms, receives 1 milliliter per kilogram per hour of this antineoplastic drug.

____

14. The prescriber has ordered 500 milliliters of 5% D/W with 100 units of Humulin R insulin (1 milliliter). Infuse at a rate of 0.7 milliliter per minute. How many hours will it take to complete this infusion?

____

15. Read the second medication order in Figure 11.8 (page 221). Calculate the flow rate in milliliters per hour. ________

16. An infusion of 1000 milliliters of 5% D/W is started at 11 A.M. The flow rate is 20 drops per minute, and the drop factor is 20 drops per milliliter. At what time will this infusion finish? ________

Notes/Workspace

Notes/Workspace

17. The prescriber ordered: Vibramycin 200 mg in 50 mL lactated Ringer's solution, 0.08 mg/kg/min. The patient weighs 74 kilograms, and the drop factor is 10 drops per milliliter. Calculate the flow rate in drops per minute. _________

18. Calculate the flow rate in milliliters per hour for a patient receiving an IV of 250 milliliters of 5% D/W with 200 milligrams of methyldopa (Aldomet), 0.005 milligram per kilogram per minute. The patient weighs 200 pounds. _________

19. Read the information in the third medication order in Figure 11.8 (page 221). Calculate the flow rate in drops per minute when the drop factor is 10 drops per milliliter. _________

20. The prescriber ordered: amikacin sulfate 120 mg/m^2/hr. The package insert directions are as follows: Add 250 mg to 100 mL 5% D/W. Calculate the flow rate in milliliters per hour if the patient's BSA is 0.9 square meter. _________

Additional Exercises

Now, on your own, test yourself! Ask your instructor to check your answers.

1. The prescriber ordered: acyclovir sodium 5 mg/kg/hr IV. The directions are as follows: Add 500 mg (10 mL) to 100 mL 5% D/W. Calculate the flow rate in milliliters per hour for a patient who weighs 160 pounds. _________

110 mL

2. Read the first medication order in Figure 11.10 (page 225). How many milliliters per hour will this IV infuse if your patient weighs 80 kilograms? _________

3. Read the second medication order in Figure 11.10. Calculate the flow rate for the infusion ordered. The drop factor is 10 drops per milliliter. _________

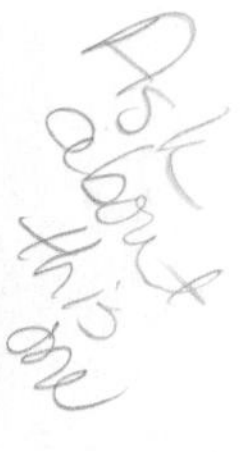

⊕ GENERAL HOSPITAL ⊕

PRESS HARD WITH BALLPOINT PEN. WRITE DATE & TIME AND SIGN EACH ORDER

DATE	TIME	A.M. (circled) / P.M.	IMPRINT
11/28/94	7:30		316413 11/28/94 James Hassad 6/3/66 4151 Geary Street Muslim San Francisco, CA 94071 BCBS June Olsen, M.D.

1. aminophylline 0.375 g in 500 mL 5% D/W, infuse 0.3 mg/kg/hr IV
2. 750 mL 5% D/0.45% NS in 8h IV
3. 250 mL 5% D/W c̄ 2g Mefoxin IVPB q12h

SIGNATURE J. Olsen M.D.

ORDERS NOTED A.M. (circled) P.M.
DATE 11/28/94 TIME 7:30
❑ MEDEX ❑ KARDEX
NURSE'S SIG. L. Ablon

FILLED BY DATE

PHYSICIAN'S ORDERS

Figure 11.10 *Physician's order sheet*

Notes/Workspace

4. Read the third medication order in Figure 11.10. How would you administer the medication if the drop factor is 15 drops per milliliter?

____

5. A patient is to receive 600 units of heparin per hour. The drop factor is 60 drops per milliliter. The order states that 12,500 units of heparin are to be added to 250 milliliters of 5% D/W. How many microdrops per minute will you infuse? ________

6. A patient has an IV of 1000 milliliters of 5% D/W. The flow rate is 36 drops per minute. If the drop factor is 10 drops per milliliter, how many hours will it take this IV to finish? ________

? **7.** An infusion of 1000 milliliters of lactated Ringer's solution is infusing at a rate of 17 drops per minute. What time will it be completed if the drop factor is 15 drops per milliliter and this infusion started at 7 A.M.? ________

Notes/Workspace

8. How many hours will an IV of 1000 milliliters of 5% D/W infuse if the order is for 125 milliliters per hour? _________

9. The thrombolytic enzyme streptokinase (Streptase) has been ordered intravenously, 1,500,000 units over 60 minutes in 50 milliliters of 0.9% NS. What will the flow rate be in microdrops per minute? _________

10. The prescriber has ordered 250 milliliters of 5% D/W with 250 milligrams of esmolol hydrochloride (Brevibloc) at a rate of 10 micrograms per kilogram per minute. What will the flow rate be in milliliters per hour if the patient weighs 75 kilograms? _________

11. If an IV is infusing at a rate of 80 microdrops per minute, how many milliliters per hour will your patient receive? _________

12. Read the mixing information on the label in Figure 11.11. The medication order reads: Solu-Medrol 1 g in 250 mL 5% D/W, 50 mg/hr. How many milliliters per hour will your patient receive? _________

NDC 0009-3389-01 8 mL Act-O-Vial®
Solu-Medrol® 1 gram *
Sterile Powder
methylprednisolone sodium succinate for injection, USP
Single-Dose Vial
For intramuscular or intravenous use

See package insert for complete product information.
Store solution at controlled room temperature 15°-30° C (59°-86° F) and use within 48 hours after mixing.
Each 8 mL (when mixed) contains:
*methylprednisolone sodium succinate equivalent to 1 gram methylprednisolone (125 mg per mL).
Lyophilized in container 814 184 001
The Upjohn Company
Kalamazoo, Michigan 49001, USA

Figure 11.11 *Drug label for Solu-Medrol*

13. The prescriber has ordered 500 milliliters of 5% D/W with 500 milligrams of lidocaine, and your patient, who weighs 80 kilograms, must receive 20 micrograms per kilogram per minute. What will the flow rate be in milliliters per hour? _________

14. The prescriber ordered: 250 mL 5% D/W with 12,500 u heparin. This is to be infused at a rate of 900 units per hour. Calculate the flow rate in milliliters per hour. _________

15. Read the information on the label in Figure 11.12.

a. How many milliliters will you add to the bottle? _________

b. Calculate the flow rate in drops per minute when the drop factor is 20 drops per milliliter and the infusion time is 30 minutes. _________

NDC 0002-7011-01
VIAL No. 7011
Rx Lilly
KEFZOL®
STERILE
CEFAZOLIN
SODIUM
USP
Equivalent to
1 g
Cefazolin

CAUTION: Federal (U.S.A.) law prohibits dispensing without prescription.
FOR INTRAVENOUS USE Protect from Light
For Dosage and Administration: See Literature
Each vial contains: 1 g of Cefazolin. The total Sodium content is approximately 48 mg (2.1 mEq Sodium ion) per g of KEFZOL.
To prepare an I.V. solution, add 100 mL of an approved isotonic diluent to the contents of this bottle. See literature. SHAKE WELL.
CAUTION: Consistent with good I.V. administration practice, to avoid the possibility of intravenous air injection, terminate the infusion before the set empties.
Prior to Reconstitution: Store at Controlled Room Temperature 59° to 86°F (15° to 30°C)
After Reconstitution: Store in a refrigerator. For Storage Time - See Accompanying Literature. If kept at room temperature, use within 24 hours.
WV 3192 AMX
ELI LILLY AND COMPANY, INDIANAPOLIS, IN 46285, U.S.A.
Exp. Date/Control No.
FOR DISPLAY ONLY

100 mL SCALE 75 mL VOLUME 50 mL APPROX 25 mL

Figure 11.12 *Drug label for Kefzol*

16. You have an order for pentamidine isethionate (Pentam 300), 300 milligrams in 250 milliliters 5% D/W at a rate of 2.5 milligrams per minute. What is the flow rate in drops per minute if the drop factor is 15 drops per milliliter? _________

17. The prescriber ordered: amphotericin B 150 mg IVPB. The directions are as follows: Add 150 mg to 250 mL, infuse in 6 h. Calculate the flow rate in drops per minute when the drop factor is 10 drops per milliliter. If medication order is changed to 20 milligrams per hour, what would the new flow rate be in drops per minute? _________

Notes/Workspace

Notes/Workspace

18. You have an order for 250 milliliters of 0.9% soduim chloride IV. Calculate the flow rate in drops per minute. The drop factor is 10 drops per milliliter, and the infusion time is 2 hours. ________

19. An infusion of 500 millliliters of lactated Ringer's solution was started at 1 P.M. The flow rate is 25 drops per minute, and the drop factor is 15 drops per milliliter. At what time will this IV finish? ________

20. A loading dose of the bronchodilator aminophylline (Aminophyllin) is ordered at 0.18 milligram per kilogram per minute. The patient weighs 70 kilograms. What will the flow rate be if 500 milligrams of aminophylline is added to 250 milliliters of 5% D/W? The drop factor is 10 drops per milliliter.

____

Cumulative Review Exercises

Review your mastery of earlier chapters.

1. The patient weighs 120 pounds. The medication order for a drug is for 200 micrograms per kilogram of body weight. The label read 2 milligrams per milliliter. How many milliliters of solution is equal to the medication order?

   ____

2. The prescriber ordered: 0.06 g ketorolac IM. How many milliliters of this NSAID are equal to 0.06 gram of this drug if the label reads 30 milligrams per milliliter? ________

3. The patient must receive 500,000 units of penicillin IM, and the vial contains 20,000,000 units (in powdered form). The directions are as follows: Add 38.7 mL to vial, 1 mL = 500,000 u. How many milliliters will equal 500,000 units? ________

4. A patient must receive grain $\frac{1}{150}$ of scopolamine, a parasympathetic depressant. The label on the ampule reads 0.6 milligram per milliliter. How many minims will you administer to this client? ________

Notes/Workspace

5. The prescriber ordered: cefprozil 0.5 g po q12. The bottle is labeled 125 mg = 5 mL. How many milliliters of this antibiotic will you give your patient? ________

6. If you have a vial labeled 25 milligrams per milliliter, how many milliliters would equal 0.025 grams? ________

7. The physician has ordered 0.25 gram of clarithromycin (Biaxin). The tablets are 250 milligrams each. How many tablets equal 0.25 gram of this antibiotic? ________

8. The prescriber has requested that you give 20 milliequivalents of potassium chloride (K-Lor) po to a patient from a bottle labeled 10 milliequivalents per 5 milliliters. How many milliliters are needed? ________

9. gr $\frac{1}{6000}$ = ________ mg

10. 0.8 mg = gr ________

11. 25 g = gr ________

12. gr $\frac{1}{120}$ = ________ g

13. 1 mL = ________ gtt

14. 2 T = ________ t

15. 30 mL = ℥ ________

chapter 12

Calculating Pediatric Dosages

Objectives

After completing this chapter, you will be able to

- *calculate pediatric dosages based on body weight.*
- *calculate pediatric dosages based on body surface area.*
- *determine body surface area using a nomogram.*

The prescriber must determine the proper kind and amount of medication for a patient. However, the dosage for infants and children is usually less than the adult dosage because they have smaller body masses and different metabolisms than adults. In this chapter, you will be introduced to methods of calculating pediatric dosages based on the recommendations of the drug's manufacturer.

For many years, pediatric dosage calculations used pediatric formulas such as Fried's rule, Young's rule, and Clark's rule (see Appendix G). These formulas are based on the weight of the child in pounds, or age of the child in months, and the normal adult dose of a specific drug. By using these formulas, one could determine how much should be prescribed for a particular child.

At the present time, the most accurate methods of determining an appropriate pediatric dose are by weight and body surface area (see Appendix F). You **must** know whether the amount of a prescribed pediatric dosage is the safe or appropriate amount for a particular patient. If this information is not on the drug label, it can be found on the package insert, in the hospital formulary, *Physician's Desk Reference* (PDR), *United States Pharmacopeia*, or in pharmacology texts.

Notes/Workspace

Calculating Drug Dosages by Body Weight

Drug manufacturers sometimes recommend a dosage based on the weight of the patient. You were introduced to this idea in Chapter 7.

Example 12.1

The medication order reads:

cefaclor 20 mg/kg po

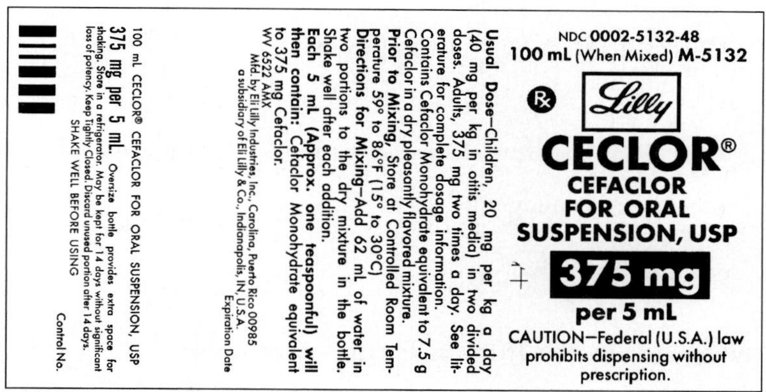

Figure 12.1 *Drug label for Ceclor*

Read the label in Figure 12.1. The child weighs 38 kilograms. How many milliliters of the drug will you administer to this child?

You want to convert body weight to dose in milliliters.

38 kg → ? mL

Notes/Workspace

Do this problem on one line as follows:

$$38 \text{ kg} \times \frac{? \text{ mg}}{? \text{ kg}} \times \frac{? \text{ mL}}{? \text{ mg}} = ? \text{ mL}$$

Since 20 mg = 1 kg, the first equivalent fraction is $\frac{20 \text{ mg}}{1 \text{ kg}}$. Since 5 mL = 375 mg, the second equivalent fraction is $\frac{5 \text{ mL}}{375 \text{ mg}}$. You cancel the kilograms and milligrams and obtain the dose in milliliters.

$$38 \cancel{\text{kg}} \times \frac{20 \cancel{\text{mg}}}{1 \cancel{\text{kg}}} \times \frac{\overset{1}{\cancel{5}} \text{ mL}}{\underset{75}{\cancel{375}} \cancel{\text{mg}}} = 10.1 \text{ mg}$$

So the child should receive 10.1 milliliters of cefaclor.

Example 12.2

How many milligrams of the antibiotic loracarbef (Lorabid) would you administer to a child with a body weight of 35 kilograms if the order is 2.9 milligrams per kilogram?

You want to convert body weight to dose in milligrams.

$$35 \text{ kg} \rightarrow ? \text{ mg}$$

$$35 \text{ kg} \times \frac{? \text{ mg}}{? \text{ kg}} = ? \text{ mg}$$

Since 2.9 mg = 1 kg, the equivalent fraction is $\frac{2.9 \text{ mg}}{1 \text{ kg}}$. You cancel the kilograms and obtain the dose in milligrams.

$$35 \cancel{\text{kg}} \times \frac{2.9 \text{ mg}}{1 \cancel{\text{kg}}} = 101.5 \text{ mg}$$

So the child would receive 101.5 milligrams of loracarbef.

Example 12.3

Compute the dose of the drug biperiden hydrochloride (Akineton), an anticholinergic drug, for a child who weighs 48 kilograms and for a prescribed order of 0.04 milligram per kilogram.

You want to convert body weight to dose in milligrams.

$$48 \text{ kg} \rightarrow ? \text{ mg}$$

$$48 \text{ kg} \times \frac{? \text{ mg}}{? \text{ kg}} = ? \text{ mg}$$

Since 0.04 mg = 1 kg, the equivalent fraction is $\frac{0.04 \text{ mg}}{1 \text{ kg}}$. You cancel the kilograms and obtain the dose in milligrams.

$$48 \cancel{\text{kg}} \times \frac{0.04 \text{ mg}}{1 \cancel{\text{kg}}} = 1.92 \text{ mg}$$

So the child should receive 1.92 milligrams of biperiden hydrochloride.

Example 12.4

Read the information on the label in Figure 12.2. The prescriber ordered:

cefaclor 20 mg/kg po bid

The child weighs 25 kilograms. How many milliliters will you prepare of this antibiotic?

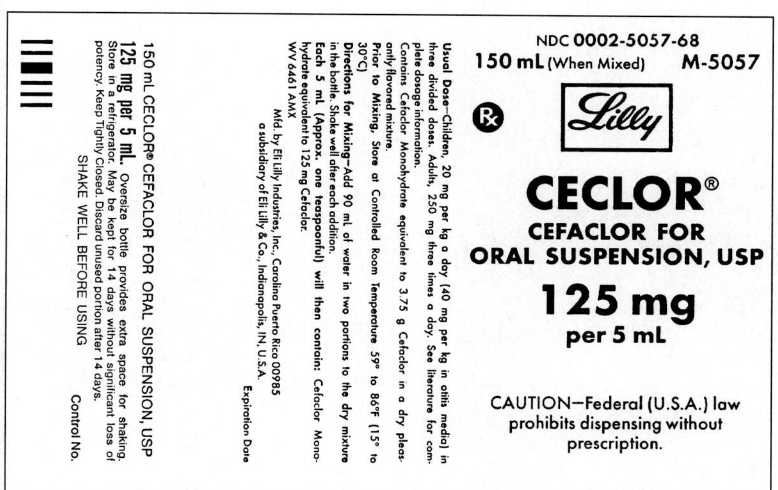

Figure 12.2 *Drug label for Ceclor*

Notes/Workspace

Notes/Workspace

You want to convert body weight to dose in milliliters.

$$25 \text{ kg} \rightarrow ? \text{ mL}$$

Do this on one line as follows:

$$25 \text{ kg} \times \frac{? \text{ mg}}{? \text{ kg}} \times \frac{? \text{ mL}}{? \text{ mg}} = ? \text{ mL}$$

Since 20 mg = 1 kg, the first equivalent fraction is $\frac{20 \text{ mg}}{1 \text{ kg}}$. Since 125 mL = 5 mL, the second equivalent fraction is $\frac{5 \text{ mL}}{125 \text{ mg}}$.

$$\overset{1}{\cancel{25}}\ \cancel{\text{kg}} \times \frac{20\ \cancel{\text{mg}}}{1\ \cancel{\text{kg}}} \times \frac{5 \text{ mL}}{\underset{5}{\cancel{125}}\ \cancel{\text{mg}}} = 20 \text{ mL}$$

So you would prepare 20 milliliters of cefaclor.

Example 12.5

You have an order for 15 milligrams per kilogram of acetaminophen (Tylenol). How many grains would you administer to a child who weighs 15 kilograms?

You want to convert body weight to dose in grains.

$$15 \text{ kg} \rightarrow \text{gr?}$$

Do this on one line as follows:

$$15 \text{ kg} \times \frac{? \text{ mg}}{? \text{ kg}} \times \frac{\text{gr ?}}{? \text{ mg}} = \text{gr ?}$$

Since 15 mg = 1 kg, the first equivalent fraction is $\frac{15 \text{ mg}}{1 \text{ kg}}$. Since 60 mg = gr 1, the second equivalent fraction is $\frac{\text{gr } 1}{60 \text{ mg}}$.

$$15\ \cancel{\text{kg}} \times \frac{\overset{1}{\cancel{15}}\ \cancel{\text{mg}}}{1\ \cancel{\text{kg}}} \times \frac{\text{gr } 1}{\underset{4}{\cancel{60}}\ \cancel{\text{mg}}} = \text{gr } \frac{15}{4} = \text{gr } 3\frac{3}{4}$$

So the dose of this analgesic drug should be grains $3\frac{3}{4}$.

Notes/Workspace

Example 12.6

The order reads:

atropine sulfate 0.04 mg IM stat

The child weighs 40 kilograms, and the recommended dose is 0.001 milligram per kilogram. Is this a safe dose for this child?

Again, you want to convert body weight to dose in milligrams.

$$40 \text{ kg} \rightarrow ? \text{ mg}$$

$$40 \text{ kg} \times \frac{? \text{ mg}}{? \text{ kg}} = ? \text{ mg}$$

You cancel the kilograms and obtain the dose in milligrams.

$$40 \cancel{\text{kg}} \times \frac{0.001 \text{ mg}}{1 \cancel{\text{kg}}} = 0.04 \text{ mg}$$

So 0.04 milligram is a safe dose for this child.

Example 12.7

The prescriber ordered 0.068 milligram po of digoxin (Lanoxin). The child weighs 45 pounds, and the recommended dose is 0.015 milligram per pound. Is this a safe dose?

You want to convert body weight to dose in milligrams.

$$45 \text{ lb} \rightarrow ? \text{ mg}$$

$$45 \text{ lb} \times \frac{? \text{ mg}}{? \text{ lb}} = ? \text{ mg}$$

You cancel the pounds and obtain the dose in milligrams.

$$45 \cancel{\text{lb}} \times \frac{0.0015 \text{ mg}}{1 \cancel{\text{lb}}} = 0.0675 \text{ mg}$$

Therefore, 0.0675 or 0.068 milligram is the correct dose, so the prescribed dose (0.068 milligrams) is correct.

Notes/Workspace

Example 12.8

The prescriber ordered:

digoxin 0.001 mg/kg po qd

The infant weighs 18 kilograms. How many milligrams would you administer to this child?

You want to convert body weight to dose in milligrams.

$$18 \text{ kg} \rightarrow ? \text{ mg}$$

$$18 \text{ kg} \times \frac{? \text{ mg}}{? \text{ kg}} = ? \text{ mg}$$

You cancel the kilograms and obtain the dose in milligrams.

$$18 \cancel{\text{kg}} \times \frac{0.001 \text{ mg}}{1 \cancel{\text{kg}}} = 0.018 \text{ mg}$$

So the infant should receive 0.018 milligram of digoxin.

Example 12.9

The prescriber ordered the antibiotic cefpodoxime (Vantin) for a child with a weight of 25 kilograms. If the label reads 50 milligrams per milliliter and the order is 4 milligrams per kilogram, what would be the dose in milliliters?

You want to convert the body weight to dose in milliliters.

$$25 \text{ kg} \rightarrow ? \text{ mL}$$

Do this on one line as follows:

$$25 \text{ kg} \times \frac{? \text{ mg}}{? \text{ kg}} \times \frac{? \text{ mL}}{? \text{ mg}} = ? \text{ mL}$$

You cancel the kilograms and milligrams and obtain the dose in milliliters.

$$\overset{1}{\cancel{25}} \cancel{\text{kg}} \times \frac{4 \cancel{\text{mg}}}{1 \cancel{\text{kg}}} \times \frac{1 \text{ mL}}{\underset{2}{\cancel{50}} \cancel{\text{mg}}} = 2 \text{ mL}$$

So, the prescribed dose is 2 milliliters of Vantin.

Notes/Workspace

Example 12.10

The prescriber ordered:

Retrovir 2.5 mg/kg po qd

The child weighs 42 kilograms. Read the information on the label in Figure 12.3 and calculate the dose in milliliters for this antiviral drug.

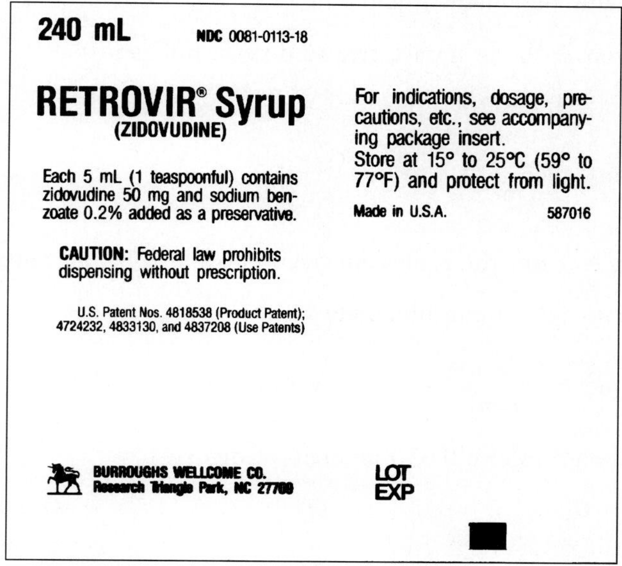

240 mL
NDC 0081-0113-18
RETROVIR® Syrup
(ZIDOVUDINE)
Each 5 mL (1 teaspoonful) contains zidovudine 50 mg and sodium benzoate 0.2% added as a preservative.
CAUTION: Federal law prohibits dispensing without prescription.
U.S. Patent Nos. 4818538 (Product Patent); 4724232, 4833130, and 4837208 (Use Patents)
For indications, dosage, precautions, etc., see accompanying package insert.
Store at 15° to 25°C (59° to 77°F) and protect from light.
Made in U.S.A.
587016
BURROUGHS WELLCOME CO.
Research Triangle Park, NC 27709
LOT
EXP

Figure 12.3 *Drug label for Retrovir*

You want to convert the body weight to dose in milliliters.

$$42 \text{ kg} \rightarrow ? \text{ mL}$$

Do this on one line as follows:

$$42 \text{ kg} \times \frac{? \text{ mg}}{? \text{ kg}} \times \frac{? \text{ mL}}{? \text{ mg}} = ? \text{ mg}$$

The order is 2.5 milligrams per kilogram, so the first equivalent fraction is $\frac{2.5 \text{ mg}}{1 \text{ kg}}$. Since 50 mg = 1 mL, the second equivalent fraction is $\frac{5 \text{ mL}}{50 \text{ mg}}$.

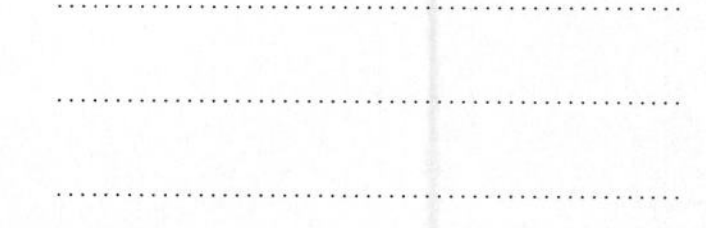

$$42 \cancel{\text{kg}} \times \frac{2.5 \cancel{\text{mg}}}{1 \cancel{\text{kg}}} \times \frac{5 \text{ mL}}{50 \cancel{\text{mg}}} = 10.5 \text{ mL}$$

So the prescribed dose is 10.5 milliliters of Retrovir.

Notes/Workspace

Calculating Drug Dosages by Body Surface Area

Drug manufacturers sometimes recommend a dosage based on body surface area (BSA). You were introduced to this idea in Chapter 2.

Example 12.11

The prescriber ordered: digoxin 0.72 mg/m^2 po qd. The child's BSA is 0.9 square meter. How many milligrams would you administer to this child?

You want to convert body surface area to dose in milligrams.

$$0.9 \text{ m}^2 \rightarrow ? \text{ mg}$$

$$0.9 \text{ m}^2 \times \frac{? \text{ mg}}{? \text{ m}^2} = ? \text{ mg}$$

Since 0.72 mg = 1 m^2, the equivalent fraction is $\frac{0.72 \text{ mg}}{1 \text{ m}^2}$. You cancel the square meter and obtain the dose in milligrams.

$$0.9 \cancel{\text{m}^2} \times \frac{0.72 \text{ mg}}{1 \cancel{\text{m}^2}} = 0.648 \text{ or } 0.65 \text{ mg}$$

So the child should receive 0.65 milligram of digoxin.

Example 12.12

If a child has a BSA of 0.5 square meter and the medication order is for 1.25 milligrams per square meter of vinblastine sulfate (Velban), then how many milligrams of this antineoplastic drug should the child receive?

You want to convert body surface area to dose in milligrams.

$$0.5 \text{ m}^2 \rightarrow ? \text{ mg}$$

$$0.5 \text{ m}^2 \times \frac{? \text{ mg}}{? \text{ m}^2} = ? \text{ mg}$$

Since the order is for 1.25 mg = 1 m^2, the equivalent fraction is $\frac{1.25 \text{ mg}}{1 \text{ m}^2}$. You cancel the square meters and obtain the dose in milligrams.

$$0.5 \cancel{\text{m}^2} \times \frac{1.25 \text{ mg}}{1 \cancel{\text{m}^2}} = 0.625 \text{ mg}$$

So the child should receive 0.625 milligram of vinblastine sulfate.

BSA Nomogram

If you do not know the BSA of a child, you can determine it from a chart called a *nomogram* (see Figure 12.4).

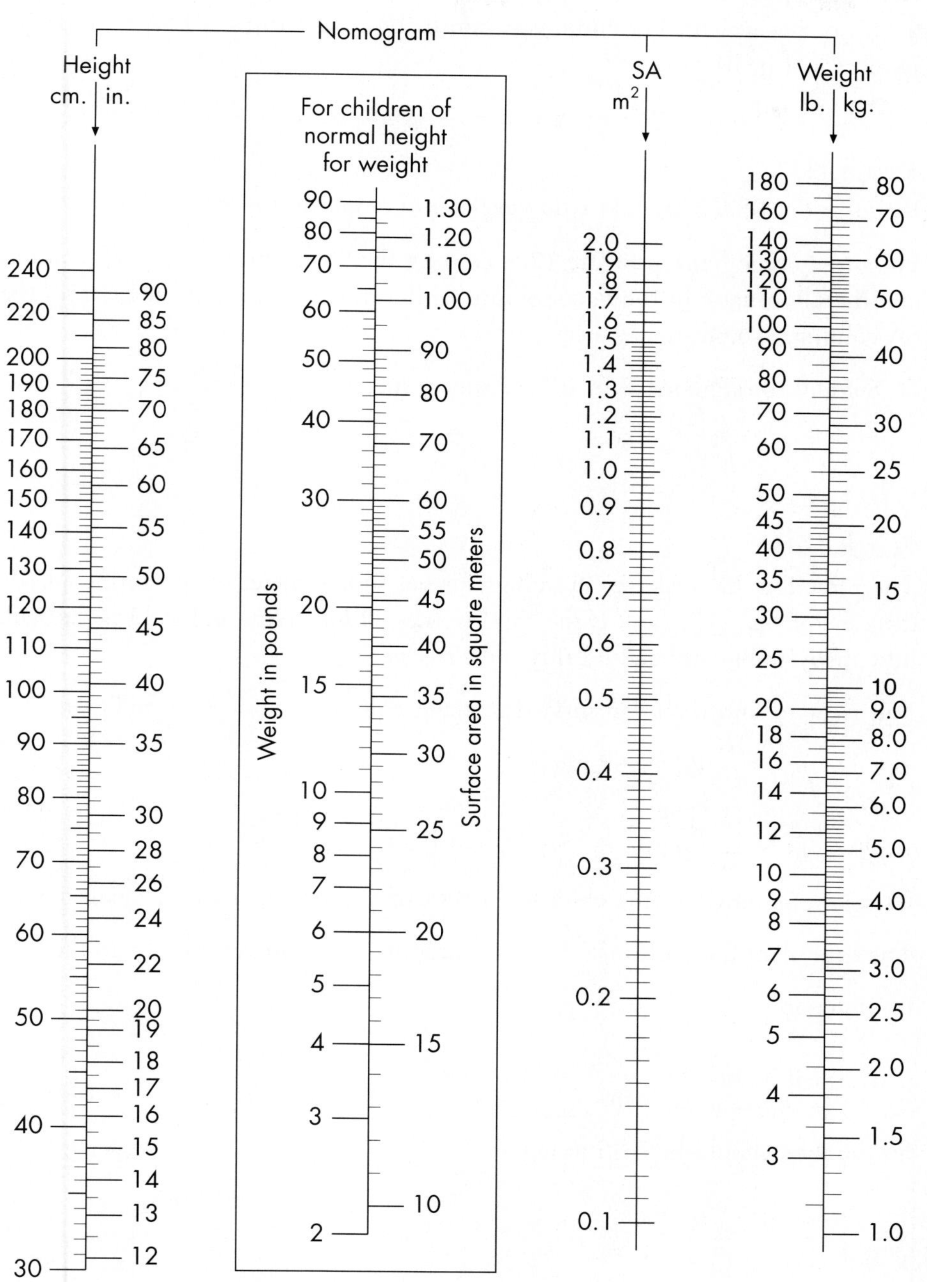

Figure 12.4 *Pediatric nomogram for determining BSA*

Notes/Workspace

Notes/Workspace

The body surface area is shown in the column labeled SA in Figure 12.4. A straight line is drawn between the child's height (first column) and the child's weight (last column). The point at which the line crosses the SA column is the estimated *BSA in square meters.* The boxed column listing weight on the left and surface in square meters on the right can be used when a child is of normal height for his or her weight. For additional information concerning a BSA nomogram, see a text of pediatrics.

Example 12.13

Estimate the BSA of a child who weighs 40 pounds and is 90 centimeters tall.

Using the nomogram in Figure 12.4, connect the 90 cm mark in the left column and the 40 lb mark in the right column with a straight line. This line crosses the SA column at 0.68 square meter.

So the child's estimated BSA is 0.68 square meter.

Example 12.14

The prescriber has ordered 30 milligrams per square meter of the antineoplastic drug melphalan (Alkeran). If the child weighs 20 kilograms and is 35 inches tall, how many milligrams should this child receive?

You want to find the body surface area and convert it to dose in milligrams.

$$\text{BSA} \rightarrow ?\ \text{mg}$$

$$\text{BSA} \times \frac{?\ \text{mg}}{?\ \text{m}^2} = ?\ \text{mg}$$

Using the nomogram, the child has a BSA of approximately 0.72 square meter. The equivalent fraction is $\frac{30\ \text{mg}}{1\ \text{m}^2}$. You cancel the square meter and obtain the dose in milligrams.

$$0.72\ \cancel{\text{m}^2} \times \frac{30\ \text{mg}}{1\ \cancel{\text{m}^2}} = 21.6\ \text{mg}$$

So the dose should be 21.6 milligrams.

Example 12.15

Hydroxine HCl (Vistaril), a skeletal muscle relaxant, has been ordered for a child. How many milliliters will you administer to a child 50 inches in height with a weight of 75 pounds if the order is for 25 milligram per square meter IM? The label reads 50 milligrams per milliliter.

You want to convert body surface area to dose in milliliters. According to the nomogram, the child's BSA is 1.05 square meters.

$$1.05 \text{ m}^2 = ? \text{ mL}$$

Do this on one line as follows:

$$1.05 \text{ m}^2 \times \frac{? \text{ mg}}{? \text{ m}^2} \times \frac{? \text{ mL}}{? \text{ mg}} = ? \text{ mL}$$

$$1.05 \cancel{\text{m}^2} \times \frac{\overset{1}{\cancel{25}} \cancel{\text{mg}}}{1 \cancel{\text{m}^2}} \times \frac{1 \text{ mL}}{\underset{2}{\cancel{50}} \text{ mg}} = 0.5 \text{ mL}$$

So you will administer 0.5 milliliter of Vistaril to the child.

Example 12.16

The prescriber has ordered 250 milligrams po qid of the antiviral drug zidovudine (AZT, Retrovir). Is this a safe dose for a child whose BSA is 1.11 square meter and the recommended dose for the drug is 100–180 milligrams per square meter?

You want to convert body surface area to dose in milligrams.

$$11.2 \text{ m}^2 \rightarrow ? \text{ mg}$$

First, use the *minimum* recommended dose of 100 milligrams per square meter.

$$1.11 \cancel{\text{m}^2} \times \frac{100 \text{ mg}}{1 \cancel{\text{m}^2}} = 111 \text{ mg}$$

Second, use the *maximum* recommended dose of 180 milligrams per square meter.

$$1.11 \cancel{\text{m}^2} \times \frac{180 \text{ mg}}{1 \cancel{\text{m}^2}} = 199.8 \text{ or } 200 \text{ mg}$$

Therefore, any prescribed amount in the range of 111–200 milligrams would be acceptable. So 250 milligrams is not a safe dose.

Notes/Workspace

Practice Sets

You will find the answers to the Try These for Practice, Exercises, and Cumulative Review Practice Sets in the Answer Section at the back of the book. Your instructor has the answers to the Additional Exercises.

Try These for Practice

Test your comprehension after reading this chapter.

1. The following order has been given for a child with a weight of 25 kilograms:

Humulin R insulin 0.11 u/kg sc bid

How many units will this child receive of this low-dose insulin? ________

2. Read the information on the label in Figure 12.5. What would the prescribed dose of Augmentin be for a patient who weighs 40 pounds if the order is for 7.5 milligrams per kilogram? ________

AUGMENTIN®
Tear along perforation
Directions for mixing: Tap bottle until all powder flows freely. Add approximately 2/3 of total water for reconstitution (total = 67 mL); shake vigorously to wet powder. Add remaining water; again shake vigorously.
Dosage: See accompanying prescribing information.
Important: Use safety closures when dispensing this product unless otherwise directed by physician or requested by purchaser.
Tear along perforation
Keep tightly closed.
Shake well before using.
Must be refrigerated.
Discard after 10 days.
125mg/5mL
NDC 0029-6085-39
AUGMENTIN®
AMOXICILLIN/
CLAVULANATE POTASSIUM
FOR ORAL SUSPENSION
When reconstituted, each 5 mL contains:
AMOXICILLIN, 125 MG,
as the trihydrate
CLAVULANIC ACID, 31.25 MG,
as clavulanate potassium
75 mL (when reconstituted)
SB SmithKline Beecham
NSN 6505-01-340-0847
Use only if inner seal is intact.
Net contents: Equivalent to 1.875 g amoxicillin and 0.469 g clavulanic acid.
Store dry powder at room temperature.
Caution: Federal law prohibits dispensing without prescription.
SmithKline Beecham Pharmaceuticals
Philadelphia, PA 19101
EXP.
LOT
9405804-C

Figure 12.5 *Drug label for Augmentin*

3. A child must receive meperidine hydrochloride (Demerol). The child's BSA is 0.8 square meter. How many milliliters will you administer to the child if the order is for 30 milligrams per square meter and the label reads 50 milligrams per milliliter? ________

4. Read the information on the label in Figure 12.6 (page 243). How many milliliters of Lanoxin would you administer to a child who weighs 40 kilograms when the order is for 0.0006 milligram per kilogram? ________

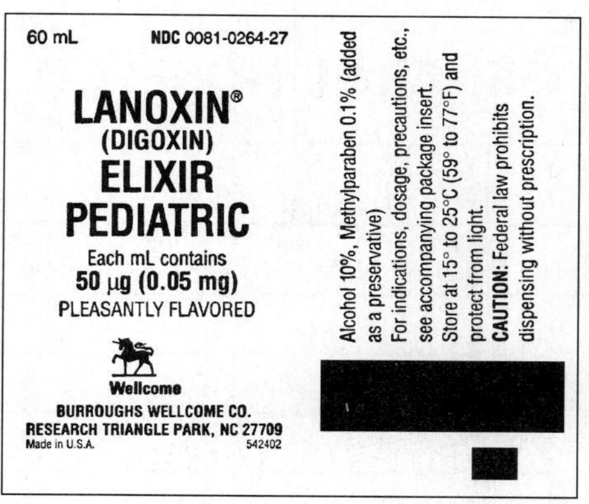

60 mL
NDC 0081-0264-27
LANOXIN®
(DIGOXIN)
ELIXIR
PEDIATRIC
Each mL contains
50 µg (0.05 mg)
PLEASANTLY FLAVORED
Wellcome
BURROUGHS WELLCOME CO.
RESEARCH TRIANGLE PARK, NC 27709
Made in U.S.A.
542402
Alcohol 10%, Methylparaben 0.1% (added
as a preservative)
For indications, dosage, precautions, etc.,
see accompanying package insert.
Store at 15° to 25°C (59° to 77°F) and
protect from light.
CAUTION: Federal law prohibits
dispensing without prescription.

Figure 12.6 *Drug label for pediatric Lanoxin*

Notes/Workspace

5. The order reads: zidovudine 180 mg/m^2 po q6h. How many milligrams would you administer to a child whose BSA is 1.2 square meters? ________

Exercises

Reinforce your understanding in class or at home.

1. Read the first order in the medication administration record shown in Figure 12.7 (page 244). The label reads 25 milligrams per 5 milliliters. How many teaspoons will you administer? ________

2. Read the second order in the MAR shown in Figure 12.7. The label on the bottle of acetaminophen reads 325 milligrams per tablet. How many tablets will you administer to this patient? ________

3. Read the third order in Figure 12.7. The child weighs 40 kilograms. How many milliliters of Keflex will you give the child if the label reads 125 milligrams per 5 milliliters? ________

4. The prescriber has ordered 3.3 micrograms per kilogram IM of fentanyl citrate (Sublimaze) as a pre-operative medication. The label on the vial reads 50 micrograms per milliliter. How many milliliters will you administer to this child whose weight is 30 kilograms? ________

5. The normal dose of a drug for a child is 0.2 milligram per square meter. If the child's BSA is 0.45 square meter, how many milligrams should this child receive? ________

Notes/Workspace

GENERAL HOSPITAL

Year 19 94 · Month 11 · Day		24	25	26			
Medication Dosage and Interval		Initials* and Hours	Initials and Hours	Initials and Hours	Initials and Hours	Initials and Hours	Initials and Hours
Date started: 11/24/94 Vistaril 0.025 g qid	I	JO	AG JO	AG JO			
	AM	10	10	10			
	I	LD LD	LD LD	LD LD			
Discontinued: 11/30/94	PM	2 6 10	2 6 10	2 6 10			
Date started: 11/24/94 acetaminophen 650 mg po q4h prn	I	JO	AG JO	AG JO			
	AM	10	1 9	7 11			
	I	JO LD	JO LD LD	LD LD			
Discontinued: 11/30/94	PM	2 8	2 6 11	8 12:00			
Date started: 11/24/94 Keflex 6.25 mg/kg po qid	I	JO	AG JO	AG JO			
	AM	10	10	10			
	I	LD LD	LD LD	LD LD			
Discontinued: 11/30/94	PM	2 6 10	2 6 10	2 6 10			

Allergies: (Specify)

Init*	Signature
JO	June Olsen
LD	Larissa Dingman
AG	Anthony Giangrasso

MEDICATION ADMINISTRATION RECORD

PATIENT IDENTIFICATION

0312578 11/24/94

Mary Johnson 6/21/89
2183 Avantlar Ave Prot
Phoenix, AR Aetna
10357

Leon Ablon, M.D.

Figure 12.7 *Medication administration record*

6. A child's BSA is 1.2 square meters, and 100 milligrams per square meter of the antineoplastic drug procarbazine HCl (Matulane) has been ordered. How many milligrams should this child receive? ________

7. If a child's BSA is 1.1 square meters, how many milligrams of the antibiotic gentamicin sulfate (Garamycin) should the child receive if the prescribed amount is 45 milligrams per square meter? ________

8. A long-acting anti-inflammatory medication, dexamethasone (Decadron), has been ordered for a child with a BSA of 1.2 square meters. How many milligrams should this child receive if the prescribed amount is 50 milligrams per square meter? ________

9. The anticholinergic medication scopolamine (Triptone) has been ordered for a child with a BSA of 0.8 square meter. How many milliliters will you prepare if the order is for 0.2 milligram per square meter and the ampule reads 0.2 milligram per milliliter? ________

10. Atropine sulfate has been ordered for a child who weighs 20 kilograms. The prescribed dose is 0.01 milligram per kilogram. Read the medication label in Figure 12.8. How many milliliters equal the prescribed dose? ________

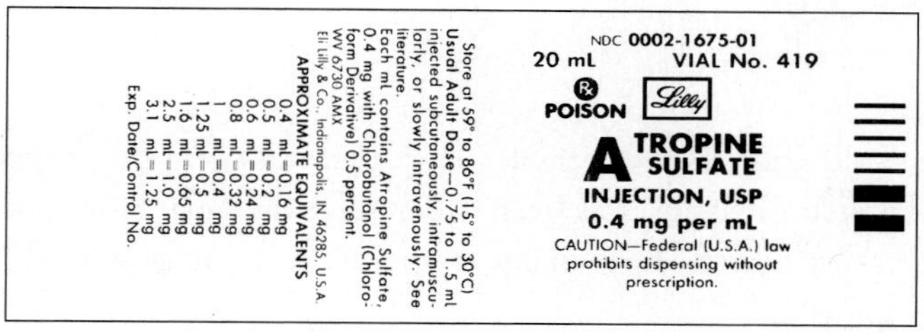

Figure 12.8 *Drug label for atropine sulfate*

11. The anticonvulsant medication phenytoin sodium (Dilantin) is ordered for a child with a BSA of 0.7 square meter. The prescribed dose is 250 milligrams per square meter. How many milliliters should this child receive if the oral suspension is 125 milligrams per milliliter? ________

12. The order states that a child is to receive: 1% lidocaine 0.5 mg/kg IV bolus. How many milliliters will you prepare for this child whose weight is 50 kilograms? ________

Notes/Workspace

Notes/Workspace

13. The prescriber orders 0.54 unit per kilogram of NPH insulin (Humulin N). If the child weighs 44 kilograms, how many milliliters will you prepare of the insulin in Figure 12.9? ________

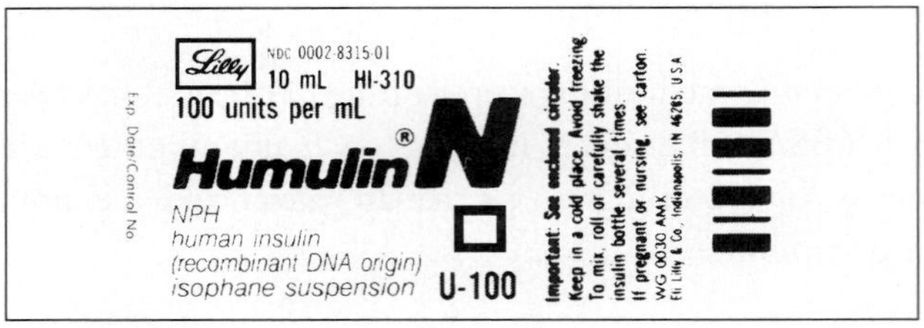

Figure 12.9 *Drug label for Humulin N insulin*

14. The prescriber ordered: Lasix 2 mg/kg po. If the child weighs 24 kilograms and the label reads 8 milligrams per milliliter, how many milliliters will you give to the child? ________

15. A 10-year-old child has a fever of 101°F, and 0.4 gram po of the antipyretic acetaminophen (Tylenol) has been ordered. If the elixir is labeled 160 milligrams per 5 milliliters, how many teaspoons will you give to the child?

____

16. A child has to receive an IV bolus of 1% lidocaine, 1 milligram per kilogram. How many milliliters will you prepare for a child with a weight of 30 kilograms? ________

17. Read the information on the label in Figure 12.10. The prescriber has ordered hydroxyzine HCl (Vistaril) IM for a child. If the child weighs 42 kilograms and the prescribed dose is 0.6 milligram per kilogram, how many milliliters will you administer to this child? ________

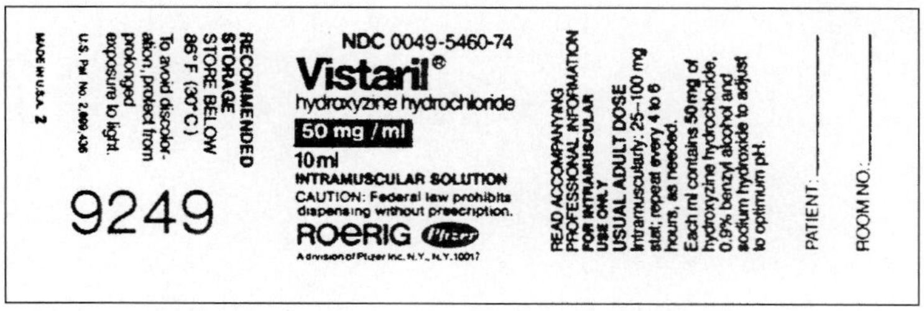

Figure 12.10 *Drug label for Vistaril*

18. The prescriber has ordered a stat dose of the gastrointestinal stimulant metoclopramide HCl (Reglan) IV, 0.1 milligram per kilogram direct IV push. If the vial is labeled 5 milligrams per milliliter and the child weighs 60 kilograms, how many milliliters will you prepare? __________

19. Meperidine HCl (Demerol) has been prescribed for a child whose weight is 60 pounds. The label on the vial reads 100 milligrams per milliliter. How many milliliters would you prepare of this narcotic analgesic if the prescribed amount is 1.04 milligrams per kilogram? __________

20. A child must receive the antineoplastic drug melphalan (Alkeran). The scored tablets are 2 milligrams each. What would be the correct dose if the order is 3 milligrams per square meter and the child's BSA is 1 square meter?

____

Notes/Workspace

Additional Exercises

Now, on your own, test yourself! Ask your instructor to check your answers.

1. The order reads: Vistaril 1.4 mg/kg IM q12h. The child weighs 48 kilograms. Read the information in Figure 12.11 and calculate the milliliters in this prescribed dose. __________

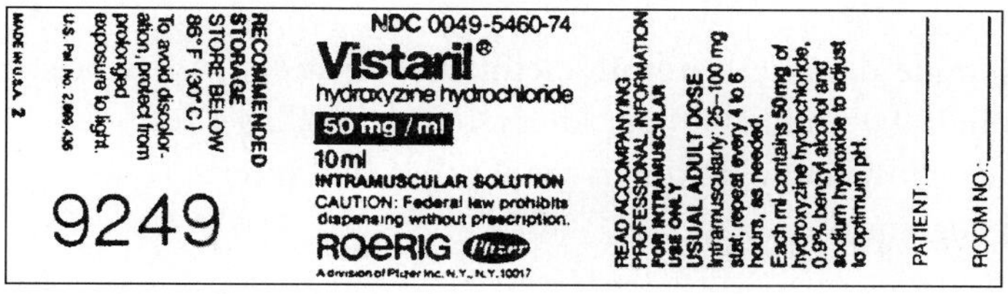

Figure 12.11 *Drug label for Vistaril*

2. The prescribed order for a child is 12 milligrams per kilogram of the sulfonamide sulfasalazine (Azulfidine), and the medication is available in 500 mg tablets. How many tablets would you give a child with a weight of 88 pounds?

____

3. Cyanocobalamin (vitamin B_{12}) is available in vials labeled 1 milligram per milliliter. How many micrograms would you give a child if the order is 2 micrograms per kilogram and the child's weight is 50 kilograms? How many milliliters would you administer to this child IM? __________

Notes/Workspace

4. The order reads: diphenhydramine 125 mcg/kg IM stat. The child weighs 25 kilograms and the medication label reads 5 milligrams per milliliter. How many milliliters will you administer to this child? ________

5. The antispasmodic drug tincture of belladonna has been prescribed for a child with nocturnal enuresis; the child is to receive 0.033 milligram per kilogram at bedtime. The label reads 0.3 milligram per milliliter. How many milliliters will you administer to this child whose weight is 45 pounds?

____

6. Read the information in Figure 12.12 and calculate the amount of atropine sulfate you would administer to a child if the order is 0.2 milligram per square meter and the child's BSA is 1.2 square meters. ________

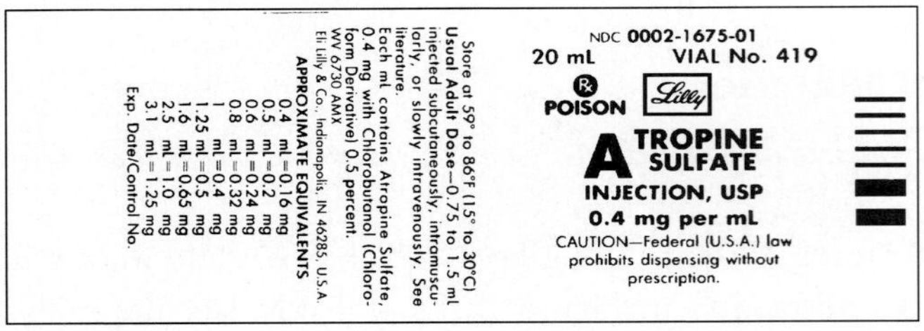

Figure 12.12 *Drug label for atropine sulfate*

7. The thiazide diuretic bendroflumethiazide (Naturetin) has been prescribed for a child, 0.05 milligram per kilogram tid. The label reads 1 milligram per milliliter. How many milliliters would the child receive if the child's weight is 34 kilograms? ________

8. The prescriber has written an order for the anti-inflammatory medication dexamethasone (Decadron) for a child with a BSA of 0.64 square meter. How many milligrams should the child receive if the order is for 0.05 gram per square meter? ________

9. The order reads: benzthiazide 0.75 mg/kg po tid. Each tablet contains 25 milligrams. If the child weighs 77 pounds, how many tablets will you administer to this child? ________

Notes/Workspace

10. A prescriber orders loracarbef (Lorabid) for a child who has a BSA of 0.9 square meter. If the label reads 100 milligrams per 5 milliliters and the recommended dose is 100 milligrams per square meter, how many milliliters will the child receive of this broad-spectrum antibiotic? _________

11. A prescriber orders ketamine hydrochloride (Ketalar), a drug that causes disassociative anesthesia. The label reads 10 milligrams per milliliter, and the child weighs 35 kilograms. The order is for 3.5 milligrams per kilogram. How many milliliters will the child receive IV from the anesthesiologist?

____

12. The order reads: digoxin 0.01 mg/kg po qd. The label on the vial reads 0.25 milligram per milliliter. How many minims will you administer to a child who weighs 18 kilograms? _________

13. The prescriber has ordered methohexital sodium (Brevital Sodium) IV, a general anesthetic for a short-term procedure. If 70 milligrams are prepared and the label reads 50 milligrams per 5 milliliters, how many milliliters equal the prescribed dose? _________

14. Digitoxin (Crystodigin), a cardiac glycoside, has been prescribed. The child weighs 36 kilograms and each tablet contains 0.2 milligram. How many tablets will you prepare if the order is for 0.011 milligram per kilogram?

____

15. A child is to receive 100 micrograms of digitoxin (Crystodigin). Tablets are available in 0.3 mg, 0.1 mg, and 0.15 mg increments. Determine which of these tablets should be administered to this child po. _________

16. The order reads: demeclocycline hydrochloride 0.15 g po tid. The recommended dose for children is 6 milligrams per pound. If the child's weight is 25.5 kilograms, would this be a safe dose? _________

Notes/Workspace

17. Read the label in Figure 12.13 for the expectorant Nucofed. If the prescriber gave the child $\frac{1}{2}$ teaspoon, how many milligrams of codeine will the child receive? ________

Each 5 mL (teaspoonful) contains: Codeine Phosphate, 10 mg (Warning: May Be Habit Forming); Pseudoephedrine Hydrochloride, 30 mg; Guaifenesin (glyceryl guaiacolate), 100 mg; Alcohol, 6.0%. Caution: Federal law prohibits dispensing without prescription. PROFESSIONAL PACKAGE—NOT TO BE SOLD
MB68 Exp. Aug., 1990
NDC 0029 3130 01
Physician's Started Dose
NUCOFED®
PEDIATRIC EXPECTORANT
Syrup
Expectorant-Antitussive Decongestant
15 mL
Beecham laboratories
DIV. OF BEECHAM INC. BRISTOL, TENN 37620
RECOMMENDED DOSAGE: Adults and Children 12 years of age and over: 2 teaspoonfuls every 6 hours, not to exceed 8 teaspoonfuls in 24 hours. Children: 6 to under 12 years: 1 teaspoonful every 6 hours, not to exceed 4 teaspoonfuls in 24 hours. 2 to under 6 years: ½ teaspoonful every 6 hours, not to exceed 2 teaspoonfuls in 24 hours. Do not give this product to children under 2 years, except under the advice and supervision of a physician.—Read Insert.
0938139 C88

Figure 12.13 *Drug label for Nucofed*

18. Read the first order in Figure 12.14. If the label reads 10 milligrams per milliliter, how many milliliters will you prepare for a child who weighs 75 pounds? ________

⊕ GENERAL HOSPITAL ⊕

Year 19 *94* Month *April* Day		*10*	*11*	*12*	*13*	*14*	*15*
Medication Dosage and Interval		Initials* and Hours	Initials and Hours	Initials and Hours	Initials and Hours	Initials and Hours	Initials and Hours
Date started: *4/10/94* *chlorpromazine 0.25 mg/kg q6h Im 12 noon, 6 P.M., 12 mid, 6 A.M.* Discontinued: *4/13/94*	I	*LD LD*	*LD LD*	*LD LD*	*LD LD*		
	AM	*12 6*	*12 6*	*12 6*	*12 6*		
	I	*JO JO*	*JO JO*	*JO JO*	*JO JO*		
	PM	*12 6*	*12 6*	*12 6*	*12 6*		
Date started: *4/10/94* *Alkeran 3 mg/m² qd po x 14 doses, start at 10 A.M.* Discontinued: *4/13/94 after 2 P.M.*	I	*LD*	*LD*	*LD*	*LD*		
	AM	*10*	*10*	*10*	*10*		
	I	*JO JO JO*	*JO JO JO*	*JO JO JO*	*JO*		
	PM	*2 6 10*	*2 6 10*	*2 6 10*	*2*		

Allergies: (Specify)

Init*	Signature
LD	*L. Dingman*
JO	*June Olsen*

MEDICATION ADMINISTRATION RECORD

PATIENT IDENTIFICATION

1077854 4/10/94
Johnny Davis 12/4/82
1622 Alki Dr. #43 RC
Seattle, WA 94032 US Health Care
L.Ablon, M.D.

Figure 12.14 *Medication administration record*

19. Read the second order in Figure 12.14 for the antineoplastic drug Alkeran. The child's BSA is 0.8 square meter. How many milligrams will you prepare of this drug? ________

20. The initial dose of dextrothyroxine (Choloxin), a drug used for the treatment of hyperlipidemia in euthyroid patients, is 0.05 milligram per kilogram. How many milligrams should be given to a child who weighs 42 kg?

____

Notes/Workspace

Cumulative Review Exercises

Review your mastery of earlier chapers.

1. How many milligrams of ethambutol HCl (Myambutal), an antitubercular drug, would you administer if the prescribed dose po is 15 milligrams per kilogram and the child weighs 35 kilograms? ________

2. How many milligrams of the antibiotic penicillin would you prepare for a child who weighs 40 kilograms if the order is 75 milligrams per kilogram?

____

3. The order reads: cefixime 8 mg/kg po. How many milligrams of this antibiotic would you administer to a child whose weight is 20 kilograms? ________

4. The order reads: 50 u Lente insulin sc. The vial is labeled 100 units per milliliter. How many minims would you administer to the patient?

____

5. The prescriber has ordered 1,200,000 units of penicillin G IM. The 5,000,000 u vial of powder has these instructions: Add 8 mL of sterile water, 1 mL = 500,000 u. How many milliliters equals 1,200,000 units? ________

6. The order is for 0.04 gram of nicardipine HCl (Cardene). Each tablet contains 20 milligrams. How many tablets equal the prescribed dose of this antianginal drug? ________

Notes/Workspace

7. The order reads: amrinone lactate 0.75 mg/kg IV bolus. How many milligrams will you prepare of this inotropic drug if the patient weighs 116 pounds?

____

8. The prescriber ordered: 900 mL of 5% D/W IV in 5 h. Calculate the flow rate in drops per minute when the drop factor is 20 drops per milliliter. _________

9. The order reads: dobutamine HCl 5 mcg/kg/min IV; add 250 mg to 250 mL 5% D/W. If the weight of the patient is 130 pounds, calculate the flow rate in milliliters per hour for this cardiac stimulant. _________

10. The prescriber ordered: 1000 mL 5% D/W at 14 gtt/min IV. The infusion began at 9 P.M. At what time will this solution be completed? The drop factor is 10 drops per milliliter. _________

11. 0.001 g = gr _________

12. How many milligrams of an antibiotic would you administer to an adult with a BSA of 1.9 square meters if the order is for 410 milligrams per square meter? _________

13. Describe how to prepare 100 milliliters of a $\frac{1}{4}$% solution from a $\frac{1}{2}$% solution.

____

____

14. The order is for 0.05 gram of nicardipine (Cardene) po. How many milligrams will you administer of this anti-anginal medication? _________

15. gr viiss = _________ mg

Case Studies and Comprehensive Self-Tests

Answers to Case Studies and Comprehensive Self-Tests 1–3 can be found in Appendix A at the back of the the book. Your instructor has the answers to Case Studies and Comprehensive Self-Tests 4–6.

Case Study 1: Horacio Gomez

Mr. Horacio Gomez has been admitted to Mission Hospital through the Emergency Room, after fainting at work. His admitting diagnosis is hypertension and dehydration. Vital signs are T: 100.2°F; P: 103; R: 28; BP: 190/102; weight: 50 kilograms. The attending physician, Dr. John Leebo, writes the following orders:

- 500 mL of 5% D/W with Arfonad 500 mg; infuse at rate of 0.25 mg/min, separate IV line
- 0.9% NS IV, 30 mL/hr primary IV line
- Flagyl 50 mg in 50 mL 5% D/W IVPB q8h
- Kefurox 25 mg/kg q12h, add 1250 mg to 100 mL 5% D/W

1. Calculate the flow rate for the Arfonad. The drop factor is 60 drops per milliliter. ________

2. Calculate the flow rate for the Flagyl and the Kefurox. Each IV will infuse in 30 minutes. The drop factor is 10 drops per milliliter. ________

3. What is the flow rate in drops per minute for the 0.9% normal saline? The drop factor is 10 drops per milliliter. ________

4. How many milligrams of Arfonad will the patient receive in 24 hours? ________

Notes/Workspace

5. Calculate the total amount of fluid the patient will receive IV in 24 hours. (Remember, 0.9% normal saline does not infuse when IVPB medication is given.) ________

Comprehensive Self-Test 1

1. The prescriber has ordered ursodiol (Actigall), a drug for dissolving gallstones, for Mr. Jones. The usual range for the dosage of this drug is 8–10 milligrams per kilogram per day in two or three divided doses. If the patient weighs 70 kilograms and the prescribed dose is 300 milligrams bid, is this a correct dose? ________

2. The nonsteroidal anti-inflammatory drug diclofenac sodium (Voltaren) is ordered for a patient with rheumatoid arthritis. The usual dose is 50 milligrams tid. Each enteric-coated tablet contains 50 milligrams of the drug. How many tablets should the patient receive each day? ________

3. An anti-infective medication, amoxicillin (Amoxil), has been ordered by the prescriber for Mary Johnson, 0.25 gram q8h. How many capsules will you require for 24 hours if each capsule contains 250 milligrams? ________

4. Read the information for the first medication order in Figure ST1.1. Each Cardizem tablet is labeled 30 milligrams. How many tablets will you administer to Mrs. Olsen? ________

5. In the second order on the medication sheet in Figure ST1.1, Mrs. Olsen must receive Humulin N (NPH insulin). How many minims contain 45 units when the label reads 100 units per milliliter? ________

6. The medication order in Figure ST1.1 is to be prepared from an ampule labeled Vistaril 50 mg/2 mL. How many minims should the patient receive? ________

7. The fourth order on the medication order sheet in Figure ST1.1 is for folic acid. Convert this order to grains. ________

8. Read the fifth order on the medication order sheet in Figure ST1.1 and calculate the number of tablets you will administer to the patient if each tablet is labeled 0.25 milligram. ________

9. Ranitidine HCl (Zantac), an H_2 receptor antagonist, is frequently ordered to inhibit gastric acid secretion. If the order is 0.15 gram po and each tablet contains 150 milligrams, how many tablets will you administer to this patient? ________

Notes/Workspace

⊕ GENERAL HOSPITAL ⊕

Year 19 *94/95* Month *Dec/Jan* Day		*31*	*1*	*2*	*3*	*4*	*5*
Medication Dosage and Interval		Initials* and Hours	Initials and Hours	Initials and Hours	Initials and Hours	Initials and Hours	Initials and Hours
Date started: *12/31* *Cardizem 0.03 g bid po*	I	*JO*	*JO*	*JO*			
	AM	*10*	*10*	*10*			
	I	*LA*	*LA*	*LA*			
Discontinued:	PM	*6*	*6*	*6*			
Date started: *12/31* *Humulin N 45 u sc q A.M. 8 A.M.*	I	*JO*	*JO*	*JO*			
	AM	*8*	*8*	*8*			
	I						
Discontinued:	PM						
Date started: *12/31* *Vistaril 45 mg IM hs*	I						
	AM						
	I	*LA*	*LA*	*LA*			
Discontinued:	PM	*10*	*10*	*10*			
Date started: *12/31* *folic acid 0.001 g qd po 10 A.M.*	I	*JO*	*JO*	*JO*			
	AM	*10*	*10*	*10*			
	I						
Discontinued:	PM						
Date started: *12/31* *vitamin C 500 mg bid po*	I	*JO*	*JO*	*JO*			
	AM	*10*	*10*	*10*			
	I	*LA*	*LA*	*LA*			
Discontinued:	PM	*6*	*6*	*6*			

Allergies: (Specify)

Init*	Signature
JO	*June Olsen*
LA	*Leon Ablon*

MEDICATION ADMINISTRATION RECORD

PATIENT IDENTIFICATION

6056812 12/31/94
Marianne Olsen 7/10/42
Rt 1 Box 456 Prot
Essex MT 60514 BCBS
Dr. Giangrasso

Figure ST1.1 *Medication order sheet*

Notes/Workspace

10. The injectable form of Zantac is labeled 25 milligrams per milliliter. If the order requires that 50 milligrams be diluted to 20 milliliters, how many milliliters of Zantac is required and how many milliliters of diluent?

____

11. You are told to infuse 20 milliliters of a solution in 20 minutes. The drop factor is 60 microdrops per milliliter. Find the flow rate. _________

12. An infusion of 5% D/W has 800 milliliters left in bag (LIB). The flow rate is 31 drops per minute, and the drop factor is 15 drops per milliliter. How many hours will it take for this IV to infuse? _________

13. Calculate the number of milliliters per minute for an IV of 250 milliliters of 5% D/W with 0.5 gram of lidocaine when the order is to administer 2 milligrams per minute. _________

14. The patient has an order for 30 milliliters po of the laxative lactulose (Chronulac). The oral solution label reads 10 grams per 15 milliliters. How many grams of this drug is the patient receiving? _________

15. The patient requires 20 milligrams IV of labetalol (Normodyne, Trandate) in 2 minutes. The vial is labeled 5 milligrams per milliliter. How many milliliters of this antihypertensive drug will the patient receive? _________

16. The order in Problem 15 has been changed to read:

Add 80 mg to 100 mL 5% D/W, infuse at rate of 2 mg/min

Calculate the flow rate in microdrops. _________

17. The prescriber has ordered 500 milligrams of bretylium tosylate (Bretylate, Bretylol), an adrenergic blocking agent, in 500 milliliters of normal saline solution, to be infused at a rate of 1 milligram per minute. The total amount of IV solution is 510 milliliters. Calculate the flow rate in milliliters per hour. _________

18. The patient was admitted with unstable ventricular tachycardia. The order reads:

500 mg bretylium tosylate (10 mL) to 50 mL 5% D/W IV

The total amount of solution is 60 milliliters; it is to be infused at a rate of 0.1 milligram per kilogram per minute. The patient weighs 120 pounds, and the drop factor is 15 drops per milliliter. Calculate the flow rate.

____

19. The order reads: vitamin C 500 mg IV daily in 100 mL 5% D/W for 120 min. The vial is labeled 500 milligrams per milliliter. Calculate the flow rate when the drop factor is 15 drops per milliliter. ________

20. If an IV of 5% D/W is started at 6:20 P.M. and is infusing at a rate of 8 drops per minute with a drop factor of 15 drops per milliliter, how many milliliters per hour is the patient receiving? ________

21. An IV of 0.9% NS has 120 milliliters LIB. If the infusion rate is 50 drops per minute and the drop factor is 15 drops per milliliter, how long will it take to complete this infusion? ________

22. Read the information on the label in Figure ST1.2. If the order is for 200 micrograms of clonidine HCl po, how many tablets will you prepare?

____

Figure ST1.2 *Drug label for clonidine*

23. A patient must have an IV infusion of 500 milliliters of 5% D/W with 50,000 units of heparin. Read the information in Figure ST1.3.

a. How many milliliters of heparin must be added to the 5% D/W?

____

b. Calculate the flow rate in milliliters per hour. The order is 500 units per hour. ________

Figure ST1.3 *Drug label for heparin*

Notes/Workspace

24. The patient must receive 150 milligrams per square meter of EES po. Read the information on the label in Figure ST1.4 and calculate the amount of milliliters you will administer to this patient if the patient's BSA is 1.8 square meters. ________

Do not accept if band on cap is broken or missing.
Child-resistant closure not required on containers of 200 ml (8 g erythromycin) or less; exemption approved by U.S. Consumer Product Safety Commission.
Each 5 ml (teaspoonful) contains: Erythromycin ethylsuccinate equivalent to erythromycin . . . . 200 mg in a fruit-flavored vehicle.
DOSAGE MAY BE ADMINISTERED WITHOUT REGARD TO MEALS.
Usual dose: Children— 30 - 50 mg/kg/day in divided doses.
See package enclosure for adult dose and full prescribing information.
Exp.
Lot

NDC 0074-6306-16
ONE PINT (473 ml)
E.E.S.® 200 LIQUID
ERYTHROMYCIN ETHYLSUCCINATE ORAL SUSPENSION, USP
Caution: Federal (U.S.A.) law prohibits dispensing without prescription.
ABBOTT
Abbott Laboratories
North Chicago, IL60064

SHAKE WELL BEFORE USING. Oversize bottle provides shake space.
Store in refrigerator to preserve taste until dispensed. Refrigeration by patient is not required if used within 14 days.
Dispense in a USP tight, light-resistant container.
++30074630616lX
©Abbott
07-8114-4/R7

Figure ST1.4 *Drug label for E.E.S.*

25. The prescriber ordered:

cefadyl 1 g in 50 mL 5% D/W IVPB in 30 min

Read the information on the label in Figure ST1.5 and calculate the total flow rate in drops per minute. The drop factor is 15 drops per milliliter.

____

NDC 0015-7628-28
EQUIVALENT TO
1 gram CEPHAPIRIN
CEFADYL
Sterile Cephapirin Sodium, USP
For IM or IV Use
CAUTION: Federal law prohibits dispensing without prescription.
APOTHECON®

This vial contains cephapirin sodium equivalent to 1 g cephapirin. Nitrogen in headspace.
Usual Dosage: Adults—500 mg to 1 g q. 6h.
For IM use, add 2 mL Sterile or Bacteriostatic Water for Injection, USP. Each 1.2 mL contains 500 mg of cephapirin.
For IV use, add 10 mL Sterile or Bacteriostatic Water for Injection, USP. Each mL contains 100 mg of cephapirin.
Following reconstitution, the solution is stable for 12 hours at room temperature or 10 days under refrigeration.
READ ACCOMPANYING CIRCULAR for detailed indications, Intermittent IV use, IM or IV dosage, and precautions.
Distributed by APOTHECON®
A Bristol-Myers Squibb Company
Princeton, NJ 08540
Made in USA
762828DRL-2

Figure ST1.5 *Drug label for cefadyl*

Notes/Workspace

Case Study 2: Ann Jackson

Mrs. Ann Jackson has been running a low-grade fever of 100.6°F for the past 3 days, accompanied by a dry hacking cough and a general feeling of malaise. She has also been having a burning sensation in her chest after eating. Her physician, Dr. Jed Anthony, ordered a chest X ray that revealed a hiatal hernia and pneumonia. He admitted her to Suburban General Hospital and wrote the following orders:

- Procardia 0.02 g po tid (each capsule contains 10 mg)
- Feldene 20 mg qd po (each tablet contains 0.02 g)
- Digoxin 0.125 mg qd po (each scored tablet contains 0.25 mg)
- Eryc 250 mg qid (each capsule contains 0.25 g)
- Zantac 50 mg in 50 mL 5% D/W q6h; infuse in 30 min
- 2000 mL 5% D/W q24h

1. How many milligrams of Procardia will Mrs. Jackson receive in 1 day? How many capsules equal 0.02 gram? ________

2. Calculate the total number of tablets and/or capsules the patient will receive at 10 A.M., assuming the first time of day for po drugs is 10 A.M. ________

3. Calculate the flow rate in drops per minute for the Zantac; the drop factor is 60 microdrops per milliliter. ________

4. What is the total amount of fluid received by the patient IVPB in 1 day? ________

5. Calculate the flow rate for the 2000 milliliters of 5% D/W IV. The drop factor is 20 drops per milliliter. ________

6. The patient is restricted to 2450 milliliters per day. How many milliliters of po fluid can this patient receive in 24 hours? ________

Comprehensive Self-Test 2

1. The order is for 0.05 gram of amitriptyline HCl (Elavil, Amitril). How many milligrams of this antidepressant drug equals 0.05 gram? ________

2. The prescriber's order reads:

   Add 125 mg morphine SO_4 to 250 mL of 5% D/W;
   infuse at a rate of 1.5 mg/h

Notes/Workspace

The drop factor is 60 microdrops per milliliter. How many microdrops per minute will the patient receive? _________

3. The patient is to receive 1 milligram per minute of a solution ordered by the prescriber, which is 1 gram of lidocaine added to 500 milliliters of 5% D/W. Calculate the flow rate in microdrops per minute. _________

4. The first order in Figure ST2.1 is for 20 milligrams bid of Feldene. If each tablet is labeled 0.02 gram, how many tablets would you administer to this patient? _________

5. The second order in Figure ST2.1 is changed to 0.1 milligram of Cytotec. How many micrograms would you administer to this patient if each scored tablet contains 200 micrograms? _________

6. Read the third order in Figure ST2.1. Each tablet is labeled 0.5 gram. How many tablets will the patient receive for each dose, and how many tablets will the patient receive in 7 days? _________

7. Prednisone tablets contain grain $\frac{1}{24}$. How many scored tablets are equal to the fourth order in Figure ST2.1? _________

8. Read the information in the fifth order in Figure ST2.1 and calculate the number of tablets you will give the patient if the label reads digoxin, 125 micrograms per tablet. _________

9. The order reads:

   vitamin B_{12} 2 mcg/kg IM

   The patient weighs 88 pounds. How many milligrams of the vitamin equal this prescribed dose? _________

10. The order reads:

    cimetidine 10 mg/kg po

    The patient weighs 20 kilograms. The label on the bottle reads 300 mg/5 mL. How many milliliters contain the prescribed dose of this anti-ulcer agent? _________

11. The nonsteroidal anti-inflammatory drug ibuprofen (Motrin, Advil, Nuprin, Rufin) has been prescribed for Mr. James. He is to receive 900 milligrams per day in divided doses or tid. Each tablet contains 0.3 gram of medication. How many tablets will you need for the daily prescribed dose? _________

GENERAL HOSPITAL

Year 19 *94* Month *December* Day		*20*	*21*	*22*	*23*	*24*	*25*
Medication Dosage and Interval		Initials* and Hours	Initials and Hours	Initials and Hours	Initials and Hours	Initials and Hours	Initials and Hours
Date started: *12/20* *Feldene 20 mg po bid* *10–6*	I	*AG*	*AG*	*AG*	*AG*	*AG*	
	AM	*10*	*10*	*10*	*10*	*10*	
	I	*JO*	*JO*	*JO*	*JO*	*JO*	
Discontinued:	PM	*6*	*6*	*6*	*6*	*6*	
Date started: *12/20* *Cytotec 200 mcg po bid* *10–6*	I	*AG*	*AG*	*AG*	*AG*		
	AM	*10*	*10*	*10*	*10*		
	I	*JO*	*JO*	*JO*	*JO*		
Discontinued: *12/24*	PM	*6*	*6*	*6*	*6*		
Date started: *12/20* *Carafate 1000 mg po ac meals and hs* *8–12–5–10*	I	*AG*	*AG*	*AG*	*AG*	*AG*	
	AM	*8*	*8*	*8*	*8*	*8*	
	I	*AG JO JO*	*AG JO JO*	*AG JO JO*	*AG JO JO*	*AG JO JO*	
Discontinued:	PM	*12 5 10*	*12 5 10*	*12 5 10*	*12 5 10*	*12 5 10*	
Date started: *12/20* *prednisone 10 mg bid for 5 days po* *10–6*	I	*AG*	*AG*	*AG*	*AG*	*AG*	
	AM	*10*	*10*	*10*	*10*	*10*	
	I	*JO*	*JO*	*JO*	*JO*	*JO*	
Discontinued: *12/24*	PM	*6*	*6*	*6*	*6*	*6*	
Date started: *12/20* *digoxin 0.25 mg qd po* *10 A.M.*	I	*AG*	*AG*	*AG*	*AG*	*AG*	
	AM	*10*	*10*	*10*	*10*	*10*	
	I						
Discontinued:	PM						
Date started: *12/24* *Cytotec 0.1 mg po bid* *10–6*	I					*JO*	
	AM					*10*	
Discontinued:	I						
	PM						

Allergies: (Specify)

Init*	Signature
AG	*Anthony Giangrasso*
JO	*June Olsen*

MEDICATION ADMINISTRATION RECORD

PATIENT IDENTIFICATION

534011 12/20/94
June Jones 4/19/22
543 Main Street RC
Hobbs, NM 102453 Aetna
Leon Ablon, M.D.

Figure ST2.1 *Medication order sheet*

Notes/Workspace

Notes/Workspace

12. If a patient has an order for 0.075 gram of the tricyclic antidepressant imipramine pamoate (Tofranil) and each tablet contains 25 milligrams, how many tablets will you prepare for the patient? ________

13. A child has a BSA of 1.2 square meters and the order is for 30 milligrams per square meter IV of the antihypertensive drug methyldopa (Aldomet). The vial reads 250 milligrams per 5 milliliters. How many milliliters will equal this prescribed dose? ________

14. The antineoplastic drug lomustine (CeeNU) is ordered for a child with a BSA of 1 square meter. The prescribed dose is 0.1 gram per square meter, and each tablet is labeled 100 milligrams. How many tablets equal this prescribed dose? ________

15. The order reads:

    liothyronine sodium 0.1 mg po

    Each tablet is labeled 50 micrograms. How many tablets will you administer to the child? ________

16. A child has an order for 1 milligram per kilogram of the diuretic furosemide (Lasix, Novosemide). The child weighs 40 kilograms. The tablets are 20 milligrams each. How many tablets will you prepare for this child? ________

17. The usual dose of the antiviral drug acyclovir (Zovirax) is 0.25 gram per square meter and the child's BSA is 0.4 square meter. How many milliliters should you prepare for the child when the label on the vial reads 500 milligrams per 2 milliliters? ________

18. A child with a BSA of 0.64 square meter is to receive 150 micrograms per square meter po of the anticonvulsant drug mephenytoin (Mesantoin). Available tablets contain 100 milligrams each. How many tablets equal the prescribed dose? ________

19. Read the label in Figure ST2.2 and calculate the milliliters required for the order:

    Ticar 350 mg IM q12h

    ____

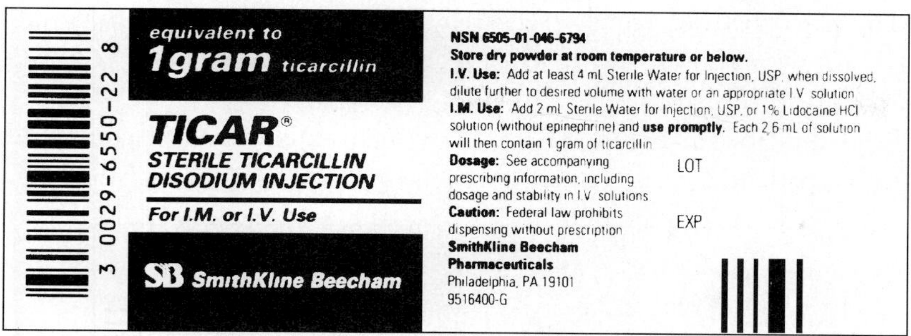

Figure ST2.2 *Drug label for Ticar*

20. The prescriber's order reads:

> Add 275 u Humulin R insulin to 500 mL 0.9% NS;
> infuse at rate of 10 u/h

Determine the flow rate and the amount of insulin that must be added to the 500 milliliters of 0.9% NS solution. Read the information on the label in Figure ST2.3. ________

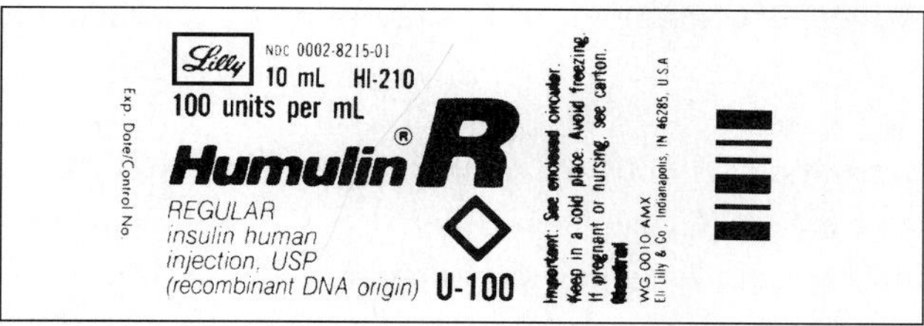

Lilly
NDC 0002-8215-01
10 mL HI-210
100 units per mL
Humulin R®
REGULAR
insulin human
injection, USP
(recombinant DNA origin)
U-100
Exp. Date/Control No.
Important: See enclosed circular.
Keep in a cold place. Avoid freezing.
If pregnant or nursing, see carton.
WG 0010 AMX
Eli Lilly & Co., Indianapolis, IN 46285, U.S.A.

Figure ST2.3 *Drug label for Humulin R*

21. The prescriber has written an order for 900 milligrams of clindamycin phosphate (Cleocin) to be added to 150 milliliters of 5% D/W IVPB and infused in 90 minutes. The drop factor is 15 drops per milliliter. Read the label in Figure ST2.4. How many milliliters of Cleocin will you add to the 150 milliliters of 5% D/W? Calculate the flow rate. ________

NDC 0009-0728-05
6505-01-246-8718
60 ml Pharmacy Bulk Package
Not for direct infusion
Cleocin Phosphate®
Sterile Solution
clindamycin phosphate injection, USP
Equivalent to clindamycin
150 mg per ml
For intramuscular or intravenous use
Caution: Federal law prohibits dispensing without prescription.
Upjohn The Upjohn Company Kalamazoo, MI 49001, USA

See package insert for complete product information.
Warning—If given intravenously, dilute before use.
Swab vial closure with an antiseptic solution. Dispense aliquots from the vial via a suitable dispensing device into infusion fluids under a laminar flow hood using aseptic technique. DISCARD VIAL WITHIN 24 HOURS AFTER INITIAL ENTRY.
Store at controlled room temperature 15°-30° C (59°-86° F)
Each ml contains: clindamycin phosphate equivalent to clindamycin 150 mg; also disodium edetate, 0.5 mg; benzyl alcohol 9.45 mg added as preservative. When necessary, pH was adjusted with sodium hydroxide and/or hydrochloric acid.
813 718 201 DATE/TIME ENTERED ....
150 mg per ml
Equivalent to clindamycin
clindamycin phosphate injection, USP
Cleocin Phosphate Sterile Solution

Figure ST2.4 *Drug label for Cleocin*

Notes/Workspace

Notes/Workspace

22. The prescriber ordered:

atropine sulfate 0.2 mg IV push stat

Read the label in Figure ST2.5. How many milliliters will you administer to the patient? ________

NDC 0002-1675-01
20 mL VIAL No. 419
POISON
Lilly
ATROPINE SULFATE
INJECTION, USP
0.4 mg per mL
CAUTION—Federal (U.S.A.) law prohibits dispensing without prescription.

Figure ST2.5 *Drug label for atropine sulfate*

23. The physician has ordered 0.15 gram po qid of aspirin. The scored tablets are 300 milligrams each. How many tablets equal 0.15 gram? ________

24. If you have an order for 200 milligrams of chloroprocaine HCl (Nesacaine) and you have a 2% solution, how many milligrams would equal 200 milligrams? ________

25. An IV preparation of 500 milligrams of lidocaine HCl (Xylocaine) in 250 milliliters of 5% D/W has been ordered at 0.2 milligram per kilogram per minute for a patient weighing 66 kilograms. If the drop factor is 10 drops per milliliter, what will be the flow rate in drops per minute? ________

Case Study 3: Lucy Shihab

Mrs. Lucy Shihab has an emergency admission to the hospital for removal of a ruptured ovarian cyst. Her vital signs are T: 103.4°F, P: 120, R: 32, BP: 100/70. Her initial assessment data includes flushed face, diaphoresis, abdominal distention, board-like abdomen, pain 7+. Following the surgical procedure, the surgeon, Dr. Lorraine Gatt, wrote the following orders:

- Demerol 50 mg IM q4h prn for pain
- Versed 0.18 mg/kg IM q4h prn for pain (patient weight: 60 kg)
- Nembutal gr $\overline{\text{iss}}$ po hs
- 1000 mL Ringer's lactate IV at a rate of 75 mL/h (drop factor 20 gtt/mL)
- Ticarcillin disodium (Ticar) 6.2 g in 250 mL 5% D/W q12h IVPB; infuse in 2 h (drop factor 10 gtt/mL)
- Ranitidine HCl (Zantac) IVPB 50 mg in 100 mL 5% D/W q6h IVPB; infuse in 20 min (drop factor 10 gtt/mL)

1. Calculate the flow rate for each IVPB medication. ________

2. How many milligrams equal the prescribed dose of Nembutal? ________

3. If Demerol is labeled 100 milligrams per 2 milliliters and Versed is labeled 10 milligrams per 2 milliliters, how many milliliters of Demerol and how many milliliters of Versed equal the prescribed dosages? ________

4. What is the total amount of IVPB fluids received by the patient in 24 hours? ________

5. Calculate the total amount of IV fluid received by the patient in 24 hours. (Remember, in this situation, the primary line is not infusing when the patient is receiving the ticarcillin disodium and ranitidine HCl.) ________

Notes/Workspace

Comprehensive Self-Test 3

1. An IV of 1000 milliliters of Ringer's lactate in 12 hours is ordered. The drop factor is 10 drops per milliliter. What will be the flow rate in drops per minute? ________

2. How would you prepare 100 milliliters of a 2.5% solution from a 10% solution? ________

3. The prescriber has ordered 7500 units IV push of the anticoagulant heparin sodium (Liquaemin). The vial is labeled 10,000 units per milliliter. How many milliliters equal 7500 units? ________

4. Read the label in Figure ST3.1 and calculate the milliliters of Ceclor that should be administered if the order is for 250 milligrams per square meter and the patient's BSA is 1.7 square meters. ________

NDC 0002-5130-48
100 mL (When Mixed) M-5130
℞ Lilly
CECLOR®
CEFACLOR FOR ORAL SUSPENSION, USP
187 mg per 5 mL
CAUTION—Federal (U.S.A.) law prohibits dispensing without prescription.

Usual Dose—Children, 20 mg per kg a day (40 mg per kg in otitis media) in two divided doses. Adults, 375 mg two times a day. See literature for complete dosage information. Contains Cefaclor Monohydrate equivalent to 3.74 g Cefaclor in a dry pleasantly flavored mixture. Prior to Mixing, Store at Controlled Room Temperature 59° to 86°F (15° to 30°C) Directions for Mixing—Add 62 mL of water in two portions to the dry mixture in the bottle. Shake well after each addition. Each 5 mL (Approx. one teaspoonful) will then contain: Cefaclor Monohydrate equivalent to 187 mg Cefaclor.
WV 6502 AMX
Mfd. by Eli Lilly Industries, Inc., Carolina, Puerto Rico 00985 a subsidiary of Eli Lilly & Co., Indianapolis, IN, U.S.A.
Expiration Date

100 mL CECLOR® CEFACLOR FOR ORAL SUSPENSION, USP
187 mg per 5 mL. Oversize bottle provides extra space for shaking. Store in a refrigerator. May be kept for 14 days without significant loss of potency. Keep Tightly Closed. Discard unused portion after 14 days.
SHAKE WELL BEFORE USING
Control No.

Figure ST3.1 *Drug label for Ceclor*

Notes/Workspace

5. The order for a patient is 1 milligram per 35 kilograms of Alkeran qd. Read the label in Figure ST3.2 and calculate the number of tablets you would administer to a patient who weighs 70 kilograms. ________

Store at 15°-25°C (59°-77°F) in a dry place, protect from light. Dispense in glass, tight, light-resistant container as defined in the U.S.P. 403916 Made in U.S.A.

50 Tablets NDC-0081-0045-35

ALKERAN®
(MELPHALAN)
Each scored tablet contains
2 mg

CAUTION: Federal law prohibits dispensing without prescription.
For indications, dosage, precautions, etc., see accompanying package insert.

BURROUGHS WELLCOME CO.
Research Triangle Park, NC 27709

WARNING—This drug is only to be taken under close medical supervision. Do not take in larger doses or more frequently or for a longer time than specifically directed by the physician. Periodic blood counts are necessary to determine proper dose and to avoid ill effects.

Figure ST3.2 *Drug label for Alkeran*

6. The prescriber ordered:

Vibramycin 60 mg/m^2 po bid

Read the information on the label in Figure ST3.3 and determine the amount of milliliters you will prepare for a patient with a BSA of 0.9 square meter.

____

MADE IN USA 9

RECOMMENDED STORAGE
STORE BELOW 86°F. (30°C.)
SHAKE WELL
This prescription, when in suspension, will maintain its potency for two weeks when kept at room temperature. Discard unused portion after two weeks.

For oral use only
Mixing Directions: Tap bottle lightly to loosen powder. Add 47.6 ml of water to the bottle to make a total volume of 60 ml. Shake well.
†When reconstituted, each teaspoonful (5 ml) contains doxycycline monohydrate equivalent to 25 mg of doxycycline.
doxycycline U.S. Pat. No. 3,200,149

6277

NDC 0069-0970-65
Vibramycin®
monohydrate
doxycycline monohydrate
FOR ORAL SUSPENSION
This package contains doxycycline monohydrate equivalent to 300 mg of doxycycline in a raspberry-flavored mixture.†
60 ml BOTTLE
RASPBERRY FLAVORED
CAUTION: Federal law prohibits dispensing without prescription.
Pfizer LABORATORIES DIVISION
PFIZER INC NEW YORK N.Y. 10017

READ ACCOMPANYING PROFESSIONAL INFORMATION
USUAL DOSAGE:
Adults: 200 mg on the first day (100 mg every 12 hours) followed by a maintenance dose of 100 mg a day.
Children above eight years of age: Under 100 lbs.—2 mg/lb. of body weight daily divided in two doses on the first day, followed by 1 mg/lb. of body weight on subsequent days in one or two doses.
Over 100 lbs.—See adult dosage.

Figure ST3.3 *Drug label for Vibramycin*

7. The order reads:

Mycostatin oral suspension 350,000 u tid

Read the information on the label in Figure ST3.4 and determine the amount of drug you will administer to this patient po. ________

Notes/Workspace

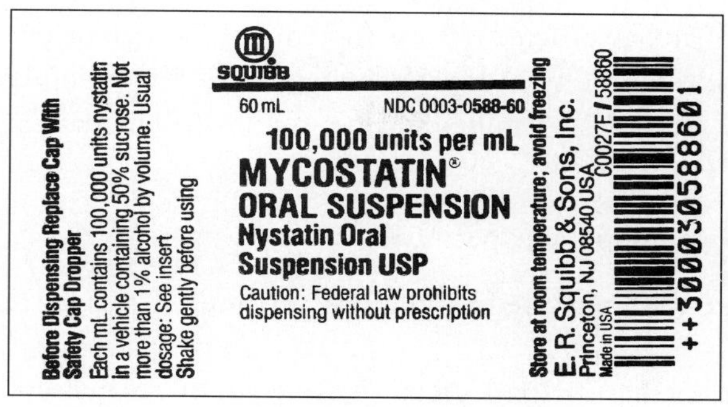

Figure ST3.4 *Drug label for Mycostatin*

8. Read the information in the label in Figure ST3.5 and calculate the strength of the lidocaine hydrochloride solution in grams per milliliter. Change this ratio to a percentage. _________

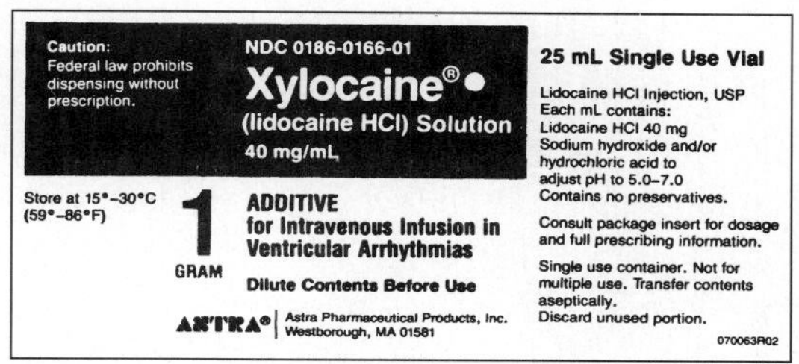

Figure ST3.5 *Drug label for Xylocaine*

9. An IV of 0.9% NS is infusing at a rate of 30 drops per minute. There are 360 milliliters LIB. The drop factor is 15 drops per milliliter. Calculate the number of hours this IV will infuse. _________

10. The order reads:

probucol 0.5 g po

Available tablets of this antilipophilic drug are 250 milligrams each. How many tablets will you administer? _________

11. A 1-million-unit vial of penicillin G potassium powder has the following instructions for dilution: Add 9.6 mL of diluent, then 1 mL = 100,000 u. If the prescriber orders 250,000 units IM, how many milliliters will you prepare? _________

12. A child with a BSA of 0.8 square meter has an order for 100 milligrams per square meter po of the anti-arrhythmic agent amiodarone hydrochloride (Cordarone). How many milligrams equal the prescribed dose? _________

13. How would you prepare 1 pint (500 milliliters) of a 25% solution from a pure drug in powdered form? _________

Notes/Workspace

14. The prescriber has ordered 10 micrograms per kilogram per minute IV of dobutamine (Dobutrex). Add 250 milligrams to 500 milliliters of 5% D/W. Each vial is labeled 12.5 milligrams per milliliter. The patient's weight is 70 kilograms.

    a. How many milligrams per hour will the patient receive? ________

    b. Calculate the flow rate in milliliters per hour. ________

15. The prescriber has ordered grain $\frac{1}{300}$ of ergonovine maleate, po. Available tablets are 0.2 milligram each. How many tablets of this oxytoxic drug equal the ordered dose? ________

16. The amebicide drug iodoquinol (Amebaquin) has been ordered po for a patient in the amount of 630 milligrams. The available tablets are 210 milligrams each. How many tablets will you administer? ________

17. A patient weighing 54 kilograms is to receive 150 micrograms per kilogram per day po of the antineoplastic preparation melphalan (Alkeran). The scored tablets are 2 milligrams each. How many tablets will you administer? ________

18. The order is for 500 milliliters of an IV solution with 25 milligrams of a drug. The patient is to receive 0.05 milligram per minute. The drop factor is 60 microdrops per milliliter. What will the flow rate be in microdrops per minute? ________

19. The first order in Figure ST3.6 is for cefazolin. If the patient weighs 90 kilograms, how many milligrams will you prepare? Calculate the milliliters equivalent to this dose if the label reads 1 milliliter per 500 milligrams. ________

20. Read the second order in Figure ST3.6. If the medication is available in 5-mg scored tablets, how many Coumadin tablets will you administer to the patient? ________

21. The drug Quibron from the third order in Figure ST3.6 is available in an oral suspension labeled 0.3 gram per 10 milliliters. How many milliliters will you administer to the patient? ________

⊕ GENERAL HOSPITAL ⊕

Year 19 *94* Month *March* Day		*12*	*13*	*14*	*15*	*16*	*17*
Medication Dosage and Interval		Initials* and Hours	Initials and Hours	Initials and Hours	Initials and Hours	Initials and Hours	Initials and Hours
Date started: *3/12*	I	*LA*	*LA*				
cefazolin 8 mg/kg IM q12h	AM	*10*	*10*				
10 A.M. 10 P.M.	I	*AG*	*AG*				
Discontinued:	PM	*10*	*10*				
Date started: *3/12*	I	*LA*	*LA*				
Coumadin 2 $\frac{1}{2}$ mg qd po *10 A.M.*	AM	*10*	*10*				
	I						
Discontinued:	PM						
Date started: *3/12*	I	*LA*	*LA*				
Quibron 300 mg po bid *10 A.M.*	AM	*10*	*10*				
6 P.M.	I	*AG*	*AG*				
Discontinued:	PM	*6*	*6*				
Date started: *3/12*	I	*LA*	*LA*				
prednisone 20 mg po bid for 5 days	AM	*10*	*10*				
10 A.M. 6 P.M.	I	*AG*	*AG*				
Discontinued: *3/16*	PM	*6*	*6*				
Date started: *3/12*	I	*LA*	*LA*				
Diuril 0.5 g qd po *10 A.M.*	AM	*10*	*10*				
	I						
Discontinued:	PM						
Date started: *3/12*	I	*LA*	*LA*				
Xanax 0.25 mg po tid *10 A.M.*	AM	*10*	*10*				
2 P.M. 6 P.M.	I	*LA AG*	*LA AG*				
Discontinued:	PM	*2 6*	*2 6*				

Allergies: (Specify)

Init*	Signature
LA	*Leon Ablon*
AG	*Anthony Giangrasso*

MEDICATION ADMINISTRATION RECORD

PATIENT IDENTIFICATION

7810056 3/12/94

Jonathan Dingmen 6/6/41
451 Seaside Rd Buddhist
Tallahassee FA 10023 BCBS

Dr. Olsen

Figure ST3.6 *Medication order sheet*

Notes/Workspace

Notes/Workspace

22. The fourth order in Figure ST3.6 is for 20 milligrams of prednisone. How many 10-mg tablets will you need for a 5-day supply? ________

23. If the medication in the fifth order in Figure ST3.6 for Diuril is changed to 1.5 grams po of Diuril, how many milligrams would you administer to the patient? ________

24. The drug available for the fifth medication order in Figure ST3.6 is 0.5-mg tablets of Xanax. How many scored tablets will you give this patient? ________

25. An initial dose (2 grams po) of sulfisoxazole suspension (Gantrisin) is ordered. The bottle is labeled 500 milligrams per 5 milliliters. How many milliliters of this antibiotic equal the prescribed dose? ________

Case Study 4: Mr. Aziz

Mr. Aziz, 45 years old, is admitted to the hospital for a closure of a colostomy. His original surgery was 3 months previous. At that time, his diagnosis was intestinal obstruction. A colostomy was performed. His admission vital signs are T: 98.6°F, P: 88, R: 18, and BP: 132/82. He weighs 70 kilograms. His surgeon, Dr. James Chou, has written the following orders.

Orders for the Day of Surgery:

- Demerol 50 mg and Versed 0.005 g IM at 7 A.M.
- gr $\frac{1}{150}$ atropine sulfate IM at 7 A.M.

Postoperative Orders:

- Demerol 50 mg and Vistaril 0.8 mg/kg IM q4h prn for relief of pain
- 1000 mL 5% D/W in 0.45% NS IV at the rate of 125 mL/h
- Mefoxin 1 g in 100 mL 5% D/W IVPB q6h; infuse in 60 min
- Pepcid 50 mg in 100 mL 5% D/W IVPB q8h; infuse in 30 min

The drop factor for all IV solutions and medications is 10 drops per milliliter.

1. Calculate the flow rate for all IVPB solutions. ________

2. How many milliliters equal the prescribed dose of atropine sulfate if the ampule reads 0.4 milligram per milliliter? ________

3. If the label for Demerol reads 50 milligrams per milliliter and the label for Versed reads 0.005 gram per milliliter, how many milliliters will you administer to this patient? ________

4. What is the total amount of fluid the patient will receive from the IVPB medications in 24 hours and the solution of 5% D/0.45% NS? ________

5. Calculate the amount of Vistaril the patient will receive with 50 milligrams of Demerol if the ampule of Vistaril reads 25 milligrams per milliliter. ________

Notes/Workspace

Comprehensive Self-Test 4

1. The order is for 0.25 gram of ticlopidine (Ticlid). Calculate the number of tablets of this platelet aggregation inhibitor that you would administer if each tablet contains 250 milligrams. ________

2. A client has a history of migraine headaches, and the physician has ordered 0.02 gram bid of the beta-adrenergic blocker timolol maleate (Timoptic). Each tablet contains 10 milligrams. How many tablets will you administer to this patient? ________

3. A prescriber ordered 50 units per kilogram sc of epoetin alfa (Epogen). The label reads 2000 units per milliliter. The patient weighs 90 pounds. How many milliliters will you administer to this patient? ________

4. The antineoplastic drug cisplatin (Platinol) has been ordered IV for your patient, who is to receive 25 milligrams per square meter in 1000 milliliters of 0.9% NS, to be infused in 8 hours. The patient's BSA is 1.5 square meters, and the label reads 25 milligrams per 25 milliters.

   a. Calculate the total amount of solution with drug added. ________

   b. Calculate the flow rate in milliliters per hour. ________

5. If the drug available for the first order in Figure ST4.1 contains 1.2 milligrams of colchicine per tablet, how many tablets will you administer to the patient? ________

6. Read the second order in Figure ST4.1 and determine how many tablets you will administer to the patient if 0.12 g tablets of Cardizem SR is available. ________

Notes/Workspace

7. Read the third order in Figure ST4.1 and calculate the number of tablets you will administer if each tablet contains grain $1\frac{1}{2}$. ________

GENERAL HOSPITAL

Year 19 94 / Month October / Day		14	15	16	17	18	19
Medication Dosage and Interval		Initials* and Hours	Initials and Hours	Initials and Hours	Initials and Hours	Initials and Hours	Initials and Hours
Date started: 10/14 colchicine gr $\frac{1}{50}$ po bid 10 A.M. 6 P.M.	I	AG	AG	AG	AG		
	AM	10	10	10	10		
	I	LA	LA	LA	LA		
Discontinued:	PM	6	6	6	6		
Date started: 10/14 Cardizem SR 120 mg po qd 10 A.M.	I	AG	AG	AG	AG		
	AM	10	10	10	10		
	I						
Discontinued:	PM						
Date started: 10/14 Aldactone 100 mg po bid 10 A.M. 6 P.M.	I	AG	AG	AG	AG		
	AM	10	10	10	10		
	I	LA	LA	LA	LA		
Discontinued:	PM	6	6	6	6		
Date started: 10/14 Estromed 0.625 mg po qd	I	AG	AG	AG	AG		
	AM	10	10	10	10		
	I						
Discontinued:	PM						
Date started: 10/14 famotidine 40 mg po hs 10 P.M.	I						
	AM						
	I	LA	LA	LA	LA		
Discontinued:	PM	10	10	10	10		

Allergies: (Specify)

Init*	Signature
AG	Anthony Giangrasso
LA	Leon Ablon

MEDICATION ADMINISTRATION RECORD

PATIENT IDENTIFICATION

9906431 9/14/94

Larissa Luby 7/7/40
93120 Second Ave S.E. Prot
Detroit MI 60422 Medicare

June Olsen, MD

Figure ST4.1 *Medication order sheet*

Notes/Workspace

8. If the Estromed in the fourth order in Figure ST4.1 is available in 325-μg tablets, how many tablets will you administer to this patient? __________

9. Read the fourth order in Figure ST4.1. How many milligrams of famotidine (Pepcid) will the patient receive in 7 days? __________

10. A child has been admitted to the hospital with a diagnosis of herpes simplex viral encephalitis. The prescriber orders:

vidarabine monohydrate 15 mg/kg in 1000 mL 5% D/W

The patient weighs 75 pounds. The label reads 200 milligrams per milliliter, and the total amount is to be infused in 24 hours. Calculate the flow rate in milliliters per hour. __________

11. A patient with AIDS has been diagnosed with CMV (cytomegalovirus). The prescriber has ordered the antiviral drug ganciclovir (Cytovene); the patient will receive 5 milligrams per kilogram IV in 100 milliliters of 5% D/W. Each vial reads 500 milligrams per 2 milliliters. The weight of the patient is 50 kilograms. Calculate the flow rate in drops per minute if the drop factor is 15 drops per milliliter. Infuse in 60 minutes. __________

12. A prescriber has ordered 0.8 milligram po of folic acid (Folvite) for your patient. Each tablet contains 0.0008 gram. How many tablets will you administer to this patient? __________

13. Read the label in Figure ST4.2. If the order is for 0.0002 gram, how many tablets will you administer to the patient? __________

Clonidine Hydrochloride Tablets, USP
0.1 mg
N 3 0781-1471-01 3
Each tablet contains:
Clonidine Hydrochloride, USP 0.1 mg
Usual Dosage: See package insert.
Store at controlled room temperature 15°-30°C (59°-86°F). Dispense in a tight, light-resistant container. **KEEP THIS AND ALL DRUGS OUT OF THE REACH OF CHILDREN.**
Rev. 91-2E C92/11
Manufactured By
Geneva Pharmaceuticals, Inc.
Broomfield, CO 80020
Geneva pharmaceuticals, inc.

Figure ST4.2 *Drug label for clonidine hydrochloride*

Notes/Workspace

14. The prescriber ordered:

40 mEq potassium chloride po qd

Read the information in Figure ST4.3 and determine the number of tablets you will administer to the patient. ________

Exp.
Lot
03-1941-7/R14
Store below 86°F (30°C).
Do not accept if break-away ring on cap is broken or missing.

K·Tab
POTASSIUM CHLORIDE
EXTENDED-RELEASE
TABLETS, USP
10 mEq (750 mg)
Caution: Federal (U.S.A.) law prohibits dispensing without prescription.

6505-01-235-2629
Dispense in a USP tight container.
Each tablet contains: 750 mg potassium chloride (equivalent to 10 mEq).
Each yellow ovaloid tablet bears the a and the trademark K-TAB for identification.
See enclosure for prescribing information.
Filmtab–Film-sealed tablets, Abbott.
©Abbott
Abbott Laboratories
North Chicago, IL60064 U.S.A.

Figure ST4.3 *Drug label for K-Tab*

15. Read the information on the label in Figure ST4.4. Determine the volume of chlorpromazine HCl that you will administer to the patient if the order is for 0.15 milligram per kilogram and the patient's weight is 60 kilograms.

____

GG
Chlorpromazine
Hydrochloride
Syrup, USP
10 mg/5 mL
Each 5 mL (1 teaspoonful) contains:
Chlorpromazine Hydrochloride, USP 10 mg
This product blanketed by nitrogen.
PROTECT FROM LIGHT

Geneva
pharmaceuticals, inc.

N 3 0781-4017-04 1
Usual Dosage: See package insert.
Caution: Avoid direct contact with skin or clothes because of possibility of contact dermatitis (skin reaction). Wash thoroughly or change clothes if direct contact occurs.
Store at controlled room temperature 15°-30°C (59°-86°F).
Important: Dispense only in a tight **amber glass** container. This product is light sensitive. Never dispense in a flint, green, or blue bottle.
KEEP THIS AND ALL DRUGS OUT OF THE REACH OF CHILDREN.
Rev. 92-1E C92/7
Manufactured By
Geneva Pharmaceuticals, Inc.
Broomfield, CO 80020

Figure ST4.4 *Drug label for chlorpromazine hydrochloride*

16. Read the information on the label in Figure ST4.5. Calculate the volume of medication required if the order is for grain $\frac{1}{3}$ of elixir of phenobarbital.

____

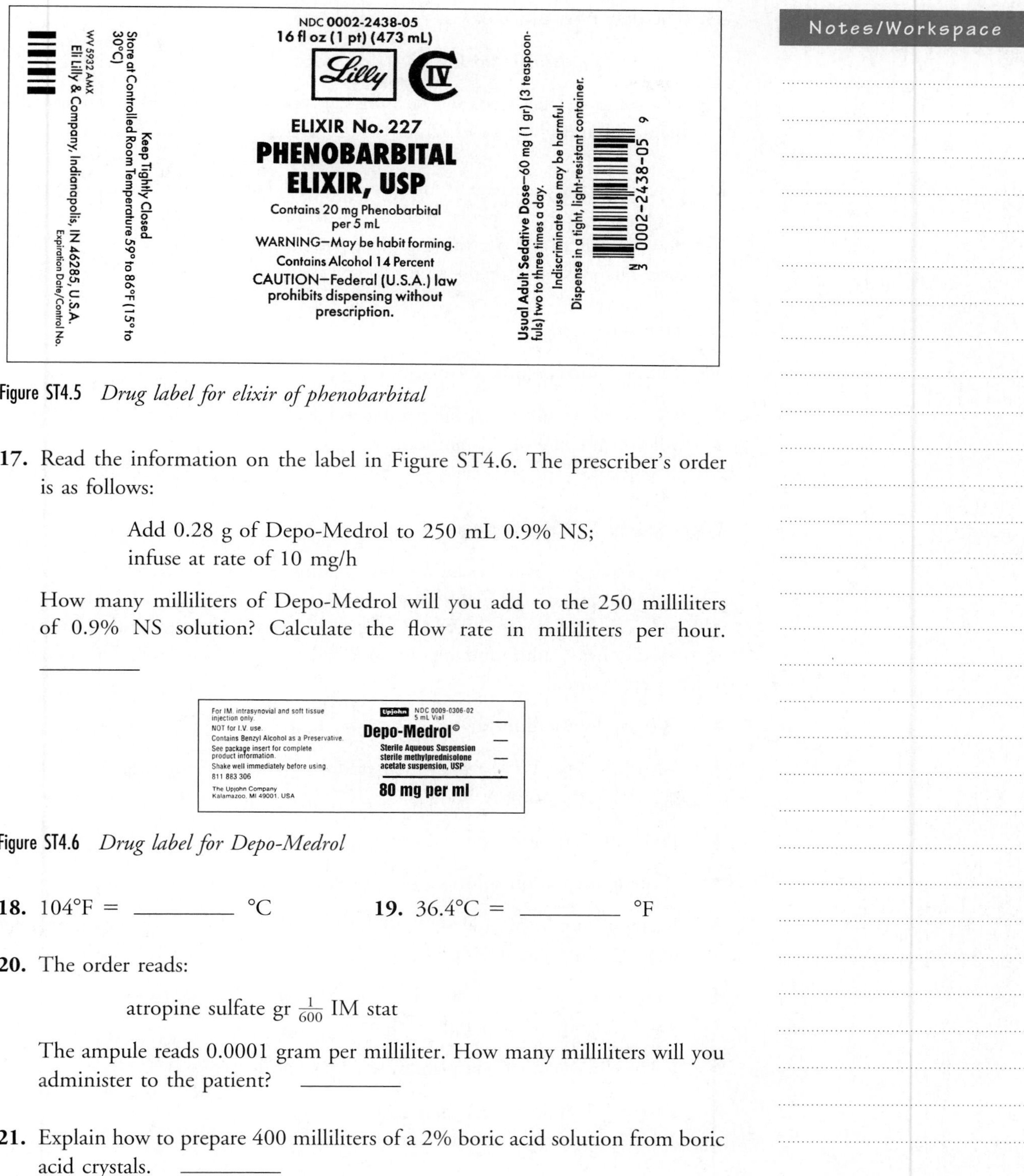

Figure ST4.5 *Drug label for elixir of phenobarbital*

17. Read the information on the label in Figure ST4.6. The prescriber's order is as follows:

> Add 0.28 g of Depo-Medrol to 250 mL 0.9% NS;
> infuse at rate of 10 mg/h

How many milliliters of Depo-Medrol will you add to the 250 milliliters of 0.9% NS solution? Calculate the flow rate in milliliters per hour.

____

Figure ST4.6 *Drug label for Depo-Medrol*

18. 104°F = ________ °C

19. 36.4°C = ________ °F

20. The order reads:

> atropine sulfate gr $\frac{1}{600}$ IM stat

The ampule reads 0.0001 gram per milliliter. How many milliliters will you administer to the patient? ________

21. Explain how to prepare 400 milliliters of a 2% boric acid solution from boric acid crystals. ________

22. A 1:10,000 solution of epinephrine contains how many milligrams of epinephrine in 1 milliliter? ________

Notes/Workspace

Notes/Workspace

23. The prescriber ordered:

digoxin 0.008 mg po

The solution label reads 0.004 milligram per 5 milliliters. How many milliliters will you give to this patient? ________

24. A patient is to receive 0.5 milligram per kilogram per minute of cefuroxime (Ceftin). The order reads: Add 0.5 g to 100 mL 5% D/W. Calculate the flow rate in drops per minute. The patient weighs 60 kilograms, and the drop factor is 10 drops per milliliter. ________

25. The order reads:

doxycycline 4.4 mg/kg po

Each 5 mL = 50 mg. If the patient weighs 64 pounds, how many milliliters will you prepare of this antibiotic? ________

Case Study 5: Chu Wang

Mr. Chu Wang is seen and examined by his family physician, Dr. Thomas Mohan. He is short of breath and diaphoretic. Vital signs are T: 99°F; P: 132; R: 34; BP: 220/142. Dr. Mohan admits Mr. Wang to Maryland Hospital with a diagnosis of congestive heart failure and hypertension. He weighs 125 pounds. The following orders were written:

- 500-mg low-sodium diet
- 500 mL 5% D/W with methyldopa 500 mg; infuse at the rate of 0.1 mg/kg/h, primary line (1)
- Procardia 0.02 g po tid
- Hyperalimentation solution 10% D/W 25 mL/h, peripheral line
- Flagyl 50 mg in 50 mL 5% D/W IVPB q8h; infuse in 60 min via primary line (2); drop factor 10 gtt = 1 mL
- Cimetidine 300 mg in 50 mL 5% D/W q6h; infuse in 20 min via primary line (2); drop factor 10 gtt = 1 mL
- 0.9% NS, 10 mL/h via primary line (2) KVO
- Restrict IV fluid to less than 1500 mL per day

1. Calculate the flow rate for each IVPB medication (Flagyl and cimetidine). _________

2. Calculate the flow rate for the IV with the methyldopa. _________

3. How many milliliters in total of the IVPB solution will the patient receive in 24 hours? _________

4. How many tablets of Procardia will you administer to the patient each day? _________

5. How many grams of dextrose will the patient receive in 24 hours? _________

6. Calculate the total amount of solution that the patient will receive in 24 hours. Is this amount within the prescribed limit of 3000 milliliters? _________

Notes/Workspace

Comprehensive Self-Test 5

1. The antineoplastic drug, bleomycin sulfate (Blenoxane), has been ordered for your patient, who will receive 4 units per square meter IV. Each vial is labeled 15 units per 2 milliliters. The patient's BSA is 1.4 square meters. How many milliliters will you prepare for your patient? _________

2. The prescriber has ordered 3 milligrams per square meter of the antineoplastic drug leucovorin calcium (Wellcovorin). The patient's BSA is 1.2 square meters. How many minims will you administer to this patient if the ampule reads 5 milligrams per milliliter? _________

3. Your patient has had an exacerbation of his rheumatoid arthritis symptoms, and the prescriber has ordered 10 milligrams per square meter IVPB of the antineoplastic drug methotrexate sodium in 50 milliliters of 0.9% NS. The patient's BSA is 1.7 square meters. The label on the vial reads 25 milligrams per milliliter.

   a. How many milliliters of this drug will you add to the 50 milliliters of 0.9% NS? _________

   b. Calculate the flow rate for the total amount of this solution, which must infuse in 30 minutes. The drop factor is 10 drops per milliliter. _________

Notes/Workspace

4. The thrombolytic agent alteplase recombinant drug (t-PA, Activase) is to be prepared for a patient who will receive 1.25 milligrams per kilogram. This patient weighs 100 kilograms. The vial directions are as follows: Add 50 mL to vial and 1 mg/mL.

   a. How many milliliters will you prepare for this patient? ________

   b. Calculate the flow rate in milliliters per hour if the IV must infuse in 90 minutes. ________

5. The order reads:

   amikacin sulfate 7.5 mg/kg in 200 mL 5% D/W IVPB

   The label on the vial reads 250 milligrams per milliliter. The patient weighs 90 kilograms.

   a. How many milliliters of the antibiotic must be added to the 200 milliliters of 5% D/W? ________

   b. Calculate the flow rate in drops per minute if the drop factor is 10 drops per milliliter and the length of time for the infusion is 2 hours. ________

6. A corticosteroid, betamethasone sodium (Celestone), has been prescribed for its anti-inflammatory action. The patient is to receive 5 milligrams in an IV push. The label on the vial reads 4 milligrams per milliliter. How many milliliters will you prepare for this patient? ________

7. A child has had an acute onset of bronchial asthma. The prescriber ordered:

   aminophylline 0.3 mg/kg IV push stat

   The patient weighs 25 kilograms, and the label on the vial reads 4 milligrams per milliliter. How many milliliters will you prepare for this child? If there is an additional order of 0.125 milligram per kilogram per hour, how many milliliters per hour will you administer if the solution is labeled 100 milligrams per 100 milliliters? ________

8. Read the first order in Figure ST5.1 and calculate the number of tablets required if each tablet contains grain $\frac{1}{60}$. ________

9. A child with acute leukemia has been prescribed 3 milligrams per kilogram po of thioguanine (Lanvis). Each scored tablet contains 40 milligrams. Calculate the number of tablets required if the child weighs 20 kilograms. ________

Notes/Workspace

⊕ GENERAL HOSPITAL ⊕

Year 19 *94* Month *June* Day		*3*	*4*	*5*	*6*	*7*	*8*
Medication Dosage and Interval		Initials* and Hours	Initials and Hours	Initials and Hours	Initials and Hours	Initials and Hours	Initials and Hours
Date started: *6/3* *bumetanide 2 mg po qd* *10 A.M.*	I	*LA*	*LA*	*LA*			
	AM	*10*	*10*	*10*			
	I						
Discontinued:	PM						
Date started: *6/3* *Procardia 20 mg po tid* *10 A.M.*	I	*LA*	*LA*	*LA*			
	AM	*10*	*10*	*10*			
2 P.M. *6 P.M.*	I	*LA JO*	*LA JO*	*LA JO*			
Discontinued:	PM	*2 6*	*2 6*	*2 6*			
Date started: *6/3* *Elavil 0.05 g po bid*	I	*LA*	*LA*	*LA*			
10 A.M. *6 P.M.*	AM	*10*	*10*	*10*			
	I	*JO*	*JO*	*JO*			
Discontinued:	PM	*6*	*6*	*6*			
Date started: *6/3* *potassium chloride*	I	*LA*	*LA*	*LA*			
20 mEq po bid *10 A.M.*	AM	*10*	*10*	*10*			
6 P.M.	I	*JO*	*JO*	*JO*			
Discontinued:	PM	*6*	*6*	*6*			
Date started: *6/3* *Paraflex 0.5 g po bid*	I	*LA*	*LA*	*LA*			
10 A.M. *6 P.M.*	AM	*10*	*10*	*10*			
	I	*JO*	*JO*	*JO*			
Discontinued:	PM	*6*	*6*	*6*			

Allergies: (Specify)

Init*	Signature
LA	*Leon Ablon*
JO	*June Olsen*

MEDICATION ADMINISTRATION RECORD

PATIENT IDENTIFICATION

754886 6/3/94

John Petogna 4/12/52
451 Oceanside Blvd Prot
Cayucas, CA 93041 Aetna

Anthony Giangrasso, MD

Figure ST5.1 *Medication order sheet*

Notes/Workspace

10. The order reads:

antihemophilic factor (Factor VIII) 25 u/kg IV

The patient weighs 175 pounds. How many units will you prepare for this patient? _________

11. You have a 50-mL vial of 25% normal serum albumin.

a. How many grams of serum albumin are contained in the vial? _________

b. If the serum is to be infused at a rate of 3 milliliters per minute, how many minutes will it take to complete this infusion? _________

12. The prescriber ordered:

ACTH 40 u sc q12h

The label on the vial reads 80 units per milliliter. How many milliliters will you administer to your patient? _________

13. You are to prepare 125 milligrams of methylprednisolone (Medrol) for IM injections. The label on the vial reads 80 milligrams per milliliter. How many milliliters will you administer to your patient? _________

14. The second order in Figure ST5.1 is for Procardia. If the available tablets are 0.01 gram each, how many tablets equal this order? _________

15. Determine the number of Elavil tablets you would administer to this patient according to the third order in Figure ST5.1 if each tablet contains 25 milligrams. _________

16. If 10 mEq of potassium chloride are equal to 750 milligrams of potassium chloride, how many milligrams would be equal to the medication in the fourth order of Figure ST5.1? _________

17. Read the fifth order in Figure ST5.1. If each Paraflex tablet contained grain $\overline{\underline{\text{VIISS}}}$, how many tablets would equal this ordered dose? _________

18. Read the label in Figure ST5.2. If the patient must receive 300 milligrams of bretylium tosylate IV, how many milliliters will the patient receive? _________

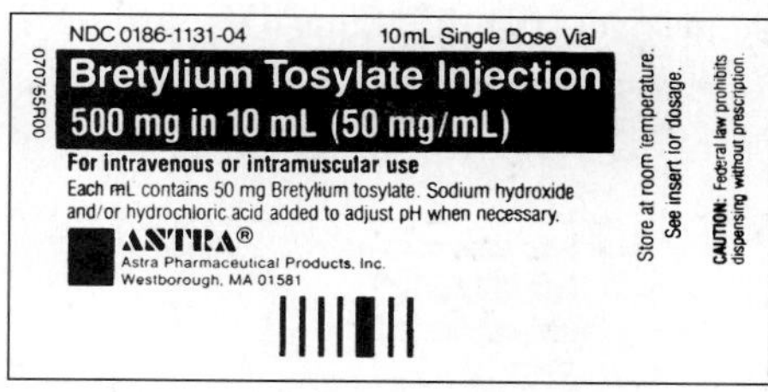

Figure ST5.2 *Drug label for bretylium tosylate*

Notes/Workspace

19. The prescriber's order reads:

Xylocaine 150 mg added to 250 mL 5% D/W, infuse in 4h

Read the label in Figure ST5.3 and calculate the milliliters of Xylocaine that you will add to the 250 milliliters of 5% D/W. What is the flow rate in milliliters per hour? ________

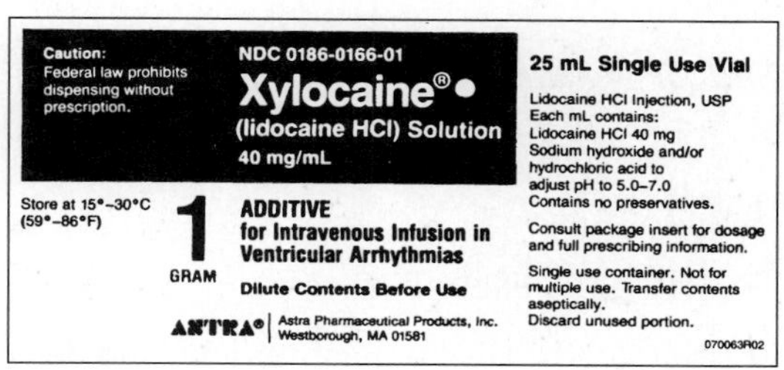

Figure ST5.3 *Drug label for Xylocaine*

20. The order reads:

amitriptyline hydrochloride 10,000 μg tid

Read the information on the label in Figure ST5.4 and determine the number of tablets you will administer to the patient. ________

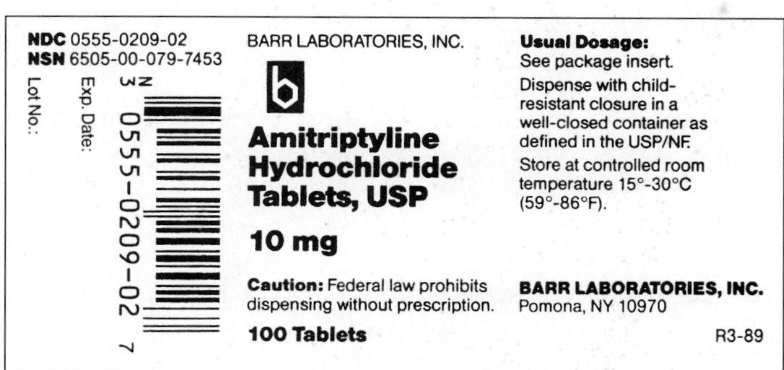

Figure ST5.4 *Drug label for amitriptyline hydrochloride*

Notes/Workspace

21. The patient must receive 10 milligrams IV push of Nubain, an analgesic, stat. Read the information on the label in Figure ST5.5. How many milliliters will you prepare for this patient? ________

NDC 0590-0399-01
NUBAIN®
(nalbuphine HCl)
20 mg/ml injection
10 ml VIAL
Each ml contains: 20 mg nalbuphine HCl, 0.94% sodium citrate hydrous, 1.26% citric acid anhydrous, 0.1% sodium metabisulfite and 0.2% of a 9:1 mixture of methyl and propylparaben, as preservatives. pH is adjusted, if necessary, with hydrochloric acid.
FOR IM, SC OR IV USE
DOSAGE: Read accompanying product information.
CAUTION: Federal law prohibits dispensing without prescription.
Store at controlled room temperature (59°-86°F, 15°-30°C).
PROTECT FROM EXCESSIVE LIGHT
Du Pont Pharmaceuticals, Inc.
Subsidiary of
E. I. du Pont de Nemours & Co. (Inc.)
Manati, Puerto Rico 00701 XB
LOT:
EXP:

Figure ST5.5 *Drug label for Nubain*

22. The prescriber ordered:

Atarax 0.05 g po at hs qd

Read the information on the label in Figure ST5.6 and determine the number of tablets that contain 0.05 gram. ________

NDC 0049-5610-66
100 Tablets
Atarax®
hydroxyzine HCl
25 mg
DISTINCTIVE TABLET SHAPE
CAUTION: Federal law prohibits dispensing without prescription.

Figure ST5.6 *Drug label for Atarax*

23. The prescriber has ordered 0.5 milligram sc of epinephrine (Adrenalin) stat. The ampule reads 1:1000. How many milliliters equals the prescribed dose?

____

24. A PICC (peripherally inserted central catheter) must be irrigated with 5,000,000 units of urokinase. If the vial reads 250,000 units per milliliter, how many milliliters equal the prescribed dose? ________

25. Epoetin alfa (Epogen), a drug that stimulates the production of red blood cells (erythropoiesis), is ordered; the patient is to receive 7500 units sc. The label on the vial reads 6,000 units per milliliter. How many minims equal the prescribed dose? ________

Case Study 6: Doris Kowalski

Notes/Workspace

Mrs. Doris Kowalski, age 54, has chronic emphysema. She has been hospitalized once for this problem. She is a heavy smoker, two packs a day. At the present time, she is admitted to the hospital with the following diagnosis: exacerbation of emphysema, rule out pneumonia. Vital signs are T: 99.6°F; P: 110; R: 36; BP: 160/92. Her admitting physician, Dr. Danielle Keefe, writes the following orders:

- 500 mL 5% D/W with 500 mg aminophylline; infuse at rate of 40 mg/h (drop factor 10 gtt/mL)
- Peripheral IV line 0.9% NS at a rate of 20 mL/h (drop factor 60 μgtt/mL)
- Penicillin 2,000,000 u in 50 mL 5% D/W q4h; infuse at rate of 50 mL in 30 min (drop factor 60 μgtt/mL)
- Elavil 0.05 g po hs

1. Calculate the flow rate for the IV orders. _________
2. How many milliliters of the three solutions will this patient receive in 24 hours? _________
3. How many units of penicillin will the patient receive in 5 days? _________
4. Calculate the number of milligrams equal to 0.05 gram of Elavil. _________
5. If the total amount of fluid is restricted to 2500 milliliters per day, how many milliliters of fluid po can the patient receive in 24 hours? _________

Comprehensive Self-Test 6

1. The order reads:

   ceftriaxone 1 g in 250 mL 5% D/W, IVPB

   The drop factor is 10 drops per milliliter, and the IVPB is to be infused in 2 hours. What is the flow rate in drops per minute? _________

2. The prescriber has ordered 400 milligrams of ciprofloxacin (Cipro) in 200 milliliters of 5% D/W. The patient is to receive 6 milligrams per kilogram per hour. The patient weighs 175 pounds, and the drop factor is 15 drops per milliliter. Calculate the flow rate in drops per minute. _________

3. The order reads: 1000 mL 5% D/W to infuse in 8 h, flow rate 41 gtt/min. After assessing the fluid intake, the nurse noted that 750 milliliters remained to be infused in 5 hours. The drop factor is 15 drops per milliliter. Recalculate the flow rate in drops per minute. _________

Notes/Workspace

4. Read the information on the drug label for Cytoxan in Figure ST6.1. If the prescriber ordered 8 milligrams per kilogram IV daily and the child weighs 32 kilograms, how many milliliters would you prepare for this child? ________

The above order has been changed to 250 milligrams per square meter, and the child's BSA is 0.9 square meter. How many milliliters will you prepare for this child now? ________

Figure ST6.1 *Drug label for Cytoxan*

5. The order reads: Add 125 mg of morphine sulfate to 250 mL 5% D/W; infuse at rate 0.005 mg/kg/min. The patient weighs 95 kilograms. Calculate the flow rate in milliliters per hour. ________

6. The prescriber ordered:

atropine sulfate 0.002 mg/kg sc 7 A.M.

The weight of the patient is 50 kilograms. Read the information on the label in Figure ST6.2. How many milliliters will you administer to this patient? ________

Figure ST6.2 *Drug label for atropine sulfate*

7. Read the information on the label in Figure ST6.3. How many capsules will you administer if the order is for 0.2 gram per 40 kilograms and the patient weighs 80 kilograms? _________

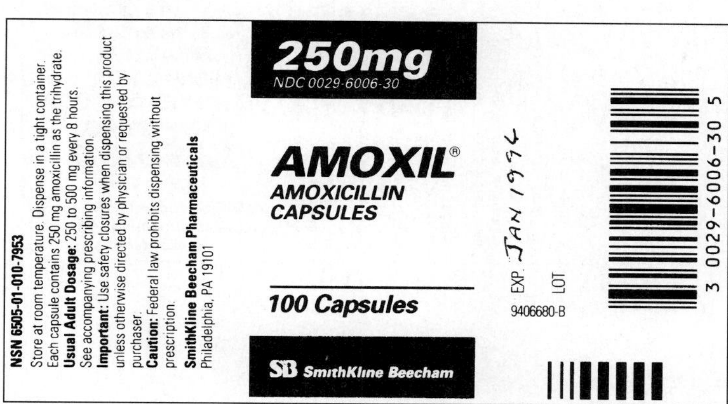

Figure ST6.3 *Drug label for Amoxil*

8. Your patient has an order for 8 milligrams per kilogram po of Ceclor. Read the information on the label in Figure ST6.4. How many milliliters will you prepare for this patient if his weight is 60 kilograms? _________

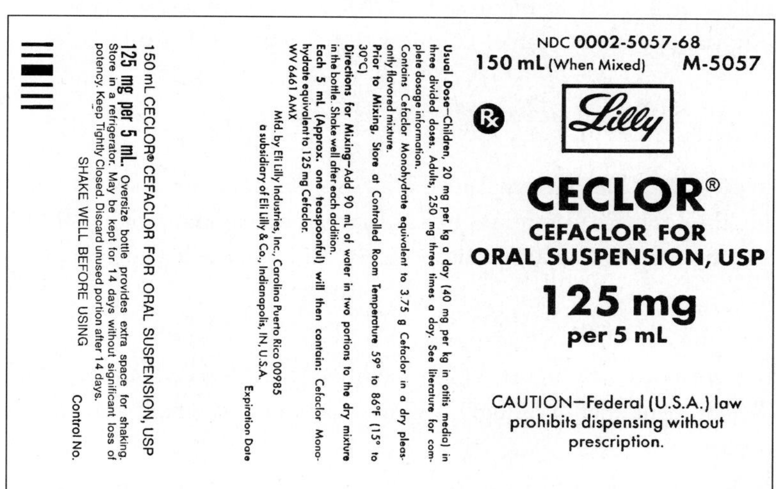

Figure ST6.4 *Drug label for Ceclor*

9. The label in Figure ST6.5 reads Ceclor, 375 milligrams per 5 milliliters. The order is for 250 milligrams bid po for 10 days.

   a. How many milliliters contain the prescribed dose? _________

   b. Calculate the amount of Ceclor you will need for 10 days. _________

   c. How many milligrams will the patient receive in 10 days? _________

Notes/Workspace

Notes/Workspace

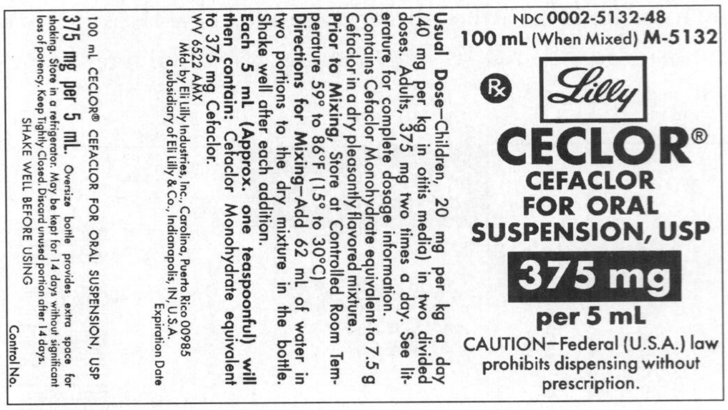

NDC 0002-5132-48
100 mL (When Mixed) M-5132
℞ Lilly
CECLOR®
CEFACLOR
FOR ORAL
SUSPENSION, USP
375 mg
per 5 mL
CAUTION—Federal (U.S.A.) law prohibits dispensing without prescription.

Figure ST6.5 *Drug label for Ceclor*

10. The order reads:

verapamil HCl 0.075 mg/kg IV push over 2 min

If the weight of the patient is 80 kilograms and the label on the vial reads 5 milligrams per 2 milliliters, how many milliliters will you prepare of this calcium channel blocker? ________

11. Read the first order in Figure ST6.6. How many tablets will you administer to the patient if each tablet contains 0.015 gram of Isordil? ________

12. Convert the second order in Figure ST6.6 to grams. ________

13. The prescriber has ordered 140 milligrams per kilogram stat of acetylcysteine as an antidote for acetaminophen toxicity. The patient weighs 70 kilograms. If you have a 20% solution, how many milliliters will you prepare?

____

14. If the third order in Figure ST6.6 was changed to 0.010 gram and each tablet of Reglan contained 5 milligrams, how many tablets would you administer to this patient? ________

15. How many tablets of Bentyl will you administer to the patient if each tablet contains grain $\frac{1}{6}$? (Refer to the fourth order in Figure ST6.6.) ________

GENERAL HOSPITAL

Year 19 *94* Month *November* Day	*10*	*11*	*12*	*13*	*14*	*15*
Medication Dosage and Interval	Initials* and Hours	Initials and Hours	Initials and Hours	Initials and Hours	Initials and Hours	Initials and Hours
Date started: *11/10* *Isordil 15 mg po tid* *10 A.M.* *2 P.M.* *6 P.M.* Discontinued: — I	*JO*	*JO*	*JO*	*JO*	*JO*	
AM	*10*	*10*	*10*	*10*	*10*	
I	*JO AG*	*JO AG*	*JO AG*	*JO AG*	*JO AG*	
PM	*2 6*	*2 6*	*2 6*	*2 6*	*2 6*	
Date started: *11/10* *Inderal 40 mg po qid* *10–2–6–10* Discontinued: — I	*JO*	*JO*	*JO*	*JO*	*JO*	
AM	*10*	*10*	*10*	*10*	*10*	
I	*JO AG AG*	*JO AG AG*	*JO AG AG*	*JO AG AG*	*JO AG AG*	
PM	*2 6 10*	*2 6 10*	*2 6 10*	*2 6 10*	*2 6 10*	
Date started: *11/10* *Reglan 5 mg po hs* *10 P.M.* Discontinued: — I						
AM						
I	*AG*	*AG*	*AG*	*AG*	*AG*	
PM	*10*	*10*	*10*	*10*	*10*	
Date started: *11/10* *Bentyl 10 mg po ac dinner 6 P.M.* Discontinued: — I						
AM						
I	*AG*	*AG*	*AG*	*AG*	*AG*	
PM	*6*	*6*	*6*	*6*	*6*	
Date started: *11/10* *digoxin 0.125 mg po qd* *10 A.M.* Discontinued: — I	*JO*	*JO*	*JO*	*JO*	*JO*	
AM	*10*	*10*	*10*	*10*	*10*	
I						
PM						
Date started: *11/10* *docusate sodium 200 mg po qd* *10 A.M.* Discontinued: — I	*JO*	*JO*	*JO*	*JO*	*JO*	
AM	*10*	*10*	*10*	*10*	*10*	
I						
PM						

Allergies: (Specify)

Init*	Signature
JO	*June Olsen*
AG	*Anthony Giangrasso*

MEDICATION ADMINISTRATION RECORD

PATIENT IDENTIFICATION

5760030 11/10/94

Marlin Anderson 1/31/07
1200 Seventh Ave #42 RC
Baltimore MD 400321 BCBS

Dr. Ablon

Notes/Workspace

Figure ST6.6 *Medication order sheet*

Notes/Workspace

16. If the available tablets of digoxin each contain 125 micrograms, how many tablets equal the fifth order in Figure ST6.6? ________

17. 102 °F = ________ °C

18. How many capsules of docusate sodium will be given to the patient for 30 days if each capsule contains 100 milligrams? (Refer to the sixth order in Figure ST6.6.) ________

19. The prescriber has written an order for the antineoplastic drug pentostatin (Nipent) for the treatment of hairy cell leukemia. The patient is to receive 4 milligrams per square meter in 50 milliliters of 5% D/W IVBP. The patient's BSA is 1.6 square meters. The medication label reads 10 milligrams per milliliter.

   a. How many milliliters of medication will you add to the 50 milliliters? ________

   b. Calculate the flow rate for this infusion in microdrops per minute when the total time for infusion is 90 minutes. ________

20. The order reads:

   phenobarbital 325 mg, added to 100 mL 5% D/W

   The label on the vial reads 250 milligrams per milliliter.

   a. How many milliliters of this drug must be added to this infusion? ________

   b. Calculate the flow rate in drops per minute when the drop factor is 10 drops per milliliter and the time for the infusion is 3 hours. ________

21. The prescriber's order reads:

   ciprofloxacin 400 mg in 200 mL 5% D/W IVPB, infuse in 90 min

   The label on the vial reads 200 milligrams per 20 milliliters.

   a. How many milliliters of ciprofloxacin will you add to the infusion? ________

   b. Calculate the flow rate in drops per minute. The drop factor is 15 drops per milliliter. ________

22. Your patient is in diabetic ketoacidosis. Calculate the flow rate of her medication in milliliters per hour for a solution of 250 milliliters of 5% D/W with 2 grams of magnesium sulfate, to be infused in 6 hours. ________

Notes/Workspace

23. The order reads:

Add 2 g lidocaine to 1000 mL; 0.02 mg/kg/min

The patient weighs 206 pounds. Calculate the flow rate for this IV in milliliters per hour. ________

24. The order reads:

500 mL 5% D/W with gr 5 phenobarbital IVPB

The patient is to receive 5 milligrams per hour. Calculate the flow rate in milliliters per hour. ________

25. The prescriber ordered:

1000 mL 0.9% NS IV 8h; flow rate 42 gtt/min

When the IV was reassessed, 150 milliliters had infused in 3 hours. The drop factor is 20 drops per milliliter. Recalculate the flow rate. ________

appendix A

Answer Section

Included in this section are answers to the Try These for Practice, Exercise, and Cumulative Review Exercise Practice Sets for all chapters. Also included are the answers to the Prerequisite Equivalent and Practice Reading Labels segments, which fall in Chapters 4 and 6, Case Studies 1–3, and Comprehensive Self-Tests 1–3. Your instructor has the answers for Additional Exercises, Case Studies 4–6 and Comprehensive Self-Tests 4–6.

Chapter 1

Try These for Practice

1. 0.875 **2.** $\frac{4}{75}$ **3.** 51.9 **4.** 1 **5.** 0.075

Exercises

1. $\frac{24}{100} = \frac{6}{25}$

2. $3\frac{24}{100} = \frac{324}{100} = \frac{81}{25}$

3. $8\overline{)5.000}$ with quotient .625; work: 4 8, 20, 16, 40, 40; so $\frac{5}{8} = 0.625$

4. $25\overline{)4.00}$ with quotient .16; work: 2 5, 150, 150; so $\frac{4}{25} = 0.16$

5. $\frac{1}{10} = 0.1$

6. $200\overline{)1.000}$ with quotient .005; work: 1 000; so $\frac{1}{200} = 0.005$

7. $300\overline{)1.0000}$ with quotient .0033; work: 900, 1000, 900; so $\frac{1}{300} = 0.003$ to the nearest thousandth

8. 45.0.0. so $\frac{4500}{100} = 45$

9. 6.25 so $\frac{6.25}{1000} = 0.00625$

10. $7\overline{)142.60}$ with quotient 20.37; work: 14, 2 6, 2 1, 50, 49; so $\frac{142.6}{7} = 20.4$ to the nearest tenth

11. $0.0.6\overline{)7.2.0.}$ with quotient 120.; work: 6, 1 2, 1 2, 00; so $\frac{7.2}{0.06} = 120$

12. $\begin{array}{r} 12000. \\ 0.006\overline{)72.000} \\ \underline{6} \\ 12 \\ \underline{12} \\ 0 \end{array}$ so $\frac{72}{0.006} = 12{,}000$

13. 123.4 so $123.4 \times 100 = 12{,}340$

14. $\begin{array}{r} 5.125 \\ \underline{\times 1.3} \\ 15375 \\ \underline{5125} \\ 6.6625 \end{array}$ so $5.125 \times 1.3 = 6.6625$

15. 36.42 so $36.42 \times 1000 = 36{,}420$

16. $\begin{array}{r} 1700 \\ 0.05\overline{)85.00} \\ \underline{5} \\ 35 \\ \underline{35} \\ 0 \end{array}$ so $\frac{85}{0.05} = 1700$

17. $\begin{array}{r} 17 \\ 0.5\overline{)8.5} \\ \underline{5} \\ 35 \\ \underline{35} \\ 0 \end{array}$ so $\frac{8.5}{0.5} = 17$

18. $\frac{\overset{2}{\cancel{4}}}{\underset{1}{\cancel{15}}} \times \frac{\overset{2}{\cancel{30}}}{1} \times \frac{1}{\underset{1}{\cancel{2}}} = 4$

19. $\frac{13}{2} \div \frac{3}{1} = \frac{13}{2} \times \frac{1}{3} = \frac{13}{6}$ or $2\frac{1}{6}$

20. $\frac{26}{1} \div \frac{13}{4} = \frac{26}{1} \times \frac{4}{13} = \frac{104}{13}$ or 8

21. $4.25 \times \frac{1}{5} = 4\frac{1}{4} \times \frac{1}{5} = \frac{17}{4} \times \frac{1}{5} = \frac{17}{20}$

22. $\frac{1}{\underset{2}{\cancel{250}}} \times \frac{\overset{1}{\cancel{125}}}{1} \times \frac{1}{0.5} = \frac{1}{1}$ or 1

23. $\frac{475}{100} \times \frac{1}{1.5} = \frac{475}{150} = \frac{19}{6} = 3\frac{1}{6}$ or $4.75 \times \frac{1}{1.5} = \frac{4.75}{1.5} = 3.2$ to the nearest tenth

24. $3 \div \frac{5}{10} = 3 \times \frac{\overset{2}{\cancel{10}}}{\underset{1}{\cancel{5}}} = 6$

25. $\left(\frac{1}{4} \div \frac{6}{1}\right) \times \frac{8}{1} = \frac{1}{\underset{1}{\cancel{4}}} \times \frac{1}{6} \times \frac{\overset{2}{\cancel{8}}}{1} = \frac{2}{6}$ or 0.3 to the nearest tenth

26. $\left(\frac{1}{4} \times \frac{160}{1}\right) \div \frac{5}{8} = \frac{1}{\underset{1}{\cancel{4}}} \times \frac{\overset{32}{\cancel{160}}}{1} \times \frac{\overset{2}{\cancel{8}}}{\underset{1}{\cancel{5}}} = 64$

27. $38\frac{2}{5}\% = 38.40\% = 38.40 = 0.384$

28. $35\% = 35 \div 100 = 0.35$

29. $6.75\% = 6\frac{3}{4}\% = 6\frac{3}{4} \div 100 = \frac{27}{4} \times \frac{1}{100} = \frac{27}{400}$

30. $1.5\% = 1\frac{1}{2} \div 100 = \frac{3}{2} \times \frac{1}{100} = \frac{3}{200}$

Chapter 2

Try These for Practice

1. Route of administration is intravenous **2.** 50 cap **3.** 10 mg **4.** Kefzol
5. Each tablet contains 25 mg

Exercises

1. lidocaine hydrochloride **2.** Xylocaine **3.** 40 mg per mL **4.** intravenous infusion
5. Antivert/25

6.

Name of Drug	Dose	Route of Administration	Time of Administration	Date Started	Date Discontinued
Clofibrate	500 mg	po	10 A.M. 2 P.M. 6 P.M.	7/18/94	7/25/94
Cardizem	60 mg	po	10 A.M. 6 P.M.	7/18/94	7/25/94
Clinoril	200 mg	po	10 A.M. 6 P.M.	7/19/94	7/26/94
Digoxin	0.125 mg	po	10 A.M.	7/19/94	7/26/94
Lasix	20 mg	po	10 A.M.	7/19/94	7/26/94
Carafate	1 g	po	7 A.M. 12 noon 5 P.M., 10 P.M.	7/20/94	7/27/94

a. Clofibrate 500 mg; Cardizem SL 60 mg
b. Clofibrate 500 mg; Cardizem SL 60 mg; Clinoril 200 mg; digoxin 0.125 mg; Lasix 20 mg; Carafate 1 g
c. one drug at 10 P.M.: Carafate 1 g

7. a. Inderal 120 mg po **b.** vitamin C two times a day **c.** 6 P.M. **d.** Inderal 120 mg
e. 10/12/94

8. a. demeclocycline hydrocloride **b.** four divided doses of 150 mg or two divided doses of 300 mg
c. 600 mg
d. capsules, two-tone, coral coloration; soft gelatin capsules, printed with LLD9 on the light side in blue ink.

Chapter 3

Try These for Practice

1. 96 oz **2.** 5 ft **3.** 4 yr **4.** 150 sec **5.** $6\frac{2}{3}$ yd

Exercises

1. $1.5\,\cancel{\text{yr}} \times \frac{12\text{ mon}}{1\,\cancel{\text{yr}}} = 18\text{ mon}$ **2.** $3\,\cancel{\text{d}} \times \frac{24\text{ h}}{1\,\cancel{\text{d}}} = 72\text{ h}$ **3.** $2\,\cancel{\text{lb}} \times \frac{16\text{ oz}}{1\,\cancel{\text{lb}}} = 32\text{ oz}$

4. $\overset{2}{\cancel{120\text{ sec}}} \times \frac{1\text{ min}}{\underset{1}{\cancel{60\text{ sec}}}} = 2\text{ min}$ **5.** $\overset{10}{\cancel{120\text{ in}}} \times \frac{1\text{ ft}}{\underset{1}{\cancel{12\text{ in}}}} = 10\text{ ft}$ **6.** $\overset{6}{\cancel{18\text{ ft}}} \times \frac{1\text{ yd}}{\underset{1}{\cancel{3\text{ ft}}}} = 6\text{ yd}$

7. $\overset{1}{\cancel{8\text{ oz}}} \times \frac{1\text{ lb}}{\underset{2}{\cancel{16\text{ oz}}}} = \frac{1}{2}\text{ lb}$ **8.** $0.5\,\cancel{\text{yd}} \times \frac{3\text{ ft}}{1\,\cancel{\text{yd}}} = 1.5 \text{ or } 1\frac{1}{2}\text{ ft}$ **9.** $1\frac{1}{2}\,\cancel{\text{yr}} \times \frac{12\text{ mon}}{1\,\cancel{\text{yr}}} = 18\text{ mon}$

10. $\frac{1}{2}\,\cancel{\text{min}} \times \frac{60\text{ sec}}{1\,\cancel{\text{min}}} = 30\text{ sec}$ **11.** $6\,\cancel{\text{ft}} \times \frac{12\text{ in}}{1\,\cancel{\text{ft}}} = 72\text{ in}$ **12.** $10\,\cancel{\text{min}} \times \frac{60\text{ sec}}{1\,\cancel{\text{min}}} = 600\text{ sec}$

13. $2.75\,\cancel{h} \times \dfrac{60\text{ min}}{1\,\cancel{h}} = 165\text{ min}$

14. $30\,\cancel{\text{mon}} \times \dfrac{1\text{ yr}}{12\,\cancel{\text{mon}}} = 2.5 \text{ or } 2\frac{1}{2}\text{ yr}$

15. $45\,\cancel{\text{min}} \times \dfrac{1\text{ h}}{60\,\cancel{\text{min}}} = \dfrac{45}{60} \text{ or } \dfrac{3}{4}\text{ h}$

16. $66\,\cancel{\text{in}} \times \dfrac{1\text{ ft}}{12\,\cancel{\text{in}}} = 5\text{ ft, }6\text{ in or }5\frac{1}{2}\text{ ft}$

17. $60\,\cancel{h} \times \dfrac{1\text{ d}}{24\,\cancel{h}} = 2.5 \text{ or } 2\frac{1}{2}\text{ d}$

18. $7\,\cancel{\text{lb}} \times \dfrac{16\text{ oz}}{1\,\cancel{\text{lb}}} = 112\text{ oz}$

19. $5\,\cancel{\text{ft}} \times \dfrac{12\text{ in}}{1\,\cancel{\text{ft}}} = 60\text{ in} + 4\text{ in} = 64\text{ in}$

20. $3\frac{1}{2}\,\cancel{\text{lb}} \times \dfrac{16\text{ oz}}{1\,\cancel{\text{lb}}} = \dfrac{112}{2} = 56\text{ oz}$

Chapter 4

Prerequisite Equivalents

Volume

1 mL = 1 cc = 1 cm^3
1 L = 1000 cc
1000 mL = 1 L

Weight

1 kg = 1000 g
1 g = 1000 mg
1 mg = 1000 μg
1 mg = 1000 mcg
1 μg = 1 mcg

Try These For Practice

1. 0.00125 g **2.** 0.04 g **3.** 5 mg **4.** 2 L **5.** 1.5 mg

Exercises

1. $75\cancel{00}\,\cancel{g} \times \dfrac{1\text{ kg}}{10\cancel{00}\,\cancel{g}} = \dfrac{75}{10} = 7.5\text{ kg}$

2. $1.5\,\cancel{L} \times \dfrac{1000\text{ cc}}{1\,\cancel{L}} = 1500\text{ cc}$

3. $2\,\cancel{L} \times \dfrac{1000\text{ mL}}{1\,\cancel{L}} = 2000\text{ mL}$

4. $75\cancel{0}\,\cancel{\text{mg}} \times \dfrac{1\text{ g}}{100\cancel{0}\,\cancel{\text{mg}}} = 0.75\text{ g}$

5. $0.005\,\cancel{g} \times \dfrac{1000\text{ mg}}{1\,\cancel{g}} = 5\text{ mg}$

6. $0.372\,\cancel{g} \times \dfrac{1000\text{ mg}}{1\,\cancel{g}} = 372\text{ mg}$

7. $0.4\,\cancel{\text{kg}} \times \dfrac{1000\text{ g}}{1\,\cancel{\text{kg}}} = 400\text{ mg}$

8. $\overset{3}{\cancel{3000}}\,\cancel{\text{cc}} \times \dfrac{1\text{ L}}{\underset{1}{\cancel{1000}}\,\cancel{\text{cc}}} = 3\text{ L}$

9. $1.75\,\cancel{\text{mg}} \times \dfrac{1\text{ g}}{1000\,\cancel{\text{mg}}} = 0.00175\text{ g}$

10. $0.0004\,\cancel{g} \times \dfrac{1000\text{ mg}}{1\,\cancel{g}} = 0.4\text{ mg}$

11. $15\cancel{000}\,\cancel{\text{mcg}} \times \dfrac{1\text{ mg}}{\cancel{1000}\,\cancel{\text{mcg}}} = 15\text{ mg}$

12. $2\cancel{00}\,\cancel{\mu g} \times \dfrac{1\text{ mg}}{10\cancel{00}\,\cancel{\mu g}} = 0.2\text{ mg}$

13. $3\cancel{0}\,\cancel{\text{mg}} \times \dfrac{1\text{ g}}{100\cancel{0}\,\cancel{\text{mg}}} = 0.03\text{ g}$

14. $0.025\,\cancel{g} \times \dfrac{1000\text{ mg}}{1\,\cancel{g}} = 25\text{ mg}$

15. $0.6\,\cancel{g} \times \dfrac{1000\text{ mg}}{1\,\cancel{g}} = 600\text{ mg}$

16. $0.8\,\cancel{L} \times \dfrac{1000\text{ mL}}{1\,\cancel{L}} = 800\text{ mL}$

17. $\overset{2}{\cancel{2000}}\,\cancel{\text{mg}} \times \dfrac{1\text{ g}}{\underset{1}{\cancel{1000}}\,\cancel{\text{mg}}} = 2\text{ g}$

18. $0.3\,\cancel{\text{mg}} \times \dfrac{1000\ \mu\text{g}}{1\,\cancel{\text{mg}}} = 300\ \mu\text{g}$

19. $5\cancel{00}\,\cancel{\mu g} \times \dfrac{1\text{ mg}}{10\cancel{00}\,\cancel{\mu g}} = 0.5\text{ mg}$

20. $25\,\cancel{\text{mg}} \times \dfrac{1\text{ g}}{1000\,\cancel{\text{mg}}} = 0.025\text{ g}$

Chapter 5

Try These for Practice

1. dr 64 **2.** 2 teacups **3.** 6 t **4.** pt $\frac{3}{4}$

5.

Apothecary	Household	Metric
pt 2	℥ 8	1 cc
℥ 16	℥ 8	1000 mg
ʒ 8	℥ 6	1000 g
♏ 60	2 T	1 mg
	3 t	
	60 gtt	
	16 oz	

Exercises

1. $\cancel{\text{♏}}\ \overset{2}{\cancel{120}}\ \frac{\text{dr } 1}{\cancel{\text{♏}}\ \underset{1}{\cancel{60}}} = \text{dr } 2$ **2.** $\cancel{\text{qt}}\ 4 \times \frac{\text{pt } 2}{\cancel{\text{qt}}\ 1} = \text{pt } 8$ **3.** $\cancel{\text{pt}}\ \overset{5}{\cancel{10}} \times \frac{\text{qt } 1}{\cancel{\text{pt}}\ \underset{1}{\cancel{2}}} = \text{qt } 5$

4. $3\ \cancel{\text{t}} \times \frac{60 \text{ gtt}}{1\ \cancel{\text{t}}} = 180 \text{ gtt}$ **5.** $\cancel{\text{℥}}\ 30 \times \frac{\text{♏ } 60}{\cancel{\text{℥}}\ 1} = \text{♏ } 1800$ **6.** $\cancel{\text{℥}}\ \frac{1}{\underset{1}{\cancel{8}}} \times \frac{\text{ʒ } \overset{1}{\cancel{8}}}{\cancel{\text{℥}}\ 1} = \text{ʒ } 1$

7. $\cancel{\text{ʒ}}\ \overset{4}{\cancel{32}} \times \frac{\text{℥ } 1}{\cancel{\text{ʒ}}\ \underset{1}{\cancel{8}}} = \text{℥ } 4$ **8.** $4\ \cancel{\text{T}} \times \frac{3 \text{ t}}{1\ \cancel{\text{T}}} = 12 \text{ t}$ **9.** $\cancel{\text{℥}}\ 24 \times \frac{\text{ʒ } 8}{\cancel{\text{℥}}\ 1} = \text{ʒ } 192$

10. $\cancel{\text{♏}}\ \overset{3}{\cancel{90}} \times \frac{\text{ʒ } 1}{\cancel{\text{♏}}\ \underset{2}{\cancel{60}}} = \text{ʒ } 1\frac{1}{2}$ **11.** apothecary: g $\frac{1}{100}$; metric: 0.6 mg **12.** 3 tsp = 1 T

13. $\cancel{\text{oz}}\ \overline{\text{ISS}} \times \frac{\text{dr } 8}{\cancel{\text{oz}}\ 1} = \text{dr } 12$ **14.** $2\frac{1}{2}\ \cancel{\text{qt}} \times \frac{2 \text{ pt}}{1\ \cancel{\text{qt}}} = 5 \text{ pt}$ **15.** $\cancel{\text{ʒ}}\ \overset{1}{\cancel{4}} \times \frac{\text{℥ } 1}{\cancel{\text{ʒ}}\ \underset{2}{\cancel{8}}} = \text{℥ } \frac{1}{2}$

16. $\cancel{\text{dr}}\ 2 \times \frac{\text{♏ } 60}{\cancel{\text{dr}}\ 1} = \text{♏ } 120$ **17.** $\overset{1}{\cancel{15}}\ \cancel{\text{gtt}} \times \frac{1 \text{ t}}{\underset{4}{\cancel{60}}\ \cancel{\text{gtt}}} = \frac{1}{4} \text{ t}$ **18.** $\cancel{\text{dr}}\ 3 \times \frac{\text{oz } 1}{\cancel{\text{dr}}\ 8} = \text{oz } \frac{3}{8}$

19. $2\ \cancel{\text{qt}} \times \frac{32 \text{ oz}}{1\ \cancel{\text{qt}}} = 64 \text{ oz}$ **20.** $\frac{1}{\underset{1}{\cancel{4}}}\ \cancel{\text{pt}} \times \frac{\overset{4}{\cancel{16}} \text{ oz}}{1\ \cancel{\text{pt}}} = 4 \text{ oz}$

Cumulative Review Exercises

1. 2500 mg **2.** 0.2 mg **3.** dr 3 **4.** dr 32 **5.** 25,000 μg **6.** 2 T **7.** 1.2 L

8. 6 g **9.** 2350 g **10.** 2500 mg **11.** $1\frac{1}{2}$ tsp **12.** 3250 mL **13.** oz $\frac{3}{4}$

14. $\frac{1}{2}$ tsp **15.** 0.24 L

Chapter 6

Prerequisite Equivalents

Metric

1 mL = 1 cc = 1 cm^3
1 L = 1000 mL
1 kg = 1000 g
1000 mg = 1 g
1000 μg = 1 mg
1 μg = 1 mcg

Apothecary

1 qt = 2 pt
1 pt = ℥ 16
℥ 1 = ʒ 8
ʒ 1 = ♏ 60

Household

1 glass = ℥ 8
1 teacup = ℥ 6
℥ 1 = 2 T
1 T = 3 t
1 t = 60 gtt
1 lb = 16 oz
1 ft = 12 in

Mixed Systems

ʒ 1 = 1 t = ♏ 60 = 60 gtt = 5 mL
℥ 1 = 2 T = ʒ 8 = 30 mL
1 measuring cup = 1 glass = ℥ 8 = $\frac{1}{2}$ pt
gr 1 = 60 mg
1 g = gr 15
1 mL = 15 gtt
1 kg = 2.2 lb
1 lb = 0.45 kg
1 in = 2.5 cm

Try These for Practice

1. 1200 mg **2.** gr $\frac{1}{240}$ **3.** 0.12 mg **4.** 27.9 kg **5.** ♏ 60

Exercises

1. $25\,\cancel{\mu g} \times \frac{1\text{ mg}}{1000\,\cancel{\mu g}} = 0.025\text{ mg}$

2. $1.5\,\cancel{kg} \times \frac{1000\text{ g}}{1\,\cancel{kg}} = 1500\text{ g}$

3. $0.0001\,\cancel{g} \times \frac{1000\text{ mg}}{1\,\cancel{g}} = 0.1\text{ mg}$

4. $0.008\,\cancel{mg} \times \frac{1000\text{ mcg}}{1\,\cancel{mg}} = 8\text{ mcg}$

5. $\cancel{gr}\,\frac{1}{\cancel{6}_{1}} \times \frac{\overset{10}{\cancel{60}}\text{ mg}}{\cancel{gr}\,1} = 10\text{ mg}$

6. $0.6\,\cancel{mg} \times \frac{\text{gr }1}{60\,\cancel{mg}} = \frac{\text{gr }0.6}{60} = \text{gr }\frac{1}{100}$

7. $0.1\,\cancel{mg} \times \frac{1\text{ g}}{1000\,\cancel{mg}} = 0.0001\text{ g}$

8. $0.2\,\cancel{mg} \times \frac{1000\text{ mcg}}{1\,\cancel{mg}} = 200\text{ mcg}$

9. $\cancel{gr}\,\frac{1}{240} \times \frac{1\text{ g}}{\cancel{gr}\,15} = \frac{1\text{ g}}{3600} = 0.00027\text{ g or }0.0003\text{ g}$

10. $\cancel{gr}\,3\frac{3}{4} \times \frac{60\text{ mg}}{\cancel{gr}\,1} = \frac{15}{\cancel{4}_{1}} \times \frac{\overset{15}{\cancel{60}}\text{ mg}}{1} = 225\text{ mg}$

11. $0.75\,\cancel{g} \times \frac{\text{gr }15}{1\,\cancel{g}} = \text{gr }11\frac{1}{4}$ or $0.75\,\cancel{g} \times \frac{\overset{40}{\cancel{1000\text{ mg}}}}{\cancel{g}} \times \frac{\text{gr }1}{\underset{3}{\cancel{60\text{ mg}}}} = \text{gr }10$

12. $\cancel{gr}\,\frac{1}{\underset{10}{\cancel{600}}} \times \frac{\overset{1}{\cancel{60}}\text{ mg}}{\cancel{gr}\,1} = 0.1\text{ mg}$

13. $\cancel{gr}\,\frac{1}{\underset{5}{\cancel{300}}} \times \frac{\overset{1}{\cancel{60}}\text{ mg}}{\cancel{gr}\,1} = 0.2\text{ mg}$

14. $\cancel{gr}\,4 \times \frac{1\text{ g}}{\cancel{gr}\,15} = \frac{4\text{ g}}{15} = 0.266\text{ g or }0.3\text{ g}$

15. $12.5\,\cancel{mg} \times \frac{1000\text{ mcg}}{1\,\cancel{mg}} = 12{,}500\text{ mcg}$

16. $\cancel{gr}\,\frac{1}{\cancel{3}_{1}} \times \frac{\overset{20}{\cancel{60}}\text{ mg}}{\cancel{gr}\,1} = 20\text{ mg}$

17. $0.75\,\cancel{g} \times \frac{1000\text{ mg}}{1\,\cancel{g}} = 750\text{ mg}$

18. $\cancel{250\text{ mg}} \times \frac{\text{gr } 1}{\cancel{60\text{ mg}}} = \text{gr } \frac{25}{6} \text{ or gr } 4\frac{1}{6}$

19. $\overset{25}{\cancel{250\text{ mg}}} \times \frac{\text{gr } 1}{\underset{6}{\cancel{60\text{ mg}}}} = \text{gr } 4\frac{1}{6}$

20. $\cancel{50\text{ mg}} \times \frac{\text{gr } 1}{\cancel{60\text{ mg}}} = \text{gr } \frac{5}{6}$

Note: 250 mg is considered to be equivalent to gr $3\frac{3}{4}$.

Cumulative Review Exercises

1. gr $\frac{3}{20}$ 2. ʒ 4 3. gr $3\frac{3}{4}$ 4. gr $\frac{3}{4}$ 5. 20 mg 6. gr 3

7. gr $\frac{9}{200}$ or gr $\frac{1}{20}$ 8. gr $\frac{1}{40}$ 9. ℥ 2 10. 1 mL 11. 0.00125 g or 0.001 g

12. gr $\frac{1}{4}$ 13. gr $\frac{1}{240}$ 14. gr $\frac{1}{6}$ 15. 0.004 g

Chapter 7

Practice Reading Labels

1. 3 cap 2. 1 tab 3. 1 cap 4. 4 cap 5. 1 cap 6. 4 cap 7. 10 mL
8. 25 mL 9. 2 tab 10. 1 cap 11. 1 cap 12. 4 tab 13. 2 tab 14. 2 tab
15. 1 tab 16. 4 cap 17. 2 tab 18. 1 tab 19. 2 tab 20. 1 tab 21. 2 tab
22. 1 cap 23. 2 tab 24. 2 tab 25. 1 tab 26. 2 tab 27. 1 tab 28. 1 tab
29. 2 tab 30. 10 mL

Try These for Practice

1. 1 tab 2. 1 tab 3. 1 tab 4. 5 mL 5. 2 cap

Exercises

1. $0.2\,\cancel{g} \times \frac{\cancel{1000\text{ mg}}}{1\,\cancel{g}} \times \frac{1\text{ cap}}{\cancel{100\text{ mg}}} = 2\text{ cap}$

2. $\overset{4}{\cancel{200\text{ mg}}} \times \frac{5\text{ mL}}{\underset{1}{\cancel{50\text{ mg}}}} = 20\text{ mL}$

3. $0.15\,\cancel{g} \times \frac{\cancel{1000\text{ mg}}}{1\text{ g}} \times \frac{1\text{ tab}}{\cancel{150\text{ mg}}} = \frac{15\text{ tab}}{15} = 1\text{ tab}$

4. $0.3\,\cancel{g} \times \frac{\cancel{1000\text{ mg}}}{1\,\cancel{g}} \times \frac{1\text{ tab}}{\cancel{300\text{ mg}}} = \frac{3\text{ tab}}{3} = 1\text{ tab}$

5. $0.1\,\cancel{g} \times \frac{\cancel{1000\text{ mg}}}{1\,\cancel{g}} \times \frac{1\text{ cap}}{\cancel{100\text{ mg}}} = 1\text{ cap}$

6. $\cancel{10\text{ mg}} \times \frac{1\,\cancel{g}}{\cancel{1000\text{ mg}}} \times \frac{1\text{ tab}}{0.005\,\cancel{g}} = \frac{1\text{ tab}}{0.5} = 2\text{ tab}$

7. $5\,\cancel{\text{mg}} \times \frac{1\,\cancel{g}}{1000\,\cancel{\text{mg}}} \times \frac{1\text{ tab}}{0.005\,\cancel{g}} = \frac{5\text{ tab}}{5} = 1\text{ tab}$

8. $0.75\,\cancel{g} \times \frac{\overset{4}{\cancel{1000\text{ mg}}}}{1\,\cancel{g}} \times \frac{1\text{ cap}}{\underset{1}{\cancel{250\text{ mg}}}} = 3\text{ cap}$

9. $0.002\,\cancel{g} \times \frac{1000\,\cancel{\text{mg}}}{1\,\cancel{g}} \times \frac{1\text{ tab}}{2\,\cancel{\text{mg}}} = \frac{2\text{ tab}}{2} = 1\text{ tab}$

10. $0.25\,\cancel{\text{mg}} \times \frac{1\text{ tab}}{0.5\,\cancel{\text{mg}}} = \frac{0.25\text{ tab}}{0.5} = \frac{25\text{ tab}}{50} = \frac{1}{2}\text{ tab}$

11. $0.01\,\cancel{g} \times \frac{\cancel{1000\text{ mg}}}{1\,\cancel{g}} \times \frac{1\text{ tab}}{\cancel{10\text{ mg}}} = \frac{1\text{ tab}}{1} \text{ or } 1\text{ tab}$

12. $1.6\,\cancel{g} \times \frac{\overset{10}{\cancel{1000\text{ mg}}}}{1\,\cancel{g}} \times \frac{1\text{ tab}}{\underset{4}{\cancel{400\text{ mg}}}} = \frac{16\text{ tab}}{4} = 4\text{ tab}$

13. $20\,\cancel{\text{mg}} \times \frac{1\,\cancel{g}}{1000\,\cancel{\text{mg}}} \times \frac{1\text{ cap}}{0.01\,\cancel{g}} = \frac{20\text{ cap}}{10} = 2\text{ cap}$

14. $0.375\,\cancel{g} \times \frac{\overset{4}{\cancel{1000\text{ mg}}}}{1\text{ g}} \times \frac{1\text{ tab}}{\underset{1}{\cancel{250\text{ mg}}}} = 1.5\text{ tab or } 1\frac{1}{2}\text{ tab}$

15. $67\,\cancel{\text{kg}} \times \frac{0.03\,\cancel{\text{mg}}}{\cancel{\text{kg}}} \times \frac{1\text{ tab}}{0.5\,\cancel{\text{mg}}} = \frac{2.01\text{ tab}}{0.5} = 4.02 \text{ or } 4\text{ tab}$

16. $0.01\,\cancel{g} \times \frac{\overset{200}{\cancel{1000\text{ mg}}}}{1\,\cancel{g}} \times \frac{1\text{ tab}}{\underset{1}{\cancel{5\text{ mg}}}} = 2\text{ tab}$

17. $\overset{4}{\cancel{100\text{ mg}}} \times \frac{5\text{ mL}}{\underset{1}{\cancel{25\text{ mg}}}} = 20\text{ mL}$

18. $0.45\cancel{\text{ mg}} \times \frac{1\text{ tab}}{0.3\cancel{\text{ mg}}} = \frac{0.45\text{ tab}}{0.3} = 1.5$ tab, give patient $1\frac{1}{2}$ tab

19. $0.001\cancel{\text{ g}} \times \frac{1000\cancel{\text{ mg}}}{1\cancel{\text{ g}}} \times \frac{1\text{ tab}}{1\cancel{\text{ mg}}} = 1$ tab

20. $154\cancel{\text{ lb}} \times \frac{0.45\cancel{\text{ kg}}}{1\cancel{\text{ lb}}} \times \frac{7.2\cancel{\text{ mg}}}{\cancel{\text{kg}}} \times \frac{1\text{ cap}}{250\cancel{\text{ mg}}} = \frac{499\text{ cap}}{250}$ or 2 cap

Cumulative Review Exercises

1. 15 mg **2.** 1 tab **3.** ℥ 80 **4.** gr 3 **5.** gr $3\frac{3}{4}$ **6.** 0.04 g **7.** gr $41\frac{3}{5}$
8. ♏ 60 **9.** 7.5 L **10.** 500 mg **11.** 3 t **12.** 3 tab **13.** 10 mL
14. 4 tab **15.** 1.25 mL

Chapter 8

Try These for Practice

1. 40 g **2.** Use 4.5 mL of sodium chloride and dilute with water to 500 mL
3. 5 g **4.** Use 40 tab and dilute with water to 4000 mL
5. Use 2000 mL of 2% neomycin solution and dilute with water to 4000 mL

Exercises

1. $\dfrac{1000\cancel{\text{ mL}} \times \dfrac{2\text{ mL}}{\cancel{100\text{ mL}}}}{\dfrac{\overset{1}{\cancel{100\text{ mL}}}}{\underset{1}{\cancel{100\text{ mL}}}}} = 20$ mL of the 100% solution and dilute with water to 1000 mL

2. $\dfrac{\overset{5}{\cancel{500}}\text{ mL} \times \dfrac{2\cancel{\text{ mL}}}{\underset{1}{\cancel{100\text{ mL}}}}}{\dfrac{\overset{1}{\cancel{50\text{ mL}}}}{\underset{2}{\cancel{100\text{ mL}}}}} = 20$ mL of the 50% solution and dilute with water to 500 mL

3. $2000\cancel{\text{ mL}} \times \frac{\cancel{10\text{ mL}}}{\cancel{100\text{ mL}}} = 200$ mL of pure Westodyne solution and dilute with water to 2000 mL

4. $1250\cancel{\text{ mL}} \times \frac{0.45\text{ g}}{100\cancel{\text{ mL}}} = 5.6$ g of sodium chloride crystals and dilute with water to 1250 mL

5. $\overset{5}{\cancel{5000\text{ mL}}} \times \frac{1\cancel{\text{ g}}}{\underset{1}{\cancel{1000\text{ mL}}}} \times \frac{1\text{ tab}}{5\cancel{\text{ g}}} = 1$ tab and dissolves with water to 1250 mL

6. $\overset{1}{\cancel{100\text{ mL}}} \times \frac{2\text{ g}}{\underset{1}{\cancel{100\text{ mL}}}} = 2$ g of boric acid crystals and dilute with water to 100 mL

7. $\overset{10}{\cancel{1000\text{ mL}}} \times \frac{1\cancel{\text{ g}}}{\underset{1}{\cancel{100\text{ mL}}}} \times \frac{1\text{ tab}}{1\cancel{\text{ g}}} = 10$ tab (1 g) of ammonium chloride and dissolve in water to 1000 mL

8. $5\cancel{\text{ mL}} \times \frac{10\text{ g}}{100\cancel{\text{ mL}}} = \frac{50}{100}\text{ g} = 0.5\text{ g}$

9. $\dfrac{\overset{10}{\cancel{1000}}\text{ mL} \times \dfrac{2.5\cancel{\text{ mL}}}{\underset{1}{\cancel{100\text{ mL}}}}}{\dfrac{3\cancel{\text{ mL}}}{100\cancel{\text{ mL}}}} = 833.3$ mL of the 3% hydrogen peroxide solution and dilute with water to 1000 mL

10. $\dfrac{\overset{1}{\cancel{100}}\ \cancel{\text{mL}} \times \dfrac{1\text{ mL}}{\cancel{100\text{ mL}}}}{\dfrac{\overset{1}{\cancel{20\text{ mL}}}}{\underset{5}{\cancel{100\text{ mL}}}}}$ = 5 mL of the 20% solution and dilute with water to 100 mL

11. $\overset{80}{\cancel{4000}}\ \cancel{\text{mL}} \times \dfrac{1\ \cancel{\text{g}}}{\underset{1}{\cancel{50\text{ mL}}}} \times \dfrac{1\text{ tab}}{0.5\ \cancel{\text{g}}}$ = 160 tab of potassium permanganate and dissolve in water to 4000 mL

12. $\dfrac{\overset{10}{\cancel{1000}}\text{ mL} \times \dfrac{10\ \cancel{\text{mL}}}{\underset{1}{\cancel{100\text{ mL}}}}}{\dfrac{\overset{1}{\cancel{25\text{ mL}}}}{\underset{4}{\cancel{100\text{ mL}}}}}$ = 400 mL of the 25% Lysol solution and dilute with water to 1000 mL

13. $3\ \cancel{\text{L}} \times \dfrac{10\text{ g}}{\cancel{100\text{ mL}}} \times \dfrac{\cancel{1000\text{ mL}}}{1\ \cancel{\text{L}}}$ = 300 g of glucose

14. $\dfrac{4000\ \cancel{\text{mL}} \times \dfrac{1\ \cancel{\text{mL}}}{\cancel{40\text{ mL}}}}{\dfrac{1\ \cancel{\text{mL}}}{20\ \cancel{\text{mL}}}}$ = 2000 mL of the 1:20 solution and dilute with water to 4000 mL

15. $\dfrac{\overset{4}{\cancel{1000}}\text{ mL} \times \dfrac{1\ \cancel{\text{mL}}}{\underset{3}{\cancel{750\text{ mL}}}}}{\dfrac{1\ \cancel{\text{mL}}}{500\ \cancel{\text{mL}}}}$ = 666.7 mL of the 1:500 solution of Zephiran Chloride and dilute with water to 5000 mL

16. $\dfrac{\overset{5}{\cancel{500\text{ mL}}} \times \dfrac{0.025\text{ mL}}{\underset{1}{\cancel{100\text{ mL}}}}}{\dfrac{1\ \cancel{\text{mL}}}{100\ \cancel{\text{mL}}}}$ = 12.5 mL of the 1% solution and dilute with water to 500 mL

17. 1:1000 or 0.1%

18. $\overset{20}{\cancel{2000\text{ mL}}} \times \dfrac{10\ \cancel{\text{g}}}{\underset{1}{\cancel{100\text{ mL}}}} \times \dfrac{1\text{ tab}}{1\ \cancel{\text{g}}}$ = 200 tab (1 g) and dissolve in water to 2000 mL

19. $\dfrac{\overset{2}{\cancel{500\text{ mL}}} \times \dfrac{1\text{ mL}}{\underset{3}{\cancel{750\text{ mL}}}}}{\dfrac{2\ \cancel{\text{mL}}}{100\ \cancel{\text{mL}}}}$ = 33.3 mL of the 2% solution and dilute with water to 500 mL

20. $250\text{ mL} \times \dfrac{0.05\ \cancel{\text{mL}}}{\underset{1}{\cancel{100\text{ mL}}}} \times \dfrac{\overset{1}{\cancel{100\text{ mL}}}}{1\ \cancel{\text{mL}}}$ = 12.5 mL of the 1% solution and dilute with water to 250 mL

Cumulative Review Exercises

1. Take 62.5 mL of the 10% boric acid solution and dilute with water to 250 mL
2. 2.5 g **3.** 25 mL of pure drug and dilute with water to 500 mL **4.** 1 tab **5.** 3 tab
6. 1 tab **7.** ♏ 60 **8.** 500 mg **9.** 0.75 g **10.** 2.5 g **11.** gr $\frac{5}{6}$
12. 8 tab **13.** 0.6 mg **14.** 300 mg **15.** 5 pt

Chapter 9

Try These for Practice

1.

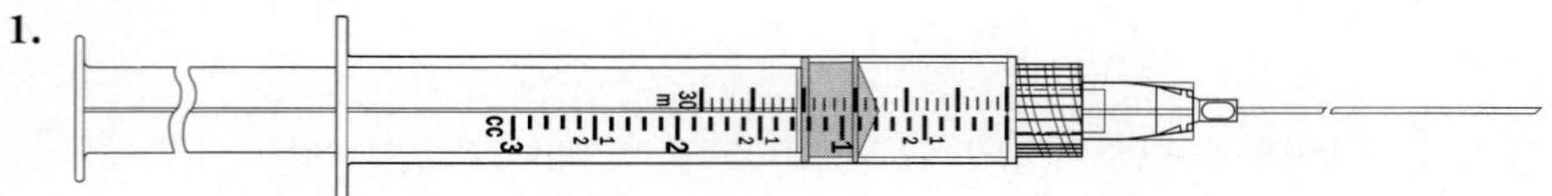

♏ 15 on a 3 cc syringe

2.

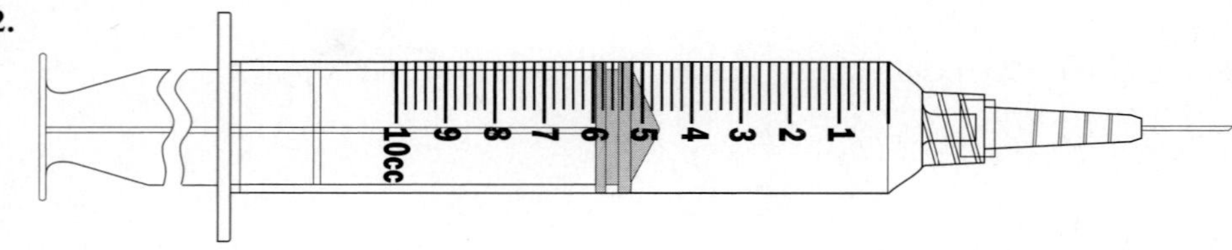

5.2 cc on a 10 cc syringe

3.

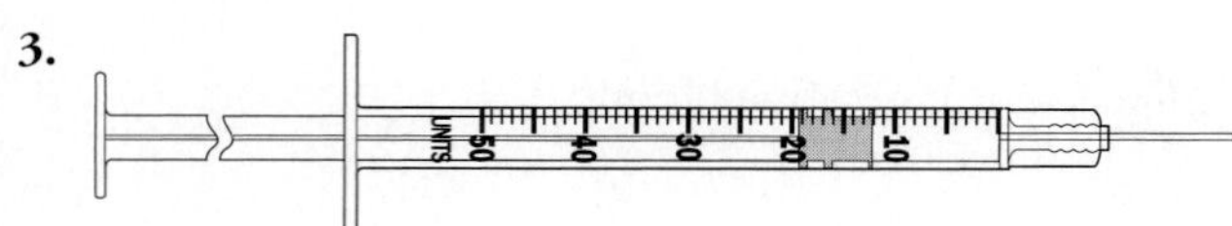

12 u on a 50 u insulin syringe

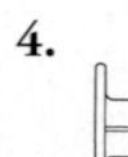
4.

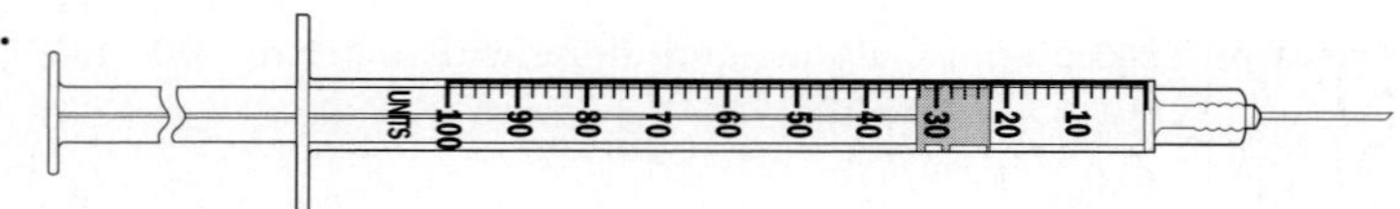

22 u on a 100 u insulin syringe

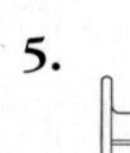
5.

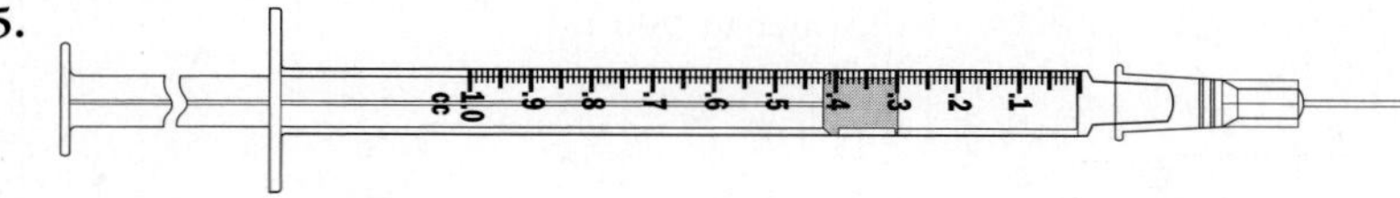

0.3 cc on a tuberculin syringe

Exercises

1.

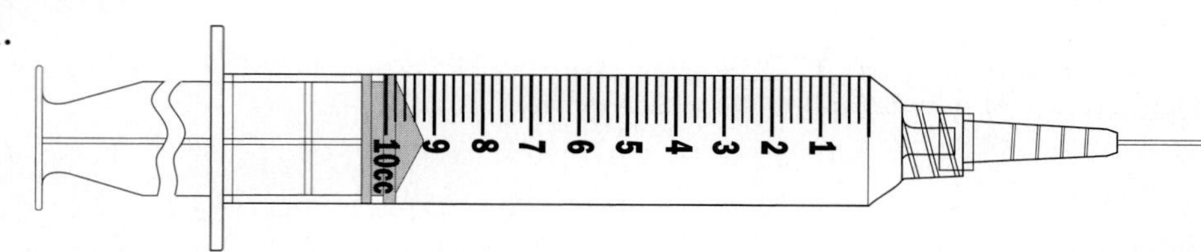

9.8 cc on a 10 cc syringe

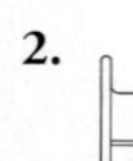
2.

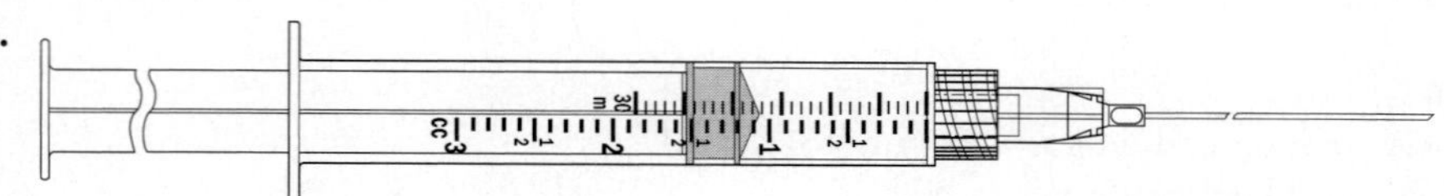

1.2 cc on a 3 cc syringe

3.

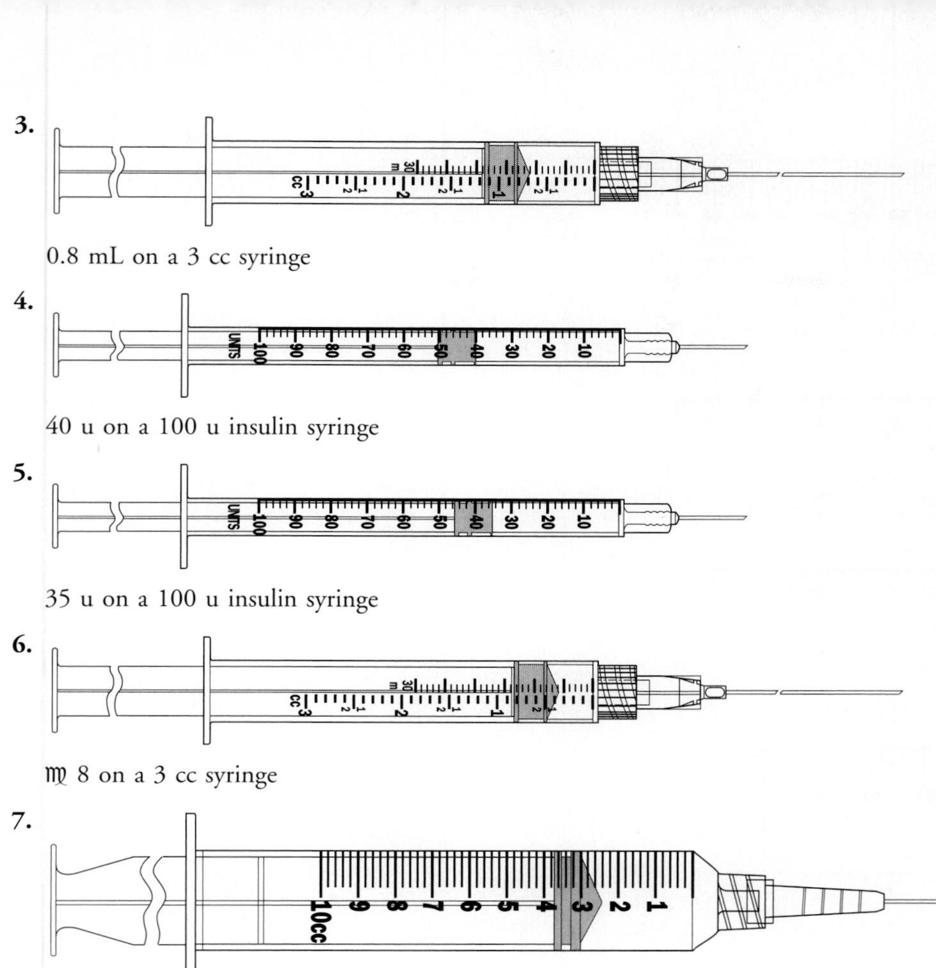

0.8 mL on a 3 cc syringe

4.

40 u on a 100 u insulin syringe

5.

35 u on a 100 u insulin syringe

6.

♍ 8 on a 3 cc syringe

7.

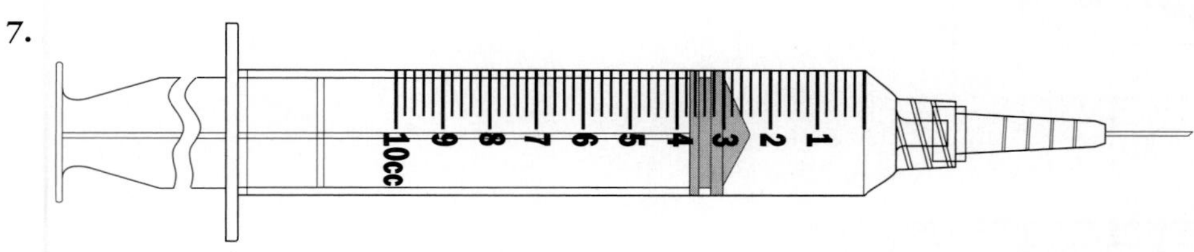

3 cc on a 10 cc syringe

8.

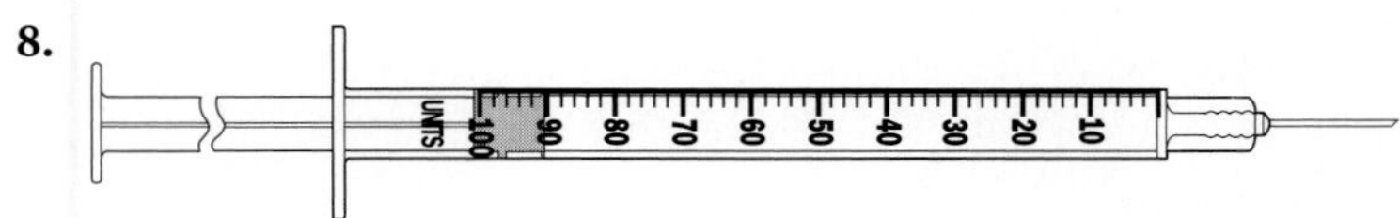

90 u on a 100 u insulin syringe

9.

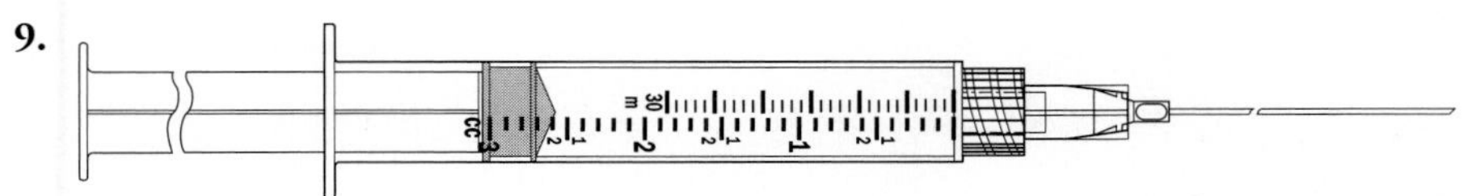

2.7 cc on a 3 cc syringe

10.

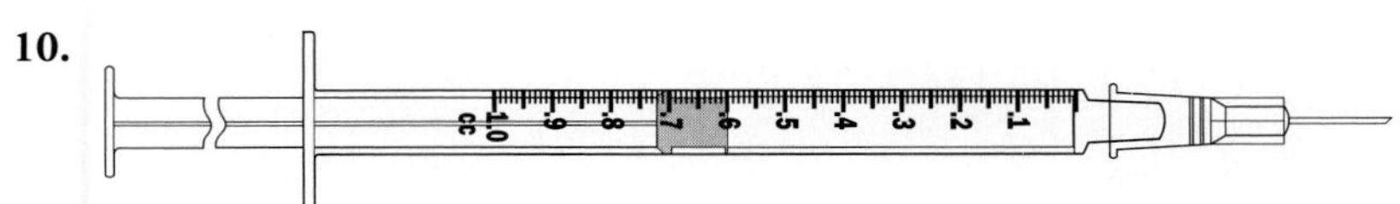

0.6 cc on a tuberculin syringe

11.

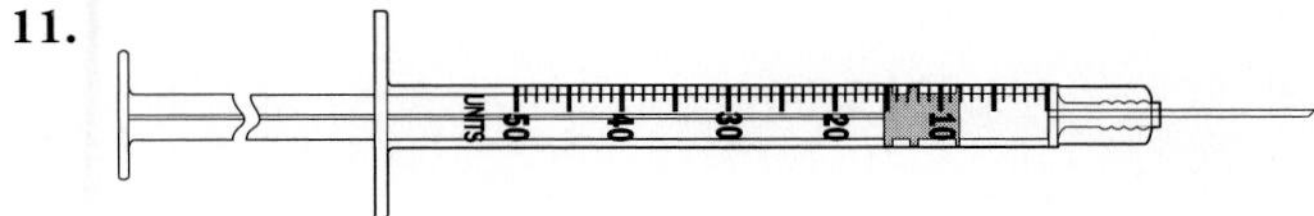

8 u on a 50 u insulin syringe

12.

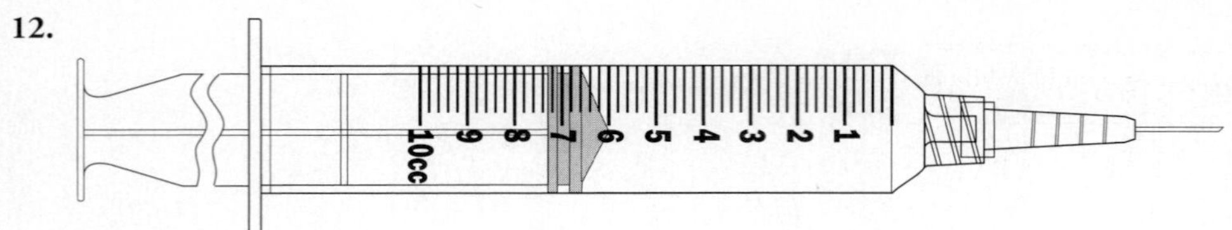

6.6 cc on a 10 cc syringe

13.

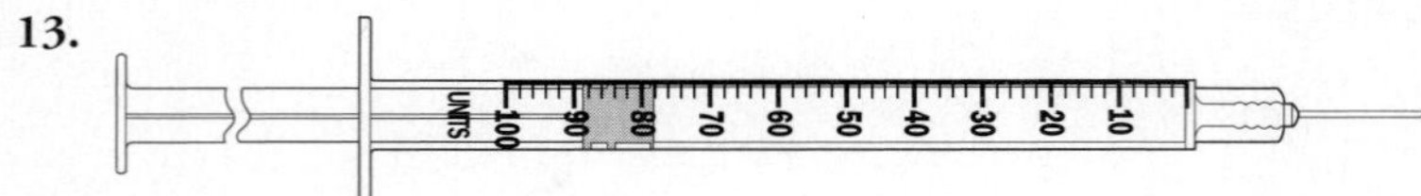

78 u on a 100 u insulin syringe

14.

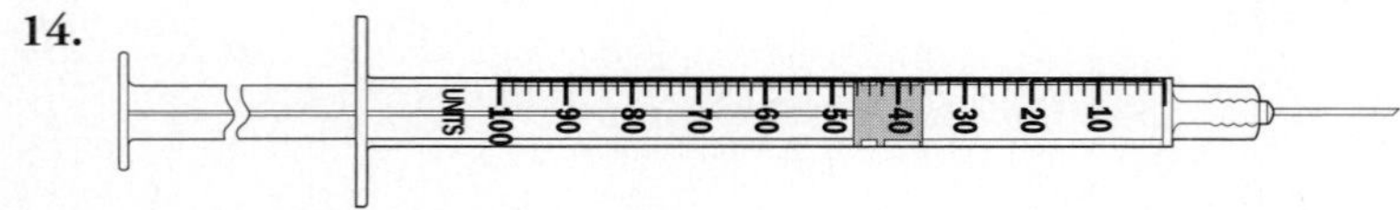

36 u on a 100 u insulin syringe

15.

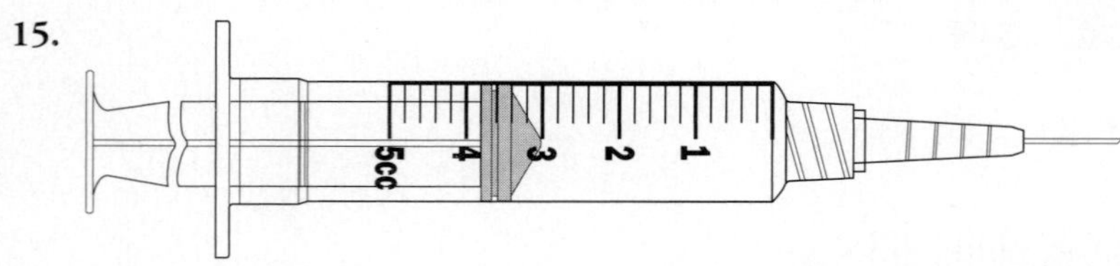

3.4 cc on a 5 cc syringe

16.

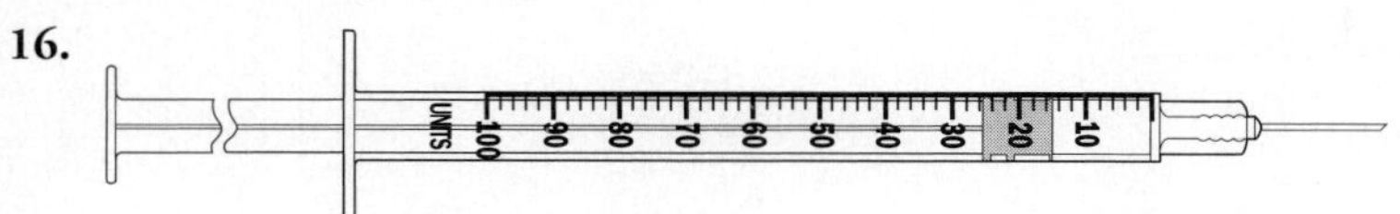

15 u on a 100 u insulin syringe

17.

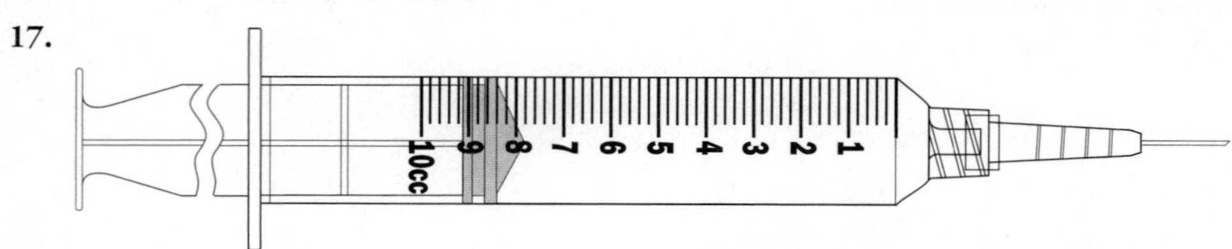

8.4 cc on a 10 cc syringe

18.

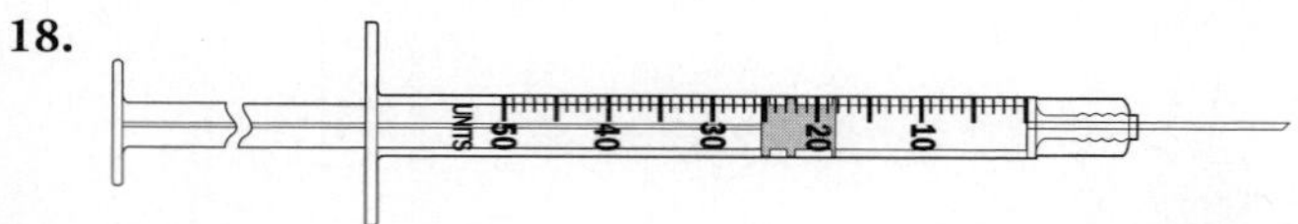

18 u on a 50 u insulin syringe

19.

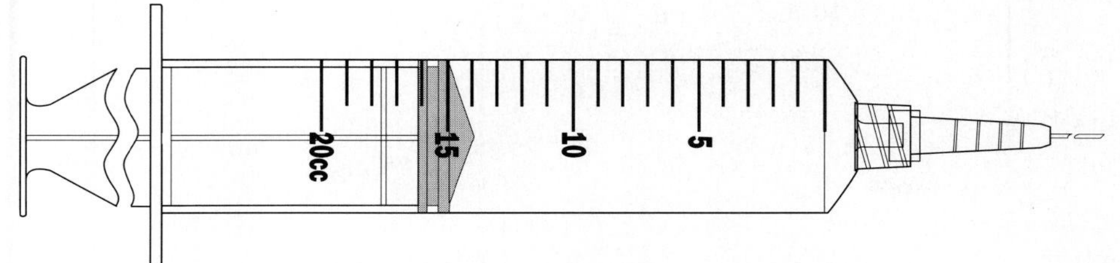

14.8 cc on a 20 cc syringe

20.

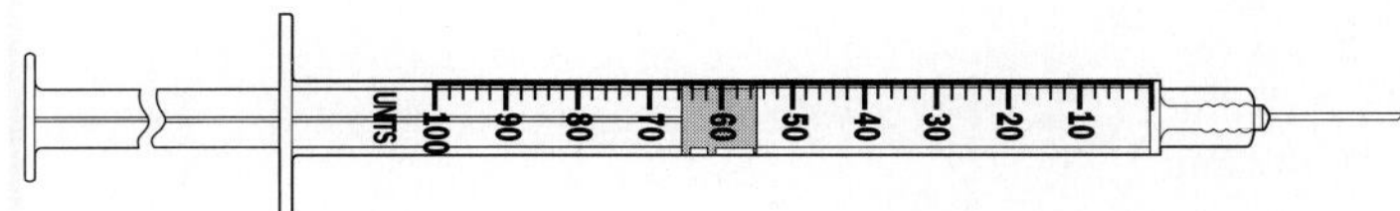

55 u on a 100 u insulin syringe

Cumulative Review Exercises

1. 600 mg **2.** 1.2 mL **3.** 1 cap **4.** 10 mg **5.** 3.3 mL **6.** 0.25 mg

7. 24 oz **8.** ℥ 2 **9.** gr $\frac{1}{100}$ **10.** gr $\frac{3}{50}$ **11.** 1 cap **12.** 3 tab

13. 2 tab **14.** 4 tab **15.** 1 tab

Chapter 10

Try These for Practice

1. 1.3 mL **2.** 0.3 mL **3.** 1.5 mL **4.** 2 mL **5.** ♏ 8

Exercises

1. $\overset{1}{\cancel{25\text{ u}}} \times \frac{2\text{ mL}}{\underset{2}{\cancel{50\text{ u}}}} = 1\text{ mL}$

2. $\overset{16}{\cancel{64\text{ kg}}} \times \frac{2\ \cancel{\text{u}}}{\cancel{\text{kg}}} \times \frac{1\text{ mL}}{\underset{25}{\cancel{100\text{ u}}}} = \frac{32\text{ mL}}{25} = 1.28 \text{ or } 1.3\text{ mL}$

3. $0.03\ \cancel{\text{g}} \times \frac{1000\ \cancel{\text{mg}}}{1\ \cancel{\text{g}}} \times \frac{1\text{ mL}}{\cancel{10\text{ mg}}} = 3\text{ mL}$

4. $\overset{5}{\cancel{500\text{ mg}}} \times \frac{1\text{ mL}}{\underset{4}{\cancel{400\text{ mg}}}} = \frac{5\text{ mL}}{4} = 1.25\text{ mL}$

5. $45\ \cancel{\text{kg}} \times \frac{1\ \cancel{\text{mg}}}{\cancel{\text{kg}}} \times \frac{1\text{ mL}}{10\ \cancel{\text{mg}}} = \frac{4.5\text{ mL}}{10} = 0.45\text{ mL or } 0.5\text{ mL}$

6. $0.05\ \cancel{\text{g}} \times \frac{\overset{20}{\cancel{1000\text{ mg}}}}{\cancel{\text{g}}} \times \frac{1\text{ mL}}{\underset{1}{\cancel{50\text{ mg}}}} = 1\text{ mL}$

7. $0.25\ \cancel{\text{mg}} \times \frac{1\ \cancel{\text{g}}}{1000\ \cancel{\text{mg}}} \times \frac{5\text{ mL}}{0.025\ \cancel{\text{g}}} = 0.05\text{ mL}$

8. $\overset{6}{\cancel{75\text{ kg}}} \times \frac{\overset{1}{\cancel{100\text{ mcg}}}}{\cancel{\text{kg}}} \times \frac{1\ \cancel{\text{mg}}}{\underset{10}{\cancel{1000\text{ mcg}}}} \times \frac{1\text{ mL}}{\underset{1}{\cancel{12.5\text{ mg}}}} = \frac{6\text{ mL}}{10}$ or 0.6 mL

9. $0.5\ \cancel{\text{mg}} \times \frac{1\text{ mL}}{0.25\ \cancel{\text{mg}}} = \frac{0.5\text{ mL}}{0.25} = 2\text{ mL}$

10. $7.5\cancel{\text{mg}} \times \frac{4\text{ mL}}{10\ \cancel{\text{mg}}} = \frac{30\text{ mL}}{10} = 3\text{ mL}$

11. $\overset{2}{\cancel{100{,}000\text{ u}}} \times \frac{1\text{ mL}}{\underset{1}{\cancel{50{,}000\text{ u}}}} = 2\text{ mL}$

12. $0.015\ \cancel{\text{g}} \times \frac{\overset{100}{\cancel{1000\text{ mg}}}}{1\ \cancel{\text{g}}} \times \frac{1\text{ mL}}{\underset{1}{\cancel{10\text{ mg}}}} = 1.5\text{ mL}$

13. $\overset{4}{\cancel{40\text{ u}}} \times \dfrac{1\text{ mL}}{\underset{10}{\cancel{100\text{ u}}}} = 0.4\text{ mL}$ **14.** $\overset{1}{\cancel{25\text{ kg}}} \times \dfrac{10\ \cancel{\text{mg}}}{\cancel{\text{kg}}} \times \dfrac{1\text{ mL}}{\underset{2}{\cancel{50\text{ mg}}}} = \dfrac{10\text{ mL}}{2} = 5\text{ mL}$

15. $\overset{5}{\cancel{250\text{ mg}}} \times \dfrac{1\ \cancel{\text{mL}}}{\underset{4}{\cancel{200\text{ mg}}}} \times \dfrac{\text{♏ } 15}{1\ \cancel{\text{mL}}} = \dfrac{\text{♏ } 75}{4} = \text{♏ } 18.75 \text{ or ♏ } 19$ **16.** $\overset{3}{\cancel{75\text{ mg}}} \times \dfrac{1\text{ mL}}{\underset{1}{\cancel{25\text{ mg}}}} = 3\text{ mL}$

17. $0.2\text{ g} \times \dfrac{\overset{5}{\cancel{1000\text{ mg}}}}{1\text{ g}} \times \dfrac{2\text{ mL}}{\underset{1}{\cancel{200\text{ mg}}}} = 2\text{ mL}$ **18.** $1.66\ \cancel{\text{m}^2} \times \dfrac{3.3\ \cancel{\text{mg}}}{\cancel{\text{m}^2}} \times \dfrac{1\text{ mL}}{25\ \cancel{\text{mg}}} = \dfrac{5.478}{25} = 0.2\text{ mL}$

19. $155\cancel{0\text{ mg}} \times \dfrac{1\text{ mL}}{20\cancel{0\text{ mg}}} = 7.75\text{ mL}$

20. $0.0002\ \cancel{\text{g}} \times \dfrac{1000\ \cancel{\text{mg}}}{1\ \cancel{\text{g}}} \times \dfrac{1\text{ mL}}{0.2\ \cancel{\text{mg}}} = 1\text{ mL};\ 1\ \cancel{\text{mL}} \times \dfrac{0.2\text{ mg}}{1\ \cancel{\text{mL}}} \times \dfrac{5}{1} = 1\text{ mg}$

Cumulative Review Exercises

1. 278 mg **2.** 2 tab **3.** 3 tab **4.** 1 tsp **5.** ♏ 4 **6.** ♏ 9 **7.** 1 tab
8. 1.5 mL **9.** 2 cap **10.** 0.48 mL or 5 mL **11.** 0.00017 g or 0.0002 g **12.** 3 mg
13. gr 3 **14.** 150 gtt **15.** gr $\dfrac{1}{1500}$

Chapter 11

Try These for Practice

1. 20.8 or 21 gtt/min **2.** 37.5 or 38 gtt/min **3.** 30 mL/hr
4. 26.3 or 26 hr 18 min
5. a. Add 1.3 mL of clindamycin phosphate to the 50 mL bag of 5% D/W **b.** 51 μgtt/min

Exercises

1. $\dfrac{250\text{ mL}}{\underset{10}{\cancel{12{,}000\text{ u}}}} \times \dfrac{\overset{1}{\cancel{1200\text{ u}}}}{\text{hr}} = 25\text{ mL/hr}$ **2.** $\dfrac{115\ \cancel{\text{mL}}}{\underset{4}{\cancel{60}}\text{ min}} \times \dfrac{\overset{1}{\cancel{15}}\text{ gtt}}{1\ \cancel{\text{mL}}} = 28.7 \text{ or } 29\text{ gtt/min}$

3. $\dfrac{\overset{25}{\cancel{500}}\text{ mL}}{\underset{1}{\cancel{20\text{ u}}}} \times \dfrac{0.002\ \cancel{\text{u}}}{\cancel{\text{min}}} \times \dfrac{60\ \cancel{\text{min}}}{\text{hr}} = 3\text{ mL/hr}$ **4.** $\dfrac{28\ \cancel{\text{gtt}}}{\cancel{\text{min}}} \times \dfrac{1\text{ mL}}{\underset{1}{\cancel{10\text{ gtt}}}} \times \dfrac{\overset{6}{\cancel{60\text{ min}}}}{\text{hr}} = 168\text{ mL/hr}$

5. $\dfrac{500\ \cancel{\text{cc}}}{\underset{8}{\cancel{120}}\text{ min}} \times \dfrac{\overset{1}{\cancel{15}}\text{ gtt}}{\cancel{\text{cc}}} = 62.5 \text{ or } 63\text{ gtt/min}$

6. $500\ \cancel{\text{mL}} \times \dfrac{\overset{1}{\cancel{15\text{ gtt}}}}{1\ \cancel{\text{mL}}} \times \dfrac{1\ \cancel{\text{min}}}{27\ \cancel{\text{gtt}}} \times \dfrac{1\ \cancel{\text{hr}}}{\underset{4}{\cancel{60\text{ min}}}} = \dfrac{500\ \cancel{\text{hr}}}{108} = 4.629\text{ hr or 4 hr 38 min}$

The infusion will end at 10:38 P.M.

7. $66\ \cancel{\text{kg}} \times \dfrac{0.06\ \cancel{\text{mg}}}{\cancel{\text{kg/min}}} \times \dfrac{\overset{1}{\cancel{250}}\text{ mL}}{\underset{1}{\cancel{250\text{ mg}}}} \times \dfrac{60\ \cancel{\text{min}}}{\text{hr}} = 23.76 \text{ or } 23.8\text{ mL/hr}$ **8.** $\dfrac{\overset{10}{\cancel{2500}}\text{ u}}{\underset{1}{\cancel{250\text{ mL}}}} \times \dfrac{50\ \cancel{\text{mL}}}{\text{hr}} = 500\text{ u/hr}$

9. $\dfrac{\overset{5}{\cancel{250}}\text{ mL}}{\underset{4}{\cancel{200\text{ mg}}}} \times \dfrac{10\ \cancel{\text{mg}}}{\text{hr}} = \dfrac{50\text{ mL}}{4\text{ hr}}$ or 12.5 mL/hr **10.** $100\ \cancel{\text{lb}} \times \dfrac{0.45\ \cancel{\text{kg}}}{1\ \cancel{\text{lb}}} \times \dfrac{0.005\text{ mg}}{1\ \cancel{\text{kg/min}}} \times \dfrac{60\ \cancel{\text{min}}}{1\text{ hr}} = 13.5\text{ mg/hr}$

11. $70\,\cancel{\text{kg}} \times \frac{\cancel{30}\,\cancel{\text{mcg}}}{1\,\cancel{\text{kg/min}}} \times \frac{1\,\cancel{\text{mg}}}{\cancel{1000}\,\cancel{\text{mcg}}} \times \frac{\overset{13}{\cancel{260}}\text{ mL}}{\underset{25}{\cancel{500}}\,\cancel{\text{mg}}} \times \frac{\cancel{60}\,\cancel{\text{min}}}{1\text{ hr}} = \frac{1638}{25} = 65.5\text{ mL/hr}$

12. $122\,\cancel{\text{lb}} \times \frac{0.45\,\cancel{\text{kg}}}{1\,\cancel{\text{lb}}} \times \frac{0.003\,\cancel{\text{mg}}}{\cancel{\text{kg/min}}} \times \frac{250\text{ mL}}{\underset{8}{\cancel{160}}\,\cancel{\text{mg}}} \times \frac{\overset{3}{\cancel{60}}\,\cancel{\text{min}}}{1\text{ hr}} = 15.5\text{ mL/hr}$

13. $60\,\cancel{\text{kg}} \times \frac{1\,\cancel{\text{mL}}}{1\,\cancel{\text{kg/hr}}} \times \frac{\overset{1}{\cancel{60}}\,\mu\text{gtt}}{1\,\cancel{\text{mL}}} \times \frac{1\,\cancel{\text{hr}}}{\underset{1}{\cancel{60}}\text{ min}} = 60\ \mu\text{gtt/min}$

14. $\overset{25}{\cancel{500}}\,\cancel{\text{mL}} \times \frac{1\,\cancel{\text{min}}}{0.7\,\cancel{\text{mL}}} \times \frac{1\text{ hr}}{\underset{3}{\cancel{60}}\,\cancel{\text{min}}} = \frac{2.5\text{ hr}}{2.1} = 11.9\text{ hr or } 11\text{ hr } 54\text{ min}$

15. $\frac{\overset{1}{\cancel{250}}\text{ mL}}{\underset{4}{\cancel{1000}}\,\cancel{\text{mg}}} \times \frac{20\,\cancel{\text{mg}}}{1\text{ hr}} = \frac{20\text{ mL}}{4\text{ hr}}$ or 5 mL/hr

16. $\frac{\cancel{1000}\,\cancel{\text{mL}}}{1} \times \frac{\overset{1}{\cancel{20}}\text{ gtt}}{1\,\cancel{\text{mL}}} \times \frac{1\,\cancel{\text{min}}}{\underset{1}{\cancel{20}}\,\cancel{\text{gtt}}} \times \frac{1\text{ hr}}{\cancel{60}\,\cancel{\text{min}}} = 16.66\text{ hr or } 16\text{ hr } 40\text{ min}$

The infusion will finish at 3:40 A.M.

17. $74\,\cancel{\text{kg}} \times \frac{0.08\,\cancel{\text{mg}}}{\cancel{\text{kg}}/\text{min}} \times \frac{\overset{1}{\cancel{50}}\,\cancel{\text{mL}}}{\underset{4}{\cancel{200}}\,\cancel{\text{mg}}} \times \frac{10\text{ gtt}}{\cancel{\text{mL}}} = 14.8\text{ or } 15\text{ gtt/min}$

18. $\overset{1}{\cancel{200}}\,\cancel{\text{lb}} \times \frac{0.45\,\cancel{\text{kg}}}{1\,\cancel{\text{lb}}} \times \frac{0.005\,\cancel{\text{mg}}}{\cancel{\text{kg/min}}} \times \frac{250\text{ mL}}{\underset{1}{\cancel{200}}\,\cancel{\text{mg}}} \times \frac{60\,\cancel{\text{min}}}{1\text{ hr}} = 33.75\text{ mL/hr or } 33.8\text{ mL/hr}$

19. $\frac{250\,\cancel{\text{mL}}}{1\,\cancel{\text{g}}} \times \frac{0.15\,\cancel{\text{g}}}{1\,\cancel{\text{hr}}} \times \frac{\overset{1}{\cancel{10}}\text{ gtt}}{1\,\cancel{\text{mL}}} \times \frac{1\,\cancel{\text{hr}}}{\underset{6}{\cancel{60}}\text{ min}} = \frac{37.5\text{ gtt}}{6\text{ min}}$ or 6 gtt/min

20. $0.9\,\cancel{\text{m}^2} \times \frac{120\,\cancel{\text{mg}}}{\cancel{\text{m}^2}/\text{hr}} \times \frac{\cancel{100}\text{ mL}}{\cancel{250}\,\cancel{\text{mg}}} = 43.2\text{ mL/hr}$

Cumulative Review Exercises

1. 5.4 mL **2.** 2 mL **3.** 1 mL **4.** ♏ 10 **5.** 20 mL **6.** 1 mL **7.** 1 tab
8. 10 mL **9.** 0.01 mg **10.** gr $\frac{1}{75}$ **11.** gr 375 **12.** 0.006 g **13.** 15 gtt
14. 6 t **15.** 1 oz

Chapter 12

Try These for Practice

1. 2.75 u **2.** 5.4 mL **3.** 0.5 mL **4.** 0.5 mL **5.** 216 mg

Exercises

1. $0.025\,\cancel{\text{g}} \times \frac{\overset{40}{\cancel{1000}}\,\cancel{\text{mg}}}{1\,\cancel{\text{g}}} \times \frac{\overset{1}{\cancel{5}}\,\cancel{\text{mL}}}{\underset{1}{\cancel{25}}\,\cancel{\text{mg}}} \times \frac{1\text{ t}}{\underset{1}{\cancel{5}}\,\cancel{\text{mL}}} = 1\text{ t}$

2. $\overset{2}{\cancel{650}}\,\cancel{\text{mg}} \times \frac{1\text{ tab}}{\cancel{325}\,\cancel{\text{mg}}} = 2\text{ tab}$

3. $40\ \cancel{\text{kg}} \times \frac{6.25\ \cancel{\text{mg}}}{1\ \cancel{\text{kg}}} \times \frac{\overset{1}{\cancel{5}}\ \text{mL}}{\underset{25}{\cancel{125}}\ \cancel{\text{mg}}} = 10\ \text{mL}$

4. $\overset{3}{\cancel{30}}\ \cancel{\text{kg}} \times \frac{3.3\ \cancel{\text{mcg}}}{\cancel{\text{kg}}} \times \frac{1\ \text{mL}}{\underset{5}{\cancel{50}}\ \cancel{\text{mcg}}} = 1.98\ \text{mL or } 2\ \text{mL}$

5. $0.45\ \cancel{\text{m}^2} \times \frac{0.2\ \text{mg}}{\cancel{\text{m}^2}} = 0.09\ \text{mg}$

6. $1.2\ \cancel{\text{m}^2} \times \frac{100\ \text{mg}}{\cancel{\text{m}^2}} = 120\ \text{mg}$

7. $1.1\ \cancel{\text{m}^2} \times \frac{45\ \text{mg}}{\cancel{\text{m}^2}} = 49.5\ \text{or}\ 50\ \text{mg}$

8. $1.2\ \cancel{\text{m}^2} \times \frac{50\ \text{mg}}{\cancel{\text{m}^2}} = 60\ \text{mg}$

9. $0.8\ \cancel{\text{m}^2} \times \frac{0.2\ \cancel{\text{mg}}}{\cancel{\text{m}^2}} \times \frac{1\ \text{mL}}{0.2\ \cancel{\text{mg}}} = 0.8\ \text{mL}$

10. $20\ \cancel{\text{kg}} \times \frac{0.01\ \cancel{\text{mg}}}{\cancel{\text{kg}}} \times \frac{1\ \text{mL}}{0.4\ \cancel{\text{mg}}} = 0.5\ \text{mL}$

11. $0.7\ \cancel{\text{m}^2} \times \frac{\overset{2}{\cancel{250}}\ \cancel{\text{mg}}}{\cancel{\text{m}^2}} \times \frac{1\ \text{mL}}{\underset{1}{\cancel{125}}\ \cancel{\text{mg}}} = 1.4\ \text{mL}$

12. $50\ \cancel{\text{kg}} \times \frac{0.5\ \cancel{\text{mg}}}{\cancel{\text{kg}}} \times \frac{\overset{1}{\cancel{100}}\ \text{mL}}{1\ \cancel{\text{g}}} \times \frac{1\ \cancel{\text{g}}}{\underset{10}{\cancel{1000}}\ \cancel{\text{mg}}} = \frac{25\ \text{mL}}{10} = 2.5\ \text{mL}$

13. $44\ \cancel{\text{kg}} \times \frac{0.54\ \cancel{\text{u}}}{\cancel{\text{kg}}} \times \frac{1\ \text{mL}}{100\ \cancel{\text{u}}} = \frac{23.76}{100} = 0.2\ \text{mL}$

14. $42\ \cancel{\text{kg}} \times \frac{\overset{1}{\cancel{2}}\ \cancel{\text{mg}}}{\cancel{\text{kg}}} \times \frac{1\ \text{mL}}{\underset{4}{\cancel{8}}\ \cancel{\text{mg}}} = \frac{42\ \text{mL}}{4} = 10.5\ \text{mL}$

15. $0.4\ \cancel{\text{g}} \times \frac{1000\ \cancel{\text{mg}}}{1\ \cancel{\text{g}}} \times \frac{5\ \cancel{\text{mL}}}{160\ \cancel{\text{mg}}} \times \frac{1\ \text{tsp}}{5\ \cancel{\text{mL}}} = 2\frac{1}{2}\ \text{tsp}$

16. $30\ \cancel{\text{kg}} \times \frac{1\ \cancel{\text{mg}}}{\cancel{\text{kg}}} \times \frac{\overset{1}{\cancel{100}}\ \text{mL}}{1\ \cancel{\text{g}}} \times \frac{1\ \cancel{\text{g}}}{\underset{10}{\cancel{1000}}\ \cancel{\text{mg}}} = 3\ \text{mL}$

17. $42\ \cancel{\text{kg}} \times \frac{0.6\ \cancel{\text{mg}}}{\cancel{\text{kg}}} \times \frac{1\ \text{mL}}{50\ \cancel{\text{mg}}} = 0.5\ \text{mL}$

18. $60\ \cancel{\text{kg}} \times \frac{0.1\ \cancel{\text{mg}}}{\cancel{\text{kg}}} \times \frac{1\ \text{mL}}{5\ \cancel{\text{mg}}} = 1.2\ \text{mL}$

19. $60\ \cancel{\text{lb}} \times \frac{0.45\ \cancel{\text{kg}}}{1\ \cancel{\text{lb}}} \times \frac{1.04\ \cancel{\text{mg}}}{\cancel{\text{kg}}} \times \frac{1\ \text{mL}}{100\ \cancel{\text{mg}}} = 0.28\ \text{mL or } 0.3\ \text{mL}$

20. $1\ \cancel{\text{m}^2} \times \frac{3\ \cancel{\text{mg}}}{\cancel{\text{m}^2}} \times \frac{1\ \text{tab}}{2\ \cancel{\text{mg}}} = \frac{3\ \text{tab}}{2}\ \text{or}\ 1\frac{1}{2}\ \text{tab}$

Cumulative Review Exercises

1. 525 mg 2. 300 mg 3. 160 mg 4. ♏ 8 5. 2.4 mL 6. 2 tab 7. 39.15 mg
8. 60 gtt/min 9. 17.55 or 18 mL/h 10. 8:54 A.M. 11. gr $\frac{1}{60}$ 12. 779 mg
13. 50 mL of the $\frac{1}{2}$ strength solution diluted to 100 mL 14. 50 mg 15. 500 mg

Case Studies and Comprehensive Self-Tests

Case Study 1

1. $\frac{\overset{1}{\cancel{500}}\ \cancel{\text{mL}}}{\underset{1}{\cancel{500}}\ \cancel{\text{mg}}} \times \frac{0.25\ \cancel{\text{mg}}}{\text{min}} \times \frac{60\ \mu\text{gtt}}{\cancel{\text{mL}}} = 15\ \mu\text{gtt/min}$

2. $$\frac{50\ \cancel{mL}}{\underset{3}{\cancel{30}}\ min} \times \frac{\overset{1}{\cancel{10}}\ gtt}{1\ \cancel{mL}} = 16.6 \text{ or } 17\ gtt/min$$

$$50\ \cancel{kg} \times \frac{\overset{1}{\cancel{25}}\ \cancel{mg}}{\cancel{kg}/\underset{3}{\cancel{30}}\ min} \times \frac{100\ \cancel{mL}}{\underset{50}{\cancel{1250}}\ \cancel{mg}} \times \frac{\overset{1}{\cancel{10}}\ gtt}{1\ \cancel{mL}} = 33.3 \text{ or } 33\ gtt/min$$

3. $$\frac{\overset{1}{\cancel{30}}\ \cancel{mL}}{\underset{2}{\cancel{60}}\ min} \times \frac{10\ gtt}{1\ \cancel{mL}} = 5\ gtt/min$$

4. The patient will receive 360 mg of Arfonad in 24 h

5. Arfonad: $$\frac{\overset{1}{\cancel{15}}\ \cancel{\mu gtt}}{\cancel{min}} \times \frac{1\ mL}{\underset{4}{\cancel{60}}\ \cancel{\mu gtt}} \times \frac{60\ \cancel{min}}{1\ \cancel{h}} \times \frac{24\ \cancel{h}}{1} = 360\ mL/d$$

Flagyl: 50 mL × 3 = 150 mL/d
Kefurox: 100 mL × 2 = 200 mL/d
So Flagyl 150 mL in 1.5 h
Kefurox 200 mL in 1.0 h
0.9% sodium chloride 30 mL/h for 21.5 h = 645 mL
Total amount of IV fluid in 24 h is 1355 mL

Comprehensive Self-Test 1

1. Prescribed is $\frac{300\ mg \times 2}{1\ d} = 600\ mg/d.$

Usual dosage: $$70\ \cancel{kg} \times \frac{8\ mg}{1\ \cancel{kg} \times 1\ d} = 560\ mg/d$$

$$70\ \cancel{kg} \times \frac{10\ mg}{1\ \cancel{kg} \times 1\ d} = 700\ mg/d$$

The prescribed dose is correct.

2. $$\overset{1}{\cancel{50}}\ \cancel{mg} \times 3 \times \frac{1\ tab}{\underset{1}{\cancel{50}}\ \cancel{mg}} = 3\ tab/d$$

3. $$\frac{0.25\ \cancel{g}}{\underset{1}{\cancel{8}}\ \cancel{h}} \times \overset{3}{\cancel{24}}\ h \times \frac{\overset{4}{\cancel{1000}}\ \cancel{mg}}{1\ \cancel{g}} \times \frac{1\ cap}{\underset{1}{\cancel{250}}\ \cancel{mg}} = 3\ cap/24\ h$$

4. $$0.03\ \cancel{g} \times \frac{1\ tab}{30\ \cancel{mg}} \times \frac{1000\ \cancel{mg}}{1\ \cancel{g}} = 1\ tab$$

5. $$45\ \cancel{u} \times \frac{\text{♏}\ 15}{100\ \cancel{u}} = \text{♏}\ 9$$

6. $$\overset{9}{\cancel{45}}\ \cancel{mg} \times \frac{\text{♏}\ \cancel{30}}{\underset{10}{\cancel{50}}\ \cancel{mg}} = \text{♏}\ 27$$

7. $$0.001\ \cancel{g} \times \frac{gr\ 15}{1\ \cancel{g}} = gr\ \frac{15}{1000} = gr\ \frac{3}{200}$$

8. $$\cancel{500}\ \cancel{mg} \times \frac{1\ \cancel{g}}{\underset{2}{\cancel{1000}}\ \cancel{mg}} \times \frac{1\ tab}{0.25\ \cancel{g}} = \frac{1}{0.5}\ tab = 2\ tab$$

9. $$0.15\ \cancel{g} \times \frac{1000\ \cancel{mg}}{1\ \cancel{g}} \times \frac{1\ tab}{150\ \cancel{mg}} = 1\ tab$$

10. $50\ \cancel{mg} \times \frac{1\ mL}{25\ \cancel{mg}} = 2$ mL of Zantac required and 18 mL of diluent

11. $$\frac{\overset{1}{\cancel{20}}\ \cancel{mL}}{\underset{1}{\cancel{20}}\ min} \times \frac{60\ \mu gtt}{1\ \cancel{mL}} = 60\ \mu gtt/min$$

12. $$800\ \cancel{mL} \times \frac{15\ \cancel{gtt}}{1\ \cancel{mL}} \times \frac{1\ \cancel{min}}{31\ \cancel{gtt}} \times \frac{1\ h}{60\ \cancel{min}} = 6.45\ h$$

$$0.45\ \cancel{h} \times \frac{60\ min}{1\ \cancel{h}} = 27\ min$$

It will take 6 hours and 27 minutes.

13. $\frac{2\ \text{mg}}{1\ \text{min}} \times \frac{1\ \text{g}}{1000\ \text{mg}} \times \frac{250\ \text{mL}}{0.5\ \text{g}} = 1\ \text{mL/min}$

14. $30\ \text{mL} \times \frac{10\ \text{g}}{15\ \text{mL}} = 20\ \text{g}$

15. $20\ \text{mg} \times \frac{1\ \text{mL}}{5\ \text{mg}} = 4\ \text{mL}$

16. $\frac{2\ \text{mg}}{1\ \text{min}} \times \frac{100\ \text{mL}}{80\ \text{mg}} \times \frac{60\ \mu\text{gtt}}{1\ \text{mL}} = 150\ \mu\text{gtt/min}$

17. $\frac{510\ \text{mL}}{500\ \text{mg}} \times \frac{1\ \text{mg}}{1\ \text{min}} \times \frac{60\ \text{min}}{1\ \text{h}} = 61\ \text{mL/h}$

18. $120\ \text{lb} \times \frac{1\ \text{kg}}{2.2\ \text{lb}} \times \frac{0.1\ \text{mg}}{\text{kg/min}} \times \frac{60\ \text{mL}}{500\ \text{mg}} \times \frac{15\ \text{gtt}}{1\ \text{mL}} = \frac{120 \times 0.1 \times 60 \times 15\ \text{gtt}}{2.2 \times 500\ \text{min}} = 10\ \text{gtt/min}$

19. $\frac{100\ \text{mL}}{120\ \text{min}} \times \frac{15\ \text{gtt}}{1\ \text{mL}} = 13\ \text{gtt/min}$

20. $\frac{8\ \text{gtt}}{1\ \text{min}} \times \frac{1\ \text{mL}}{15\ \text{gtt}} \times \frac{60\ \text{min}}{1\ \text{h}} = 32\ \text{mL/h}$

21. $\overset{2}{120}\ \text{mL} \times \frac{15\ \text{gtt}}{1\ \text{mL}} \times \frac{1\ \text{min}}{50\ \text{gtt}} \times \frac{1\ \text{h}}{\underset{1}{60}\ \text{min}} = \frac{30}{50}$ h or 36 min

22. $\overset{1}{200}\ \text{mcg} \times \frac{1\ \text{mg}}{\underset{5}{1000}\ \text{mcg}} \times \frac{1\ \text{tab}}{0.1\ \text{mg}} = \frac{1}{0.5}\ \text{tab} = 2\ \text{tab}$

23. $\overset{5}{50{,}000}\ \text{u} \times \frac{1\ \text{mL}}{10{,}000\ \text{u}} = 5\ \text{mL}$ Add 5 mL to 500 mL.

$\frac{505\ \text{mL}}{50{,}000\ \text{u}} \times \frac{500\ \text{u}}{1\ \text{h}} = \frac{2525}{500} = 5.05\ \text{mL/h}$

24. $1.8\ \text{m}^2 \times \frac{\overset{3}{150}\ \text{mg}}{\text{m}^2} \times \frac{5\ \text{mL}}{\underset{4}{200}\ \text{mg}} = 6.75\ \text{mL}$

25. Add 10 mL to the vial of Cefadyl and add total amount of drug to 50 mL of 5% D/W to equal 60 mL.

$\frac{60\ \text{mL}}{\underset{2}{30}\ \text{min}} \times \frac{15\ \text{gtt}}{1\ \text{mL}} = 30\ \text{gtt/min}$

Case Study 2

1. Procardia $0.02\ \text{g} \times \frac{1000\ \text{mg}}{1\ \text{g}} \times 3 = 60\ \text{mg/d}$

Procardia $0.02\ \text{g} \times \frac{1000\ \text{mg}}{1\ \text{g}} \times \frac{1\ \text{cap}}{10\ \text{mg}} = 2\ \text{cap}$

2. Feldene $20\ \text{mg} \times \frac{1\ \text{g}}{1000\ \text{mg}} \times \frac{1\ \text{tab}}{0.02\ \text{g}} = 1\ \text{tab}$

Digoxin $0.125\ \text{mg} \times \frac{1\ \text{tab}}{0.25\ \text{mg}} = \frac{1}{2}\ \text{tab}$

Eryc $\overset{1}{250}\ \text{mg} \times \frac{1\ \text{g}}{\underset{4}{1000}\ \text{mg}} \times \frac{1\ \text{cap}}{0.25\ \text{g}} = 1\ \text{cap}$

Total: 3 capsules and $1\frac{1}{2}$ tablets at 10 A.M.

3. Zantac: $\frac{50\ \text{mL}}{30\ \text{min}} \times \frac{60\ \mu\text{gtt}}{1\ \text{mL}} = 100\ \mu\text{gtt/min}$

4. Zantac IVPB infuses 50 mL 4 times a day = 200 mL

5. $\frac{2000\ \text{mL}}{24\ \text{h}} \times \frac{1\ \text{h}}{\underset{3}{60}\ \text{min}} \times \frac{\overset{1}{20}\ \text{gtt}}{1\ \text{mL}} = 28\ \text{gtt/min}$

6. $\begin{array}{l} \ 2000\text{ mL—5\% D/W} \\ +\ 200\text{ mL—Zantac} \\ \hline \ 2200\text{ mL—IV} \end{array}$

So patient can have 250 mL of po fluid.

Comprehensive Self-Test 2

1. $0.05\,\cancel{g} \times \dfrac{1000\text{ mg}}{1\,\cancel{g}} = 50\text{ mg}$

2. $\dfrac{1.5\,\cancel{\text{mg}}}{1\,\cancel{\text{h}}} \times \dfrac{\overset{2}{\cancel{250\text{ mL}}}}{\underset{1}{\cancel{125\text{ mg}}}} \times \dfrac{60\ \mu\text{gtt}}{1\,\cancel{\text{mL}}} \times \dfrac{1\,\cancel{\text{h}}}{60\text{ min}} = 3\ \mu\text{gtt/min}$

3. $\dfrac{1\,\cancel{\text{mg}}}{1\text{ min}} \times \dfrac{1\,\cancel{g}}{1000\,\cancel{\text{mg}}} \times \dfrac{500\,\cancel{\text{mL}}}{1\,\cancel{g}} \times \dfrac{60\ \mu\text{gtt}}{1\,\cancel{\text{mL}}} = 30\ \mu\text{gtt/min}$

4. $\overset{1}{\cancel{20}}\text{ mg} \times \dfrac{\cancel{1}\cancel{g}}{\underset{50}{\cancel{1000}}\text{ mg}} \times \dfrac{1\text{ tab}}{0.02\,\cancel{g}} = 1\text{ tab}$

5. $0.1\,\cancel{\text{mg}} \times \dfrac{1000\ \mu g}{1\,\cancel{\text{mg}}} = 100\ \mu g$

6. $\cancel{1000\text{ mg}} \times \dfrac{1\text{ g}}{\cancel{1000\text{ mg}}} \times \dfrac{1\text{ tab}}{0.5\,\cancel{g}} = 2\text{ tab}$

$\dfrac{2\text{ tab}}{1} \times \dfrac{4}{\cancel{d}} \times \dfrac{7\,\cancel{d}}{1} = 56\text{ tab}$

7. $\cancel{10}\,\cancel{\text{mg}} \times \dfrac{\cancel{\text{gr}}\ 1}{\underset{6}{\cancel{60}}\,\cancel{\text{mg}}} \times \dfrac{1\text{ tab}}{\cancel{\text{gr}}\ \dfrac{1}{24}} = \dfrac{1}{\dfrac{6}{24}} = 4\text{ tab}$

8. $0.25\,\cancel{\text{mg}} \times \dfrac{\overset{8}{\cancel{1000\ \mu g}}}{1\,\cancel{\text{mg}}} \times \dfrac{1\text{ tab}}{\underset{1}{\cancel{125\ \mu g}}} = 2\text{ tab}$

9. $88\,\cancel{\text{lb}} \times \dfrac{1\,\cancel{\text{kg}}}{2.2\,\cancel{\text{lb}}} \times \dfrac{2\,\cancel{\text{mcg}}}{1\,\cancel{\text{kg}}} \times \dfrac{1\text{ mg}}{1000\,\cancel{\text{mcg}}} = 0.08\text{ mg}$

10. $20\,\cancel{\text{kg}} \times \dfrac{\cancel{10}\,\cancel{\text{mg}}}{1\,\cancel{\text{kg}}} \times \dfrac{5\text{ mL}}{300\,\cancel{\text{mg}}} = 3.3\text{ mL}$

11. $900\,\cancel{\text{mg}} \times \dfrac{1\,\cancel{g}}{1000\,\cancel{\text{mg}}} \times \dfrac{1\text{ tab}}{0.3\,\cancel{g}} = 3\text{ tab}$

12. $0.075\,\cancel{g} \times \dfrac{1000\,\cancel{\text{mg}}}{1\,\cancel{g}} \times \dfrac{1\text{ tab}}{25\,\cancel{\text{mg}}} = 3\text{ tab}$

13. $1.2\,\cancel{m^2} \times \dfrac{30\,\cancel{\text{mg}}}{1\,\cancel{m^2}} \times \dfrac{5\text{ mL}}{250\,\cancel{\text{mg}}} = 0.7\text{ mL}$

14. $1\,\cancel{m^2} \times \dfrac{0.1\,\cancel{g}}{1\,\cancel{m^2}} \times \dfrac{1000\,\cancel{\text{mg}}}{1\,\cancel{g}} \times \dfrac{1\text{ tab}}{100\,\cancel{\text{mg}}} = 1\text{ tab}$

15. $0.1\,\cancel{\text{mg}} \times \dfrac{1000\,\cancel{\text{mcg}}}{1\,\cancel{\text{mg}}} \times \dfrac{1\text{ tab}}{50\,\cancel{\text{mcg}}} = 2\text{ tab}$

16. $40\,\cancel{\text{kg}} \times \dfrac{1\,\cancel{\text{mg}}}{1\,\cancel{\text{kg}}} \times \dfrac{1\text{ tab}}{20\,\cancel{\text{mg}}} = 2\text{ tab}$

17. $0.4\,\cancel{m^2} \times \dfrac{0.25\,\cancel{g}}{1\,\cancel{m^2}} \times \dfrac{1000\,\cancel{\text{mg}}}{1\,\cancel{g}} \times \dfrac{2\text{ mL}}{500\,\cancel{\text{mg}}} = 0.4\text{ mL}$

18. $0.64\,\cancel{m^2} \times \dfrac{150\,\cancel{\text{mg}}}{1\,\cancel{m^2}} \times \dfrac{1\text{ tab}}{100\,\cancel{\text{mg}}} = 1\text{ tab}$

19. $35\cancel{0}\,\cancel{\text{mg}} \times \dfrac{2.6\text{ mL}}{1\,\cancel{g}} \times \dfrac{1\,\cancel{g}}{100\cancel{0}\,\cancel{\text{mg}}} = \dfrac{91}{100}\text{ mL} = 0.91\text{ or }0.9\text{ mL}$

20. $275\,\cancel{\text{u}} \times \dfrac{1\text{ mL}}{100\,\cancel{\text{u}}} = 2.75$ mL of regular Humulin insulin

Add 2.75 mL to 500 mL of 0.9% NS to equal 502.75 mL.

$\dfrac{502.75}{275\,\cancel{\text{u}}} \times \dfrac{10\,\cancel{\text{u}}}{\text{h}} = 18.28\text{ or }18.3\text{ mL/h}$

21. $\overset{6}{\cancel{900}}\,\cancel{\text{mg}} \times \dfrac{1\text{ mL}}{\cancel{150}\,\cancel{\text{mg}}} = 6$ mL of Cleocin added to 150 mL 5% D/W

$\dfrac{156\,\cancel{\text{mL}}}{\underset{6}{\cancel{90}}\text{ min}} \times \dfrac{\cancel{15}\text{ gtt}}{1\,\cancel{\text{mL}}} = 26\text{ gtt/min}$

22. $0.2\,\cancel{\text{mg}} \times \dfrac{1\text{ mL}}{0.4\,\cancel{\text{mg}}} = \dfrac{0.2}{0.4}\text{ mL} = 0.5\text{ mL}$

23. $0.15\,\cancel{g} \times \dfrac{1000\,\cancel{\text{mg}}}{1\,\cancel{g}} \times \dfrac{1\text{ tab}}{300\,\cancel{\text{mg}}} = \dfrac{1}{2}\text{ tab}$

24. $200\,\cancel{\text{mg}} \times \dfrac{\cancel{100}\text{ mL}}{2\,\cancel{g}} \times \dfrac{1\,\cancel{g}}{10\cancel{00}\,\cancel{\text{mg}}} = \dfrac{200}{20} = 10\text{ mL}$

25. $66\,\cancel{\text{kg}} \times \dfrac{0.2\,\cancel{\text{mg}}}{1\,\cancel{\text{kg}}/1\text{ min}} \times \dfrac{250\,\cancel{\text{mL}}}{500\,\cancel{\text{mg}}} \times \dfrac{10\text{ gtt}}{1\,\cancel{\text{mL}}} = 66\text{ gtt/min}$

Case Study 3

1. Calculate the flow rate for each IVPB medication.

Ticarcillin: $\frac{250\ \cancel{\text{mL}}}{\cancel{120}^{12}\ \text{min}} \times \frac{\cancel{10}^{1}\ \text{gtt}}{1\ \cancel{\text{mL}}} = 21$ gtt/min Zantac: $\frac{100\ \cancel{\text{mL}}}{\cancel{20}^{2}\ \text{min}} \times \frac{\cancel{10}^{1}\ \text{gtt}}{1\ \cancel{\text{mL}}} = 50$ gtt/min

2. Nembutal: $\cancel{\text{gr}}\ \frac{3}{\cancel{2}_{1}} \times \frac{\cancel{60}^{30}\ \text{mg}}{\cancel{\text{gr}}\ 1} = 90$ mg Note: Grains $1\frac{1}{2}$ is considered to be equivalent to 100 mg.

3. Demerol: $\cancel{50}^{1}\ \cancel{\text{mg}} \times \frac{2\ \text{mL}}{\cancel{100}_{2}\ \cancel{\text{mg}}} = 1$ mL Versed: $\cancel{60}^{6}\ \cancel{\text{kg}} \times \frac{0.18\ \cancel{\text{mg}}}{\cancel{\text{kg}}} \times \frac{2\ \text{mL}}{\cancel{10}_{1}\ \cancel{\text{mg}}} = 2.2$ mL

4. Total amount of IVPB fluids received by patient in 24 h:
Ticarcillin: 250 mL × 2 (q12h) = 500 mL
Zantac: 100 mL × 4 (q6h) = 400 mL
Total: 900 mL in 24 h

5. Total amount of IV fluid received by patient in 24 h:
Ticarcillin: 250 mL in 2 h × 2 = 4 h (500 mL)

Zantac: 100 mL in 20 min × 4 = 80 min or $1\frac{1}{3}$ h (400 mL)

Total: $5\frac{1}{3}$ h = 900 mL IVPB fluid

$$\begin{array}{r} 24\ \text{h} \\ -\ 5\frac{1}{3}\ \text{h} \\ \hline 18\frac{2}{3}\ \text{h} \end{array} = 18\ \text{h} + 40\ \text{min}$$

Ringer's lactate: $\frac{75\ \text{mL}}{\cancel{\text{h}}} \times \frac{18.66\ \cancel{\text{h}}}{1} = 1399.5$ or 1400 mL

If flow rate per minute, primary line would be

$$\frac{75\ \cancel{\text{mL}}}{\cancel{60}_{3}\ \text{min}} \times \frac{\cancel{20}^{1}\ \text{gtt}}{1\ \cancel{\text{mL}}} = 25\ \text{gtt/min}$$

Ringer's lactate: 1400 mL
IVPB: 900 mL
Total: 2300 mL
So this patient received a total of 2300 mL IV fluid in 24 h.

Comprehensive Self-Test 3

1. $\frac{\cancel{1000}^{250}\ \cancel{\text{mL}}}{\cancel{12}_{3}\ \cancel{\text{h}}} \times \frac{\cancel{10}\ \text{gtt}}{1\ \cancel{\text{mL}}} \times \frac{1\ \cancel{\text{h}}}{\cancel{60}_{6}\ \text{min}} = \frac{250}{18}$ gtt/min = 13.8 or 14 gtt/min

2. $\dfrac{\cancel{100}\ \text{mL} \times \dfrac{2.5\ \cancel{\text{mL}}}{\cancel{100}\ \cancel{\text{mL}}}}{\dfrac{\cancel{10}\ \cancel{\text{mL}}}{\cancel{100}\ \cancel{\text{mL}}}} = \dfrac{2.5}{\dfrac{1}{10}} = 25$ mL of the 10% solution and dilute with water to make 100 mL

3. $7500\ \cancel{\text{u}} \times \frac{1\ \text{mL}}{10{,}000\ \cancel{\text{u}}} = 0.75$ mL

4. $1.7\ \cancel{\text{m}^2} \times \frac{250\ \cancel{\text{mg}}}{1\ \cancel{\text{m}^2}} \times \frac{5\ \text{mL}}{187\ \cancel{\text{mg}}} = \frac{2125}{187}$ mL = 11.36 or 11.4 mL

5. $\cancel{70}^{2}\ \cancel{\text{kg}} \times \frac{1\ \cancel{\text{mg}}}{\cancel{35}\ \cancel{\text{kg}}} \times \frac{1\ \text{tab}}{2\ \cancel{\text{mg}}} = 1$ tab 6. $0.9\ \cancel{\text{m}^2} \times \frac{\cancel{60}^{12}\ \cancel{\text{mg}}}{1\ \cancel{\text{m}^2}} \times \frac{5\ \text{mL}}{\cancel{25}_{5}\ \cancel{\text{mg}}} = 10.8$ mL

7. $350{,}000\,\cancel{u} \times \dfrac{1\text{ mL}}{100{,}000\,\cancel{u}} = 3.5\text{ mL}$

8. $\dfrac{\cancel{20}\,\cancel{\text{mg}}}{1\text{ mL}} \times \dfrac{1\text{ g}}{\underset{50}{\cancel{1000}}\,\cancel{\text{mg}}} = $ 1:50 solution of Xylocaine; 1 gram in 50 mL

$1 \div 50 = 0.02 = 2\%$

9. $360\,\cancel{\text{mL}} \times \dfrac{15\,\cancel{\text{gtt}}}{1\,\cancel{\text{mL}}} \times \dfrac{1\,\cancel{\text{min}}}{30\,\cancel{\text{gtt}}} \times \dfrac{1\text{ h}}{60\,\cancel{\text{min}}} = 3\text{ h}$

10. $0.5\,\cancel{\text{g}} \times \dfrac{\overset{4}{\cancel{1000}}\,\cancel{\text{mg}}}{1\,\cancel{\text{g}}} \times \dfrac{1\text{ tab}}{250\,\cancel{\text{mg}}} = 2\text{ tab}$

11. $250{,}000\,\cancel{u} \times \dfrac{1\text{ mL}}{100{,}000\,\cancel{u}} = 2.5\text{ mL}$

12. $0.8\,\cancel{\text{m}^2} \times \dfrac{100\text{ mg}}{1\,\cancel{\text{m}^2}} = 80\text{ mg}$

13. $500\,\cancel{\text{mL}} \times \dfrac{25\text{ g}}{100\,\cancel{\text{mL}}} = 125\text{ g}$

Take 125 g of the pure drug and dilute in H_20 to make 500 mL.

14. a. $70\,\cancel{\text{kg}} \times \dfrac{10\,\cancel{\text{mcg}}}{1\,\cancel{\text{kg}}/1\,\cancel{\text{min}}} \times \dfrac{1\text{ mg}}{1000\,\cancel{\text{mcg}}} \times \dfrac{60\,\cancel{\text{min}}}{1\text{ h}} = 42\text{ mg/h}$

$250\,\cancel{\text{mg}} \times \dfrac{1\text{ mL}}{12.5\,\cancel{\text{mg}}} = 20\text{ mL}$ Add this to the 500 mL.

b. $\dfrac{42\,\cancel{\text{mg}}}{1\text{ h}} \times \dfrac{52\cancel{0}\text{ mL}}{25\cancel{0}\,\cancel{\text{mg}}} = 87.4\text{ mL/h}$

15. $\cancel{\text{gr}}\,\dfrac{1}{300} \times \dfrac{60\,\cancel{\text{mg}}}{\cancel{\text{gr}}\,1} \times \dfrac{1\text{ tab}}{0.2\,\cancel{\text{mg}}} = 1\text{ tab}$

16. $\overset{3}{\cancel{630}}\,\cancel{\text{mg}} \times \dfrac{1\text{ tab}}{\underset{1}{\cancel{210}}\,\cancel{\text{mg}}} = 3\text{ tab}$

17. $\overset{27}{\cancel{54}}\,\cancel{\text{kg}} \times \dfrac{\overset{3}{\cancel{150}}\,\cancel{\text{mcg}}}{1\,\cancel{\text{kg}}} \times \dfrac{1\,\cancel{\text{mg}}}{\underset{20}{\cancel{1000}}\,\cancel{\text{mcg}}} \times \dfrac{1\text{ tab}}{\underset{1}{\cancel{2}}\,\cancel{\text{mg}}} = 4\text{ tab}$

18. $\dfrac{0.05\,\cancel{\text{mg}}}{1\text{ min}} \times \dfrac{\overset{20}{\cancel{500}}\,\cancel{\text{mL}}}{\underset{1}{\cancel{25}}\,\cancel{\text{mg}}} \times \dfrac{60\ \mu\text{gtt}}{1\,\cancel{\text{mL}}} = 60\ \mu\text{gtt/min}$

19. a. $90\text{ kg} \times \dfrac{8\text{ mg}}{1\text{ kg}} = 720\text{ mg}$

b. $72\cancel{0}\,\cancel{\text{mg}} \times \dfrac{1\text{ mL}}{50\cancel{0}\,\cancel{\text{mg}}} = \dfrac{72\text{ mL}}{50} = 1.44\text{ or }1.5\text{ mL}$

20. $2.5\,\cancel{\text{mg}} \times \dfrac{1\text{ tab}}{5\,\cancel{\text{mg}}} = \dfrac{2.5}{5}\text{ tab} = \dfrac{1}{2}\text{ tab}$

21. $\overset{3}{\cancel{300}}\,\cancel{\text{mg}} \times \dfrac{1\,\cancel{\text{g}}}{1000\,\cancel{\text{mg}}} \times \dfrac{10\text{ mL}}{0.3\,\cancel{\text{g}}} = \dfrac{30}{3}\text{ mL} = 10\text{ mL}$

22. $\overset{2}{\cancel{20}}\,\cancel{\text{mg}} \times \dfrac{1\text{ tab}}{\cancel{10}\,\cancel{\text{mg}}} \times \dfrac{2}{\cancel{\text{d}}} \times \dfrac{5\,\cancel{\text{d}}}{1} = 20\text{ tab}$

23. $1.5\,\cancel{\text{g}} \times \dfrac{1000\text{ mg}}{1\,\cancel{\text{g}}} = 1500\text{ mg}$

24. $\dfrac{1\text{ tab}}{0.5\,\cancel{\text{mg}}} \times 0.25\,\cancel{\text{mg}}\ \dfrac{0.25}{0.5}\text{ tab} = \dfrac{1}{2}\text{ tab}$

25. $2\,\cancel{\text{g}} \times \dfrac{\overset{2}{\cancel{1000}}\,\cancel{\text{mg}}}{1\,\cancel{\text{g}}} \times \dfrac{5\text{ mL}}{\underset{1}{\cancel{500}}\,\cancel{\text{mg}}} = 20\text{ mL}$

Diagnostic Test of Arithmetic

1. $\frac{5}{8}$ 2. 2.75 3. 4.8 4. 0.67 5. 40 6. 326.7
7. 4.251 8. 1300 9. 2 10. $\frac{2}{9}$ 11. $\frac{4}{3}$ or $1\frac{1}{3}$ 12. $\frac{1}{16}$
13. $\frac{7}{20}$ 14. 0.025 15. $\frac{23}{5}$

endix B

Common Abbreviations on Medication Orders

To someone unfamiliar with prescriptive abbreviations, medication orders may look like a foreign language. To interpret prescriptive orders accurately and to administer drugs safely, a qualified person must have a thorough knowledge of common abbreviations. For instance, when the prescriber writes, "**Hydromorphone 1.5 mL IM q4h pc & hs**," the administrator knows how to interpret it as "Hydromorphone, 1.5 milliliters, intramuscular, every four hours, after meals and at hour of sleep." Study the following list of common abbreviations for smooth navigation through the medication orders in this book. For measurement abbreviations, refer to the inside back cover.

Abbreviation	*Meaning*
ā	before (*abante*)
āā	of each
ac	before meals (*ante cibium*)
ad	up to (*ad*)
ad lib	as desired (*ad libitum*)
A.M., am	morning
amp	ampule
aq	aqueous water
bi	two
bid, BID	two times a day
c̄	with
C	Celsius; centigrade
cap	capsule
CVP	central venous pressure
d	day
DC, dc	discontinue
D/W	dextrose in water
D5W	5% dextrose in water
Dx	diagnosis
elix	elixir
F	Fahrenheit
h, hr, H	hour
hs, HS	hour of sleep; bedtime (*hora somni*)

Abbreviation	*Meaning*
IC	intracardia
ID	intradermal
IM	intramuscular
IV	intravenous
IVP	intravenous push
IVPB	intravenous piggyback
KVO	keep vein open
LA	long acting
LIB	left in bag, left in bottle
min	minute
mU	milliunit
n	night
NPO	nothing by mouth (*per ora*)
NS	normal saline
NSAID	nonsteroidal anti-inflammatory drug
od	every day (*omni die*)
OD	right eye (*oculus dexter*)
OS	left eye (*oculus sinister*)
OU	both eyes
p̄	after
pc	after meals (*post cibum*)

Abbreviation	Meaning
PICC	peripherally inserted central catheter
P.M., pm	afternoon, evening
po, PO	by mouth (*per os*)
postop	after surgery
preop	before surgery
prn	when required or whenever necessary
Pt	patient
p	pulse
q	every (*quaque*)
qd	every day (*quaque die*)
qh	every hour (*quaque hora*)
q2h	every two hours
q3h	every three hours
q4h	every four hours
qid, QID	four times a day (*quater in die*)
qod	every other day
qn	every night (*quaque noct*)
qs	quantity sufficient or sufficient amount (*quantitas sufficiens*)

Abbreviation	Meaning
R/O	rule out
R	respiration
$\bar{s}$	without (*sine*)
sc, SC, SQ	subcutaneous
sl, SL	under the tongue (sublingual)
SR	sustained release
$\overline{ss}$, ss	one-half
stat	immediately (*statum*)
supp	suppository
susp	suspension
tid, TID	three times a day (*ter in die*)
TPN	total parenteral nutrition
T	temperature
wt	weight
>	greater than
<	less than

appendix C Dosage Preparation Forms and Packaging

Preparation Forms

Medications are manufactured in many preparation forms. Each form serves a distinct purpose. One form might release medication into the body at a slower rate than another. One form might be manufactured to facilitate swallowing. Use the following definitions of preparation forms as a reference for understanding medication orders.

Aqueous solution One or more medications completely dissolved in water.

Capsule Gelatinous container enclosing a powder, a liquid, or time-release granules of medication.

Elixir Medication dissolved in a mixture of water, alcohol, sweeteners, and flavoring.

Metered-dose inhaler Aerosol device containing multiple doses of medication for inhalation.

Ointment Semisolid preparation of medication to be applied to the skin.

Suppository Mixture of medication with a firm base that melts at body temperature and is molded into a shape suitable for insertion into body cavities.

Suspension Finely divided particles of medication undissolved in water.

Syrup Medication in water and sugar solution.

Tablet Powdered medication compressed or molded into a small disk.

Transdermal patch Adhesive disk that attaches to the skin with a center reservoir containing medication to be slowly absorbed through the skin.

Parenteral Packaging

There are three common types of parenteral medication containers for sterile solutions.

Ampule Sealed glass container with only one dose of powdered or liquid medication.

Prefilled cartridge Small, slender single-dose vial with an attached needle. A metal or plastic holder is used to inject the medication.

Vial Sealed glass container of a liquid or powdered medication with a rubber stopper, allowing multiple-dose use.

appendix 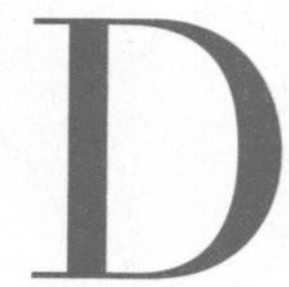 Celsius and Fahrenheit Temperature Conversions

Reading and recording a temperature is a crucial step in assessing a patient's health. Temperatures can be measured using either the Fahrenheit (F) scale, or the Celsius or centigrade (C) scale. Most health-care settings use Fahrenheit, but some are switching to Celsius. Celsius/Fahrenheit equivalency tables make it easy to convert Celsius to Fahrenheit, or vice versa. Still, it is useful to be able to make this conversion yourself.

You can use the following rules to convert from one temperature scale to the other.

Remember

$$F = \tfrac{9}{5}C + 32 \quad \text{or} \quad C = \tfrac{5}{9}(F - 32)$$

For those unfamiliar with algebra, the following rules are equivalent to the algebraic formulas.

First rule: To convert to Celsius. Subtract 32 and then divide by 1.8.

Second rule: To convert to Fahrenheit. Multiply by 1.8 and then add 32.

Note

Temperatures are rounded to the nearest tenth.

Example C.1

Convert 102.5°F to Celsius.

Using the first rule, we subtract 32.

$$\begin{array}{r} 102.5 \\ -32.0 \\ \hline 70.5 \end{array}$$

Then we divide by 1.8.

$$1.8\overline{)70.5000} = 39.17$$

So 102.5°F equals about 39.2°C.

Example C.2

Convert 3°C to Fahrenheit.

Using the second rule, we first multiply by 1.8.

$$\begin{array}{r} 1.8 \\ \times 3 \\ \hline 5.4 \end{array}$$

Then we add 32.

$$\begin{array}{r} 5.4 \\ +32.0 \\ \hline 37.4 \end{array}$$

So 3°C equals about 37.4°F.

a p p e n d i x 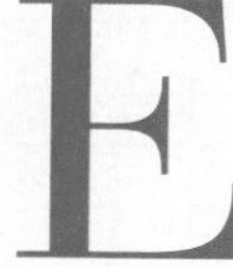

Tables of Weight Conversions

Use the following tables to convert between the metric kilogram and the household pound.

Table E.1 *Pounds to Kilograms*

lb	kg	lb	kg	lb	kg
2.2	1.0	120	54.5	240	109.1
5	2.3	125	56.8	245	111.4
10	4.5	130	59.1	250	113.6
15	6.8	135	61.4	255	115.9
20	9.1	140	63.6	260	118.2
25	11.4	145	65.9	265	120.5
30	13.6	150	68.2	270	122.7
35	15.9	155	70.5	275	125
40	18.2	160	72.7	280	127.3
45	20.5	165	75	285	129.5
50	22.7	170	77.3	290	131.8
55	25	175	79.5	295	134.1
60	27.3	180	81.8	300	136.4
65	29.5	185	84.1	305	138.6
70	31.8	190	86.4	310	140.9
75	34.1	195	88.6	315	143.2
80	36.4	200	90.9	320	145.5
85	38.6	205	93.2	325	147.7
90	40.9	210	95.5	330	150
95	43.2	215	97.7	335	152.3
100	45.5	220	100	340	154.5
105	47.7	225	102.3	345	156.8
110	50	230	104.5	350	159.1
115	52.3	235	106.8	355	161.4

Table E.2 *Kilograms to Pounds*

kg	lb	kg	lb	kg	lb
2	4.4	56	123.2	110	242
4	8.8	58	127.6	112	246.4
6	13.2	60	132	114	250.8
8	17.6	62	136.4	116	255.2
10	22	64	140.8	118	259.6
12	26.4	66	145.2	120	264
14	30.8	68	149.6	122	268.4
16	35.2	70	154	124	272.8
18	39.6	72	158.4	126	277.2
20	44	74	162.8	128	281.6
22	48.4	76	167.2	130	286
24	52.8	78	171.6	132	290.4
26	57.2	80	176	134	294.8
28	61.6	82	180.4	136	299.2
30	66	84	184.8	138	303.6
32	70.4	86	189.2	140	308
34	74.8	88	193.6	142	312.4
36	79.2	90	198	144	316.8
38	83.6	92	202.4	146	321.2
40	88	94	206.8	148	325.6
42	92.4	96	211.2	150	330
44	96.8	98	215.6	152	334.4
46	101.2	100	220	154	338.8
48	105.6	102	224.4	156	343.2
50	110	104	228.8	158	347.6
52	114.4	106	233.2	160	352
54	118.8	108	237.6	162	356.4

appendix 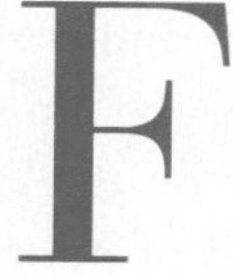 Nomogram

Dosages are sometimes based on a patient's body surface area (BSA), and nomograms are the equivalency charts used to determine the patient's BSA.

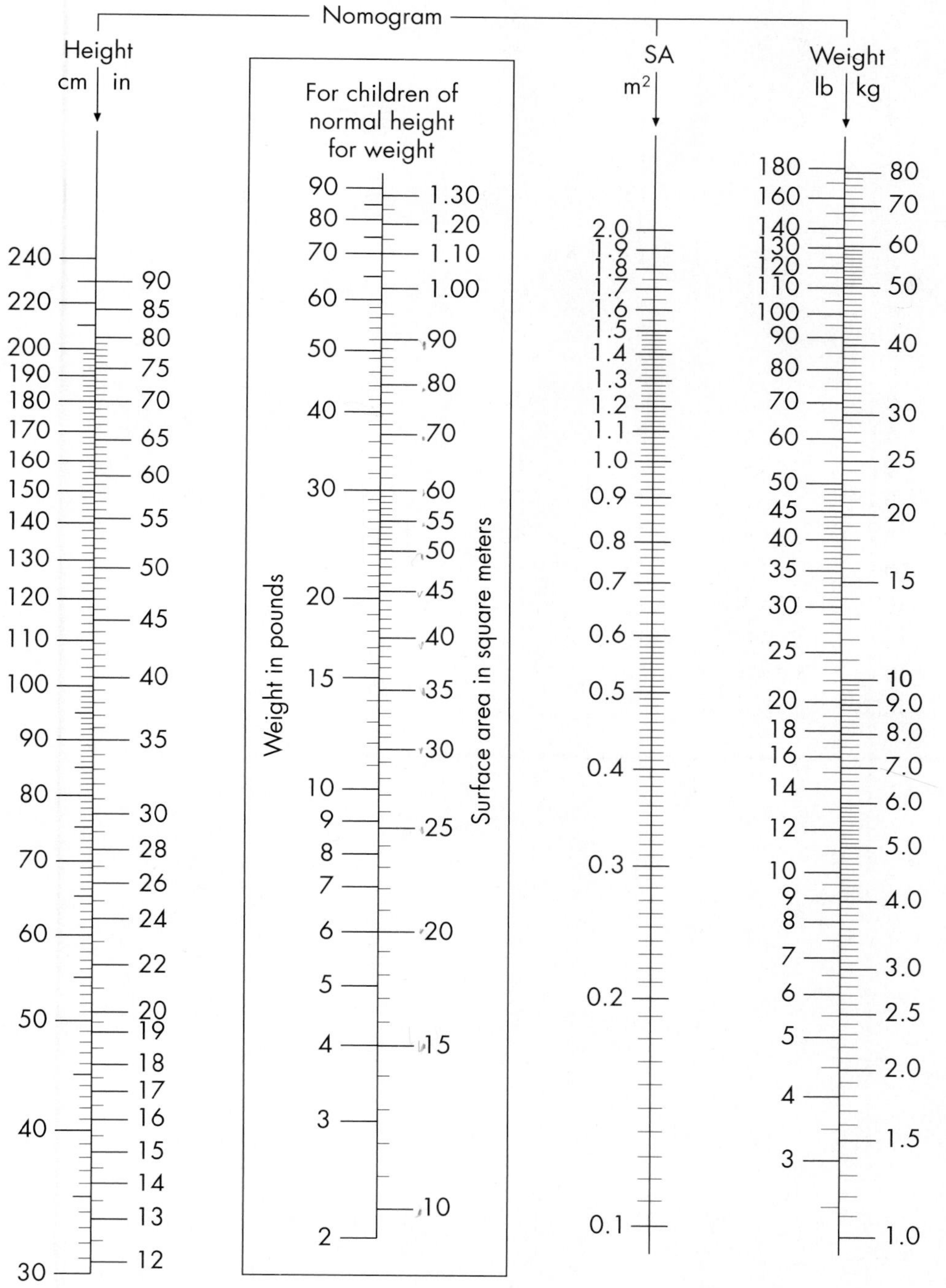

Nomogram

Height
cm | in
240, 220, 200, 190, 180, 170, 160, 150, 140, 130, 120, 110, 100, 90, 80, 70, 60, 50, 40, 30
90, 85, 80, 75, 70, 65, 60, 55, 50, 45, 40, 35, 30, 28, 26, 24, 22, 20, 19, 18, 17, 16, 15, 14, 13, 12

For children of normal height for weight
Weight in pounds
90, 80, 70, 60, 50, 40, 30, 20, 15, 10, 9, 8, 7, 6, 5, 4, 3, 2
Surface area in square meters
1.30, 1.20, 1.10, 1.00, .90, .80, .70, .60, .55, .50, .45, .40, .35, .30, .25, .20, .15, .10

SA
m²
2.0, 1.9, 1.8, 1.7, 1.6, 1.5, 1.4, 1.3, 1.2, 1.1, 1.0, 0.9, 0.8, 0.7, 0.6, 0.5, 0.4, 0.3, 0.2, 0.1

Weight
lb | kg
180, 160, 140, 130, 120, 110, 100, 90, 80, 70, 60, 50, 45, 40, 35, 30, 25, 20, 18, 16, 14, 12, 10, 9, 8, 7, 6, 5, 4, 3
80, 70, 60, 50, 40, 30, 25, 20, 15, 10, 9.0, 8.0, 7.0, 6.0, 5.0, 4.0, 3.0, 2.5, 2.0, 1.5, 1.0

To use the nomogram, you need the patient's weight and height. Draw a straight line between the patient's height (first column) and the patient's weight (last column). The point at which the line crosses the SA column is the estimated *BSA in square meters.* The boxed column listing weight on the left and surface in square meters on the right can be used when a child is of normal height for his or her weight.

appendix G Fried's Rule, Young's Rule, Clark's Rule

Pediatric dosages for children are primarily based on body surface area (BSA), weight, and/or age. Currently the preferred method is the amount of medication per kilogram of body weight or BSA. However, children's dosages can also be determined by relating the child's age in months or the child's weight in pounds to adult dosages. The formulas used to do this are known as **Fried's Rule** and **Young's Rule**, both of which use the patient's age to determine the correct pediatric dose, and **Clark's Rule**, which uses the patient's weight to determine the correct pediatric dose.

If you used **Fried's Rule** to determine a safe dose of ampicillin (Omnipen) for a 5-month-old infant, for example, you would have to know that the usual recommended adult dose of this drug is 500 milligrams and that the adult age is 150 months.

This is the formula for Fried's Rule:

$$\frac{\text{Age of infant (months)}}{\text{Adult age (months)}} \times \text{adult dose} = \text{safe dose for an infant}$$

So for the 5-month-old infant, the dose would be calculated as follows:

$$\frac{5\ \cancel{\text{mon}}}{\underset{3}{\cancel{150}}\ \cancel{\text{mon}}} \times \overset{10}{\cancel{500}}\ \text{mg} = \frac{50}{3}\ \text{mg or } 16.6\ \text{mg}$$

So 16.6 or 17 milligrams is a safe dose for a 5-month-old infant.

Young's Rule is used for the calculation of pediatric dosages for children between the ages of 1 and 12.

$$\frac{\text{Age of child (years)}}{\text{Age of child} + 12\ \text{(years)}} \times \text{adult dose} = \text{safe dose for a child}$$

So for a 5-year-old child and an adult dose of 500 milligrams, Young's Rule would be:

$$\frac{5\ \cancel{\text{yr}}}{(5 + 12)\ \cancel{\text{yr}}} \times 500\ \text{mg} = \frac{2500}{17}\ \text{mg or } 147.05\ \text{mg}$$

So 147.05 or 147 milligrams would be a safe dose for a 5-year-old child.

Clark's Rule uses the child's weight to calculate pediatric dosages. The formula is

$$\frac{\text{Child's weight (lb)}}{\text{Adult weight (lb)}} \times \text{adult dose} = \text{safe dose for child}$$

So if a child weighs 30 pounds and the adult dose is 500 milligrams, Clark's Rule would be

$$\frac{\overset{1}{\cancel{30\ \text{lb}}}}{\underset{5}{\cancel{150\ \text{lb}}}} \times 500\ \text{mg} = 100\ \text{mg}$$

Note

The weight used here is the average adult weight in pounds—that is, 150 pounds.

So, 100 milligrams is a safe dose for a 30-pound child.

As you can see, it is very similar to dimensional analysis; for example, you can use Clark's Rule with kilograms. For a child weighing 15 kilograms, the formula is

$$\frac{15\ \cancel{\text{kg}}}{70\ \cancel{\text{kg}}} \times 500\ \text{mg} = \frac{7500\ \text{mg}}{70} = 107\ \text{mg}$$

Note

The weight used here is the average adult weight in kilograms—that is, 70 kilograms.

So, 107 milligrams is a safe dose for a 15-kilogram child.

While most prescribers today base medication orders on weight or BSA, Clark's Rule, Fried's Rule, and Young's Rule are still used by some pediatricians, advanced nurse practitioners, and physician's assistants.